Hot Topics in Acute Care Surgery and Trauma

This series covers the most debated issues in acute care and trauma surgery, from perioperative management to organizational and health policy issues. Since 2011, the founder members of the World Society of Emergency Surgery's (WSES) Acute Care and Trauma Surgeons group, who endorse the series, realized the need to provide more educational tools for young surgeons in training and for general physicians and other specialists new to this discipline: WSES is currently developing a systematic scientific and educational program founded on evidence-based medicine and objective experience. Covering the complex management of acute trauma and non-trauma surgical patients, this series makes a significant contribution to this program and is a valuable resource for both trainees and practitioners in acute care surgery.

Antonio Tarasconi • Simona Bui
Mircea Chirica • Gaël Roth
Jeffry Nahmias
Editors

Oncologic Surgical Emergencies

A Practical Guide for the General Surgeon

Springer

Editors
Antonio Tarasconi
Emergency Surgery Dept.
Parma University Hospital
Parma, Italy

Simona Bui
Oncology Dept.
Parma University Hospital
Parma, Italy

Mircea Chirica
Digestive Surgery Dept
Ctr. Hosp. Univ. Grenoble Alpes
La Tronche, France

Gaël Roth
Hepato-gastroenterology and Digestive oncology Dept.
Grenoble-Alpes University Hospital
Grenoble, France

Jeffry Nahmias
Department of Surgery
University of California, Irvine
Orange, CA, USA

ISSN 2520-8284 ISSN 2520-8292 (electronic)
Hot Topics in Acute Care Surgery and Trauma

ISBN 978-3-031-36859-2 ISBN 978-3-031-36860-8 (eBook)
https://doi.org/10.1007/978-3-031-36860-8

This Springer imprint is published by the registered company Springer Nature Switzerland AG
The registered company address is: Gewerbestrasse 11, 6330 Cham, Switzerland

Contents

Emergency in Head and Neck Cancer Patients

1

A. Piccinini, M. Reale, G. P. Santoro, and E. Pasanisi

An oncological emergency can be defined as an acute condition requiring rapid intervention to avoid severe permanent damage or death. The neck is a complex anatomic region that contains many vital structures in a relatively small area. The acute event may be due to the tumor itself or may be secondary to complications arising from treatment effects.

Emergent conditions resulting from head and neck neoplasms and their treatment include acute airway obstruction and bilateral vocal cord paralysis, hemorrhage, septic complication, and thrombophlebitis. These conditions require accurate diagnosis and rapid intervention to avoid severe permanent damage or death. Successful treatment requires a coordinated response by emergency medicine physicians, otolaryngologists, vascular surgeons, and radiologists.

In this chapter, we discuss the most frequent emergencies resulting from head and neck tumors and their management.

1.1 Airway Obstruction

Acute airway obstruction refers to a blockage at the level of the upper airway or main stem bronchi.

It may result from intraluminal growth (Fig. 1.1) or extrinsic compression of the airway by head and neck tumors (Fig. 1.2).

A. Piccinini · G. P. Santoro
Department of Otorhinolaryngology and Otoneurosurgery, Azienda Ospedaliero-Universitaria di Parma, Parma, Italy

M. Reale (✉) · E. Pasanisi
University of Parma, Department of Medicine and Surgery, Department of Otorhinolaryngology and Otoneurosurgery, Parma, Italy

A. Tarasconi et al. (eds.), *Oncologic Surgical Emergencies*, Hot Topics in Acute Care Surgery and Trauma, https://doi.org/10.1007/978-3-031-36860-8_1

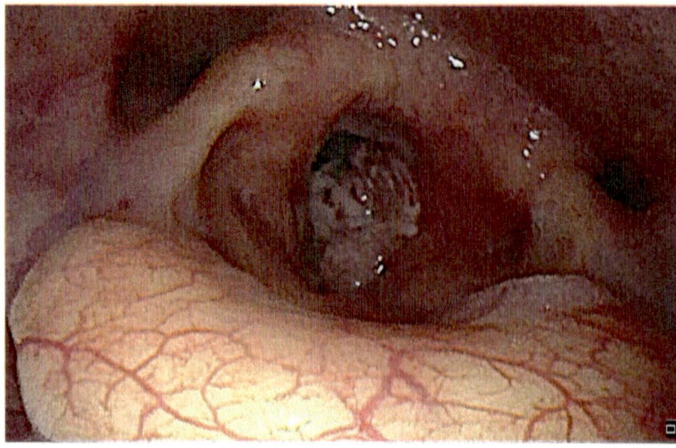

Fig. 1.1 Tumor mass obstructing the glottic plane

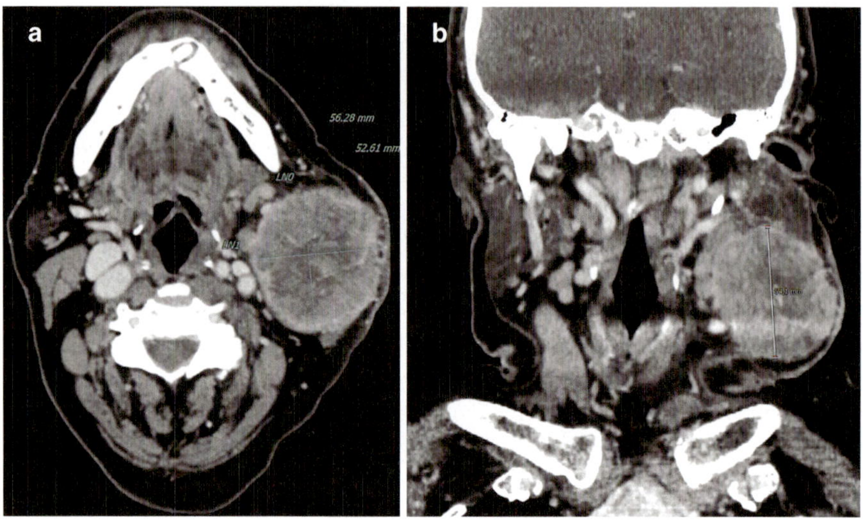

Fig. 1.2 (**a**, **b**) Laterocervical mass on CT scan, axial and coronal planes

Neoplasms of the neck and upper aerodigestive tract generally enlarge slowly, coming to clinical attention before the onset of respiratory distress [1].

Most obstructing tumors are hypopharyngeal or transglottic squamous cell carcinomas, but obstructing masses may also arise from the nasopharynx, thyroid, trachea, or esophagus. Nerve sheath tumors may result in airway obstruction, typically when large and/or multiple as in neurofibromatosis type I or II.

Dyspnea is frequently the only early symptom of airway obstruction, while stridor should be considered a very unfavorable sign (airway diameter decreased to <5 mm) [2].

Also, the chemotherapy and radiotherapy treatment can modify the respiratory space. These patients could have post-actinic edema that reduces the caliber of the upper airway.

Patients who have undergone surgical or radiochemotherapy treatment could have a tracheotomy (Fig. 1.3) or tracheal stoma (Fig. 1.4), and an obstruction of the tracheal tube or trachea could be present and leads to respiratory distress; in other cases, the tracheal tube could be dislocated.

Moreover, bilateral vocal cord paralysis is a cause of upper airway obstruction that may be seen in a variety of clinical settings, including malignancy of the thyroid, trachea, or esophagus, but also involves iatrogenic causes [1].

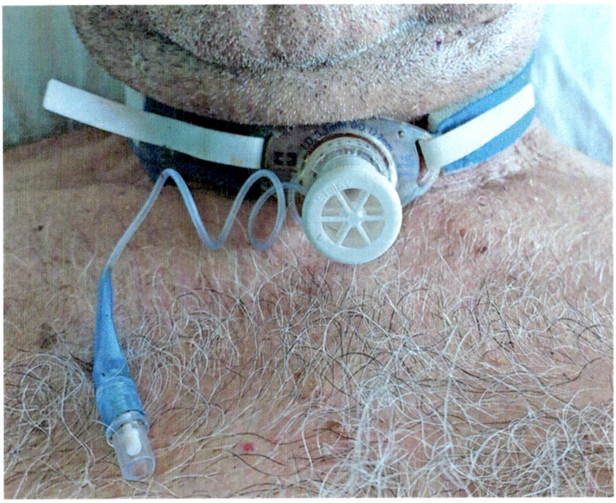

Fig. 1.3 Patient with tracheal tube

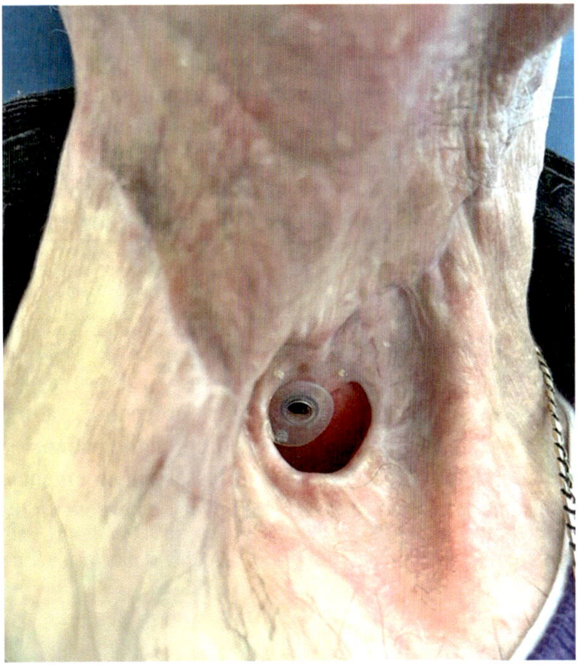

Fig. 1.4 Tracheal stoma in laryngectomy patient

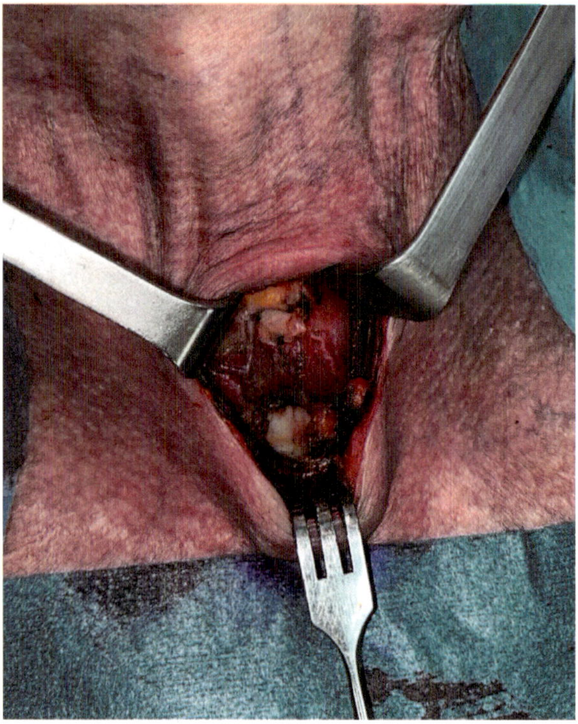

Fig. 1.8 Divarication of strap muscle

4. Separation and ligation of thyroid isthmus for a trans-isthmic tracheotomy (Fig. 1.9): The tracheotomy could be done also supra-isthmic or sub-isthmic; actually, the trans-isthmic technique is safer for accidental bleeding and facilitates the access to trachea during the change of the tracheostomy tube.
5. Recognition of the trachea, and horizontal incision between second and third tracheal rings or third and fourth tracheal rings: The inferior ring could be anchored to the skin in order to prevent some difficulties during the management of tracheostomy tube in the postoperative period (Fig. 1.10).
6. Positioning of the cuffed tracheostomy tube (Fig. 1.11).
7. Suture of the skin if the incision is large.

Every emergency physician should know the difference between tracheotomy and permanent tracheostomy (TS) in total laryngectomy patients.

In the first case, the normal connection between oropharynx, hypopharynx, larynx, and trachea is maintained (Fig. 1.3).

In case of total laryngectomy patients, the larynx is removed and an end tracheal stoma is performed; there is no connection between trachea and oropharynx, so in these patients, the risk of inhalation is not possible, and in case of emergency, they have to be intubated or ventilated through the stoma (Fig. 1.4).

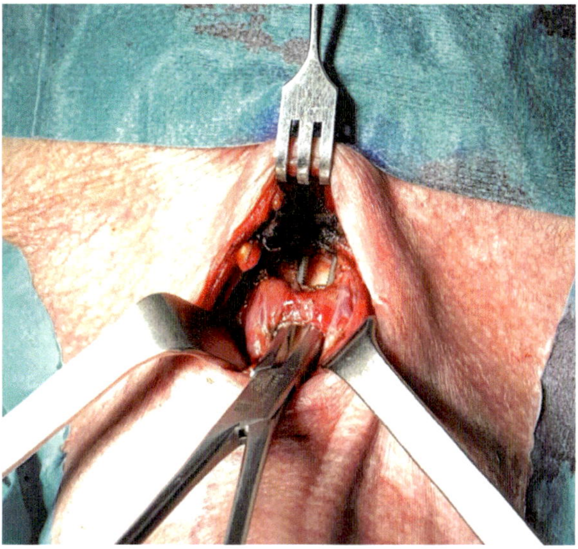

Fig. 1.9 Separation and ligation of thyroid isthmus

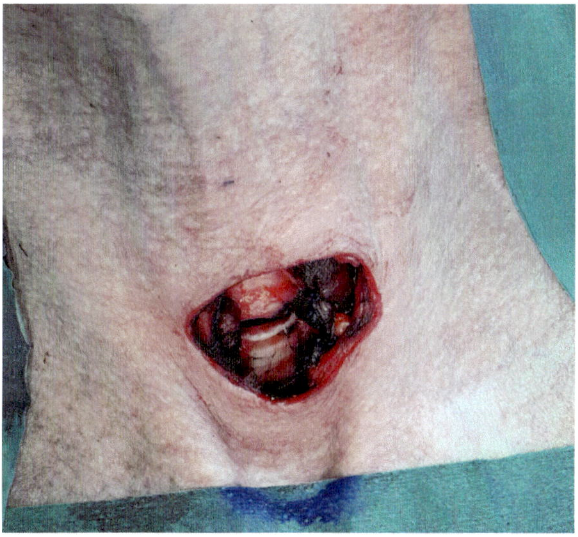

Fig. 1.10 Trachea incision

In both cases, the tracheal tube or the trachea could be obstructed by mucus or other secretions and patients could experience a breath failure.

The tracheotomy tube has another inner tube which prevents the total occlusion, and it is sufficient to remove only the inner tube to restore breath function (Fig. 1.12).

Patients in which total laryngectomy has been performed could be affected by tracheitis with formation of circumferential crusts that can lead to an obstruction of the trachea. In these cases, the trachea should be released from the obstruction with the help of a suction catheter.

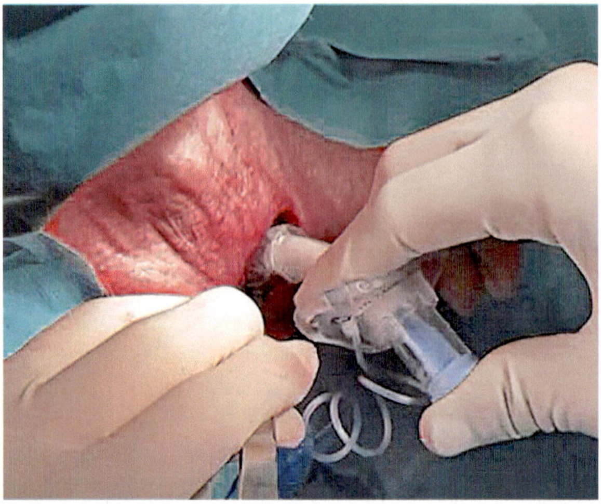

Fig. 1.11 Positioning of the tracheostomy tube

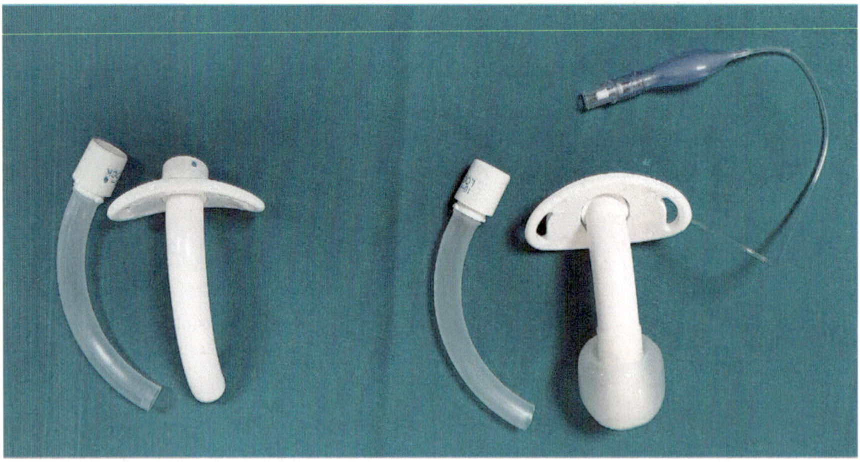

Fig. 1.12 Tracheotomy tube without and with cuff, Shiley™

In both cases, however, each maneuver must be preceded by a careful endoscopic reconnaissance of the trachea.

Another possible emergency is the dislocation of the tracheal tube: in this case, every effort should be made to replace the tube. If the original tracheostomy tube is too large for the tracheostomy stoma at the time of replacement, then the tract can be dilated with a nasal speculum or a smaller tube can be inserted.

The emergency management in tracheotomy and total laryngectomy patients with tracheostomy is highlighted in the following algorithms (Figs. 1.13 and 1.14).

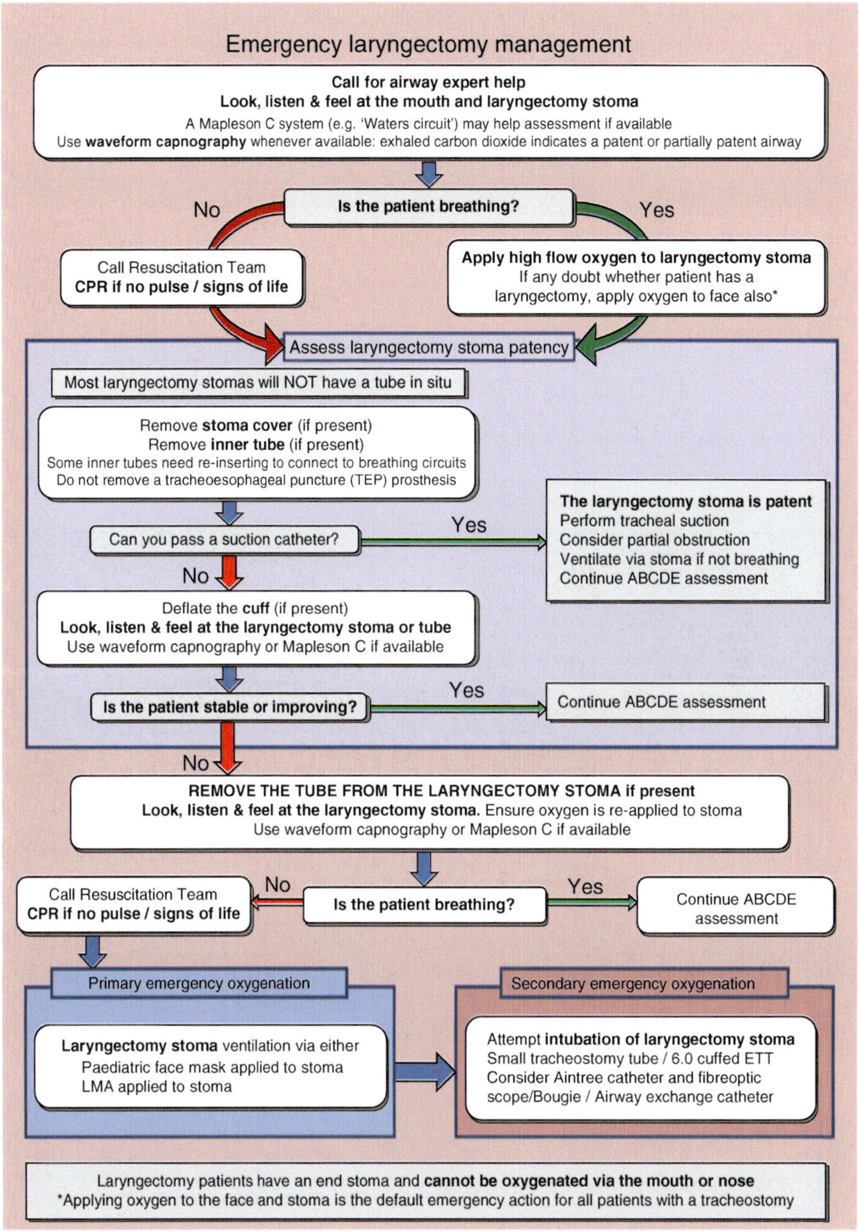

Fig. 1.13 Emergency tracheostomy management. (From [16], with permission)

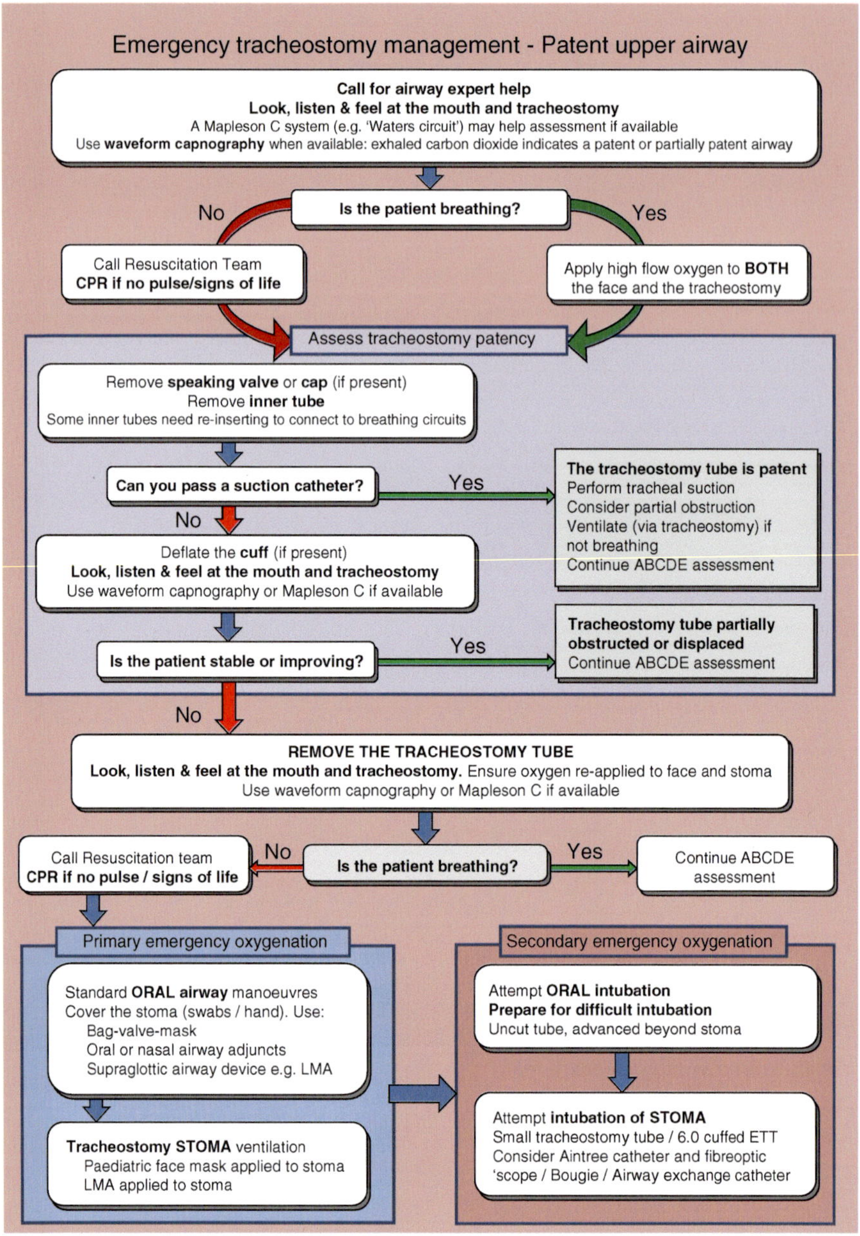

Fig. 1.14 Emergency laryngectomy management. (From [16], with permission)

1.2 Bleeding Management

Bleeding is another possible emergency in patients with head and neck cancer or treated for it. Bleeding can occur from direct tumor involvement and/or as a side effect of therapy [17]. The possible scenarios are variable: epistaxis, massive hemoptysis, neck's hematoma, and tracheoinnominate fistula.

Even in this emergency situation, the airways are at risk since in case of blood inhalation, occlusion of them can occur and/or they can collapse due to extrinsic compression. For these reasons, the management of airways is fundamental. If the patient has tracheostomy, it is important to insert a cuffed tracheostomy tube and maintain it cuffed; if the patient has no tracheostomy, all the previous considerations about the management of the airways are the same.

Furthermore, these patients often have coagulation problems, due to concomitant coagulopathies or liver diseases; these concomitant pathologies can empathize the bleeding. So, it is important to consider the necessity of a transfusion of red blood cells in the management of the bleeding and obviously take almost one intravenous line for hydration to prevent a hemorrhagic shock.

1.2.1 Epistaxis Management

The nose has a rich vascular supply, derived from both the external and internal carotid arteries, as reported in Fig. 1.15, and knowing the anatomy is important to predict the focus of bleeding and choose the best way to treat it.

Epistaxis can originate from vessels as a consequence of previous treatment and/or for other pathologies of the patient or from the tumoral mass. The bleeding may originate from the anterior part of the septum, in correspondence to the Kiesselbach's plexus, which is a network of submucosal vessels that are prone to bleeding; in this

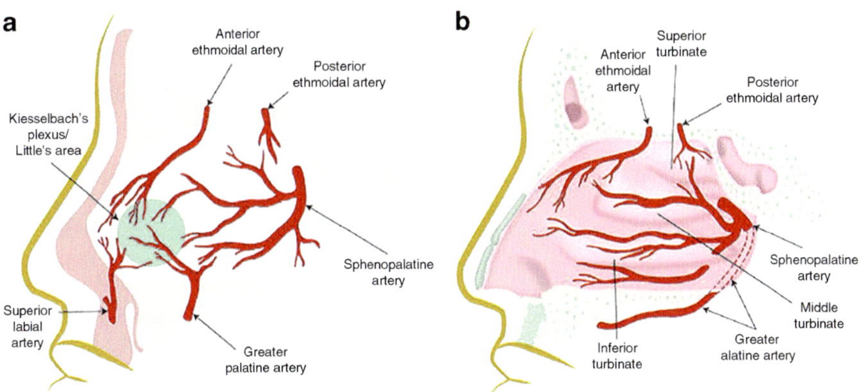

Fig. 1.15 Vascular supply of the (**a**) nasal septum and (**b**) lateral nasal wall [18]

case, the bleeding is of moderate entity. Or it may have origins posteriorly from larger caliber arteries; in this case, the epistaxis could be difficult to manage.

Severe and massive bleeding may be managed by different methods; anterior nasal packing [19] is the first attempt, followed by a posterior nasal packing [20]. If the packing is not sufficient, a surgical management of the bleeding in the operatory room is necessary, and only in selective cases can the embolization be used.

A wide variety of nasal packing techniques are available. In the author's experience, the most common are Merocel™ packing and Rapid Rhino™ for anterior nasal packing and Epi-Max™ Epistaxis Catheter for posterior nasal packing (Figs. 1.16, 1.17 and 1.18). All these types of packing can be associated with the use of hemostatic gauze (Tabotamp®/Surgicel®).

Placement of these packs should be in a direction along the floor of the nasal cavity (parallel to the ground when the patient is sitting erect with the head in neutral position) towards the nasopharynx, as opposed to the oblique direction of the nasal dorsum.

The differences between the packing are described below: Merocel is a compressed, dehydrated sponge composed of hydroxylated polyvinyl acetate; after insertion, it requires rehydration with normal saline to achieve its optimal size within the nasal cavity and compress the bleeding vessels [21]. The Rapid Rhino™ pneumatic nasal tampon (Applied Therapeutics Ltd., Glenfield, UK) consists of an inflatable nasal cuff (balloon) with a hemostatic coating (Gel Knit™ fabric; Acordis

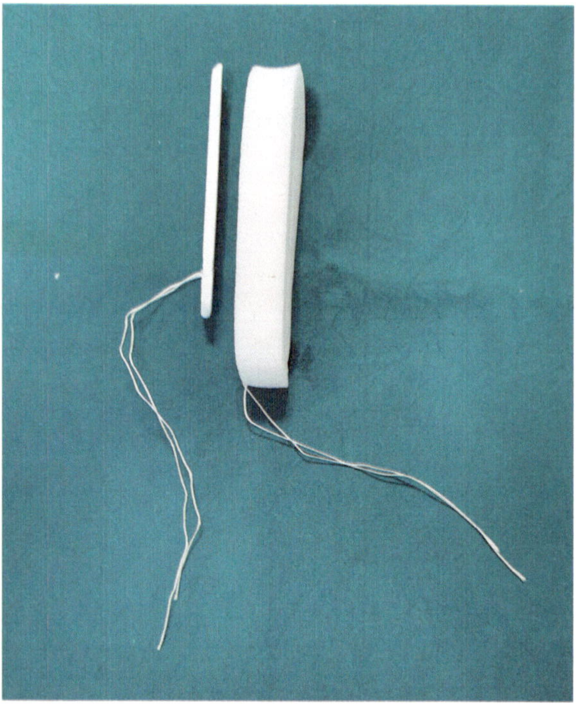

Fig. 1.16 Merocel™

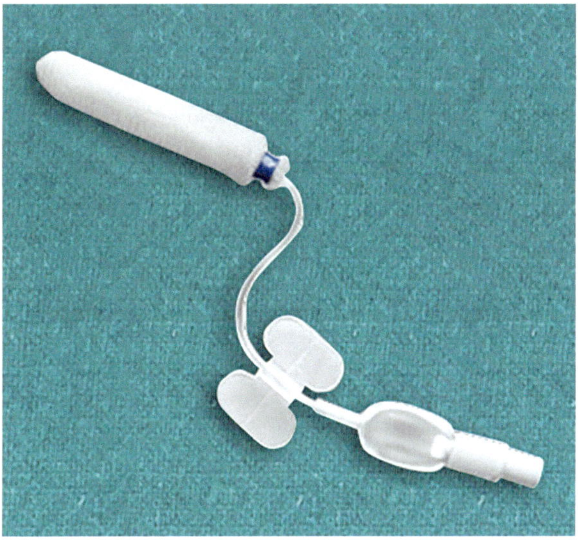

Fig. 1.17 Rapid Rhino™

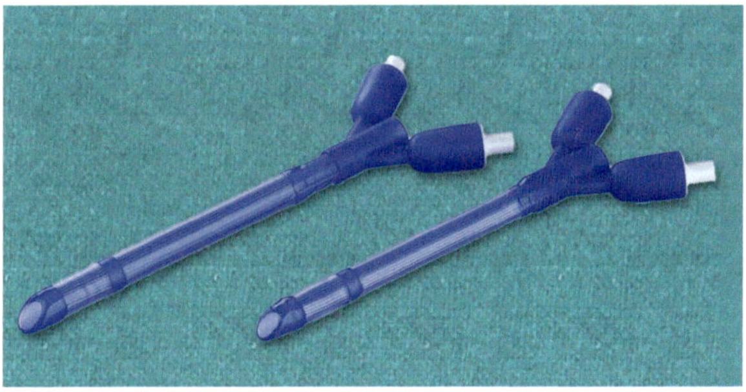

Fig. 1.18 Epi-Max™ Epistaxis Catheter

Speciality Fibres, Coventry, UK), a valve, and a pilot cuff [22]. Epi-Max™ Epistaxis Catheter is a catheter with two inflatable balloons; the proximal one has to be inflated with saline solution until maximum 30 cc, whereas the distal one has to be inflated with saline solution until maximum 10 cc. The posterior balloon occludes the choana and stops every posterior bleeding, the posterior wall of the oropharynx has to be clean after the positioning of the posterior nasal packing, and this is a sign of a well-managed bleeding.

This packaging is left in place for 48–72 h to allow the healing of the bleeding mucosa, and after this time, it has to be removed. During the removal, there is the risk of a new bleeding, so it is necessary to remove the packaging in a place where all necessaries to manage a new bleeding are present.

The second choice in management of bleeding is the surgical procedure. Nowadays, the procedure is totally endoscopic assisted: cauterization can be done in the operating room thoroughly and with greater precision, but also ligation of sphenopalatine artery or other major caliber vessels can be performed through the endoscopic approach. All these procedures must be performed by an experienced ENT surgeon.

In some selected cases, endovascular embolization has been considered an alternative treatment of severe epistaxis that has failed to respond to conservative therapy with packing or that was impossible to cauterize. There are several complications both intracranial and extracranial related to embolization of craniofacial vessels such as stroke and necrosis of nasal or palatopharyngeal soft tissues; thus, this procedure should be performed by experienced interventional radiologists.

1.2.2 Upper Aerodigestive Bleeding

Upper aerodigestive bleeding can lead to life-threatening airway obstruction, aspiration, anemia, or hypovolemic shock.

Bleeding from the upper aerodigestive tract can occur after surgery or after radiotherapy for different causes. Radiotherapy can cause obliteration of the vasa vasorum, premature atherosclerosis, adventitial fibrosis, and fragmentation of tunica media elastic fibers leading to weakening of the arterial wall [23].

Massive hemoptysis in cancer patients may also be caused by nonmalignant conditions, such as fungal infections, or may be related to thrombocytopenia or other coagulation disorders.

Usually, there is a sentinel bleed, and the entity of this bleeding can be self-limited, but immediate diagnostic workup followed by treatment should be obtained to prevent a catastrophic bleed.

When it is possible, direct pression and packing the focus of bleeding are the first things to do to stop it and then organize the next workup. Once the patient is stabilized, CT angiography (CTA) can be an effective screening tool for locating the site of hemorrhage and can also assist in procedures performed by the intervention neuroradiologist [24]. Arterial embolization offers an effective, safe, and fast method for controlling bleeding from tumors [25]. The hemostatic effect is believed to last longer in selective embolization than in ligation because embolic materials reach all the way to the periphery [26, 27]. Even if rebleeding occurs, repeat embolization is relatively easy. In the literature, the recurrence rate of hemorrhage after embolization in patients with malignant head and neck tumors is 0–33% [28–32]. Angiography alone is not without risks. It has an 8.5% incidence of complications. The incidence of neurologic complications is 2.6%, with an incidence of permanent deficit in 0.33% of the cases. Embolization introduces the added risk of thrombus propagation, inadvertent detachment of embolization materials, and complications associated with the intentional carotid occlusion. Other complications include hematoma at the catheter insertion site, infection, atheroemboli, and transient hypertension or hypotension. Atheroemboli can cause renal failure, bowel infarction, pancreatitis, and ischemia of the lower extremities [33].

The alternative to radiological management is the surgical exploration with ligation of involved vessels. The surgical procedure is difficult because of other associated problems such as recurrent tumor, postsurgical anatomical changes, fistulas, infection, and radiation necrosis. In case of surgery in addiction to neurologic complications, there are relatively high mortality rates and still high risk of bleeding due to collateral circulation [26]. During surgery, a cervical incision is performed and the focus of bleeding has to be found. When the origins of the bleeding cannot be recognized, the key to success is to ligate the external carotid artery in order to stop any possible vessel responsible for the bleeding.

1.2.3 Neck Bleeding Management

Acute neck soft tissue hemorrhage is a life-threatening emergency condition that may occur in the setting of neoplasia, particularly as delayed complication of primary or salvage therapy for extensive and/or recurrent squamous cell carcinoma of the head and neck.

Acute arterial hemorrhage is particularly dangerous when located in the upper aerodigestive tract. Airway obstruction, aspiration, and subsequent asphyxia may be lethal.

Radiotherapy is a potential causative agent for arterial erosions: Infiltrating tumor regression after radiotherapy may lead to a defect in arterial wall during or shortly after completion of the protocol. Bleeding may also result from the long-term effects of radiotherapy. Radiation-induced vascular changes vary from atherosclerosis to necrotizing vasculitis [34].

Other unusual causes of nontraumatic hemorrhage include carotid artery rupture due to infection, and massive hemorrhage from highly vascular neoplasms or thyroid nodules [1].

"Carotid blowout" is defined as an episode of acute hemorrhage from a damaged carotid in a patient who has previously undergone surgical resection for squamous cell carcinoma.

In case of acute arterial hemorrhage, the primary focus is emergency stabilization of the respiratory and cardiovascular system and cessation of bleeding by packing the pharynx, followed by surgical ligature or immediate arterial embolization, with the vessel occluded permanently if the patient tolerates a preceding balloon test occlusion.

Acute profuse hemorrhage that is not self-limited and not well controlled with surgical packing has a high morbidity and mortality rate, even with emergent endovascular or surgical therapy. Patients presenting with acute hemorrhage from carotid blowout syndrome related to advanced head and neck cancer can be effectively treated with covered stent placement, which provides immediate hemostasis; however, potential delayed ischemic or infectious complications are common in the exposed or infected neck.

In case of minor bleeding attacks, the management depends on the size and growth of the hematoma itself. The conservative choice with gentle drainage and compression dressings is enough when the hematoma seems not to be progressive. The surgical way is necessary if the hematoma enlarges rapidly, because there is a potential risk of airway compression.

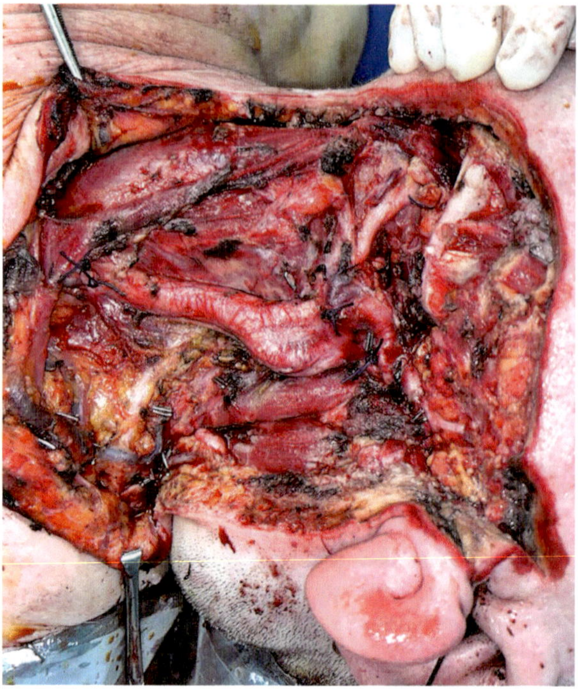

Fig. 1.19 Ligation of internal jugular vein

If the bleeding is a venous bleeding, sometimes it is self-limited, but there could be an emergency in case of rupture of the internal jugular vein. The solution for the rupture of internal jugular vein is the ligation of it (Fig. 1.19).

In the cases of postoperative bleeding of the neck in which airway compression may occur, while waiting to have access to surgery room, it is necessary to open the surgical incision in order to drain the bleeding and avoid airway compression. Obviously, in all these cases of bleeding, the airway management and intravenous support are paramount.

1.3 Tracheoinnominate Fistula

Another possible complication for patients with head and neck cancer and with tracheostomy is the formation of a tracheoinnominate fistula (TIF). It is a rare complication after tracheostomy placement ranging from 0.1 to 1% in incidence and usually occurring between postoperative days 7 and 14 [35]. TIF is caused by progressive erosion of the tracheal wall, finally communicating with the adjacent mediastinal arterial vessels, most commonly innominate artery, which is located between the trachea and the sternum in the superior mediastinum. Pressure from a constantly inflated balloon, especially at high pressures, or constant contact with the tip of the cannula causes the problem [36]. Necrosis, chronic inflammation, granulation tissue, and scarring are the hallmarks of the condition [37, 38]. The management is surgical with a sternotomy and vascular repair. Direct pressure against the anterior tracheal wall digitally with a finger or placing a cuffed tracheostomy tube can help to tamponade the bleeding, before the surgical procedure. Unluckily, the mortality rate is very high, even when surgical intervention is taken [39]. In literature, endovascular embolization or placement of a stent graft of the innominate artery is described as an alternative way of management [35].

1.4 Infectious Emergencies

Head and neck cancer patients during or after the treatment are at risk of developing infections. Deep neck infections (DNIs) and abscesses of the neck are those which require intensive care admission in 6.1% of cases [40]. They may result in life-threatening complications, such as upper airway obstruction, descending mediastinitis, jugular vein thrombosis, venous septic emboli, carotid artery rupture, adult respiratory distress syndrome, septic shock, and disseminated intravascular coagulopathy [41–43].

The mortality rate of DNI varies between 1.6 and 2.6% [44].

Chemotherapy is recorded as a risk factor [40, 45, 46]. In literature, mucositis and neutropenia are supposed to be the most responsible mechanisms [47]. Moreover, radiotherapy induces a variety of side effects on normal tissues neighboring the neoplasm, and these effects may show clinically and radiologically evident abnormalities even months or years later leading to DNI [48].

Furthermore, all these patients have a lot of comorbidities, which increases the risk of a serious infection.

Actually, in some rare cases, a DNI or an abscess could be the initial presentation of primary head and neck cancer; the incidence is unclear and may be underestimated [49, 50]. A cystic metastasis which becomes infected and presents as a neck abscess, or direct tumor which undergoes necrosis and causes DNI, could be treated as an infection, and the malignancy remains undetected [51–53]. For this reason, every patient who comes to the ENT attention for an abscess or DNI has to be investigated through a careful anamnesis in order to recognize the right origin of the disease.

In case of neck infection, the possible scenarios are a laterocervical mass which has all the characteristics of the abscesses like fluid consistence, erythema of the neck, and fever, but if it originates in the deep spaces, nothing could be appreciated in the neck and the possible signs of it are pharyngodynia, trismus, dysphagia, sialorrhea, and dyspnea.

A CT scan with contrast enhancement is necessary to evaluate the extension of the infection and to plan a correct management (Fig. 1.20).

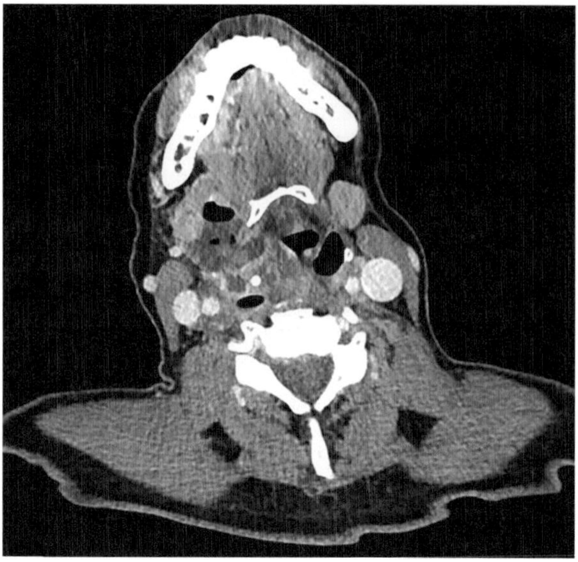

Fig. 1.20 Laterocervical abscess with extrinsic compression of the airway

In all these cases, after a careful evaluation and serum examination, it is mandatory to explore the airways through the fiberscope examination and assess their patency. In fact, the upper airways are at risk, as said above, because of extrinsic compression or secondary mucosal edema of pharynx and larynx.

The treatment of DNI and abscesses consists of, in addition to antibiotics therapy, securing the airways and, in some cases, surgical drainage. When the patient is stable, the correct treatment is endovenous large-spectrum antibiotics, possibly consulting an infectiologist, for 24–48 h with seriated serum examinations and clinical and radiological evaluations. In case of improvement, the surgical drainage might not be necessary, but if during these hours the clinical conditions worsen, surgical drainage and tracheotomy are necessary in order to avoid the complications mentioned above.

A possible vascular complication of DNI is septic thrombophlebitis of the internal jugular vein. This complication is particularly common in intravenous drug abusers, and the most common causative organisms are *S. aureus* and beta-hemolytic streptococci [1]. Septic thrombophlebitis is usually managed with hydration and antibiotics; in literature, the use of anticoagulation is controversial, but in the experience of the authors, they result helpful; surgical ligation and/or excision of the involved vessel is rarely necessary.

References

1. Fischbein N, Murr A. Imaging traumatic and nontraumatic neck emergencies in the adult. Emerg Radiol. 1999;6:94–109. https://doi.org/10.1007/s101400050033.

2. Arné J, Descoins P, Fusciardi J, Ingrand P, Ferrier B, Boudigues D, et al. Preoperative assessment for difficult intubation in general and ENT surgery: predictive value of a clinical multivariate risk index. Br J Anaesth. 1998;80(2):140–6.
3. Bansal A, Miskoff J, Lis RJ. Otolaryngologic critical care. Crit Care Clin. 2003;19(1):55–72.
4. Garantziotis S, Kyrmizakis DE, Liolios AD. Critical care of the head and neck patient. Crit Care Clin. 2003;19(1):73–90.
5. Bhatnagar S, Mishra S, Jha RR, Singhal AK, Bhatnagar N. The LMA Fastrach facilitates fibreoptic intubation in oral cancer patients. Can J Anaesth. 2005;52(6):641–5.
6. Mishra S, Bhatnagar S, Jha RR, Singhal AK. Airway management of patients undergoing oral cancer surgery: a retrospective study. Eur J Anaesthesiol. 2005;22(7):510–4.
7. Stelea C, Pătrăşcanu E, Cureniuc L, Hârtie LV, Comanescu MP, Crăcană A, et al. Airway management in head and neck cancer surgery. Roman J Oral Rehabil. 2020;12(4):5.
8. Walz JM, Zayaruzny M, Heard SO. Airway management in critical illness. Chest. 2007;131(2):608–20.
9. Mason RA, Fielder CP. The obstructed airway in head and neck surgery. Anaesthesia. 1999;54(7):625–8.
10. Benumof JL. Management of the difficult adult airway. With special emphasis on awake tracheal intubation. Anesthesiology. 1991;75(6):1087–110.
11. Johnston KD, Rai MR. Conscious sedation for awake fibreoptic intubation: a review of the literature. Can J Anaesth. 2013;60(6):584–99.
12. Varghese BT, Balakrishnan M, Kuriakose R. Fibre-optic intubation in oncological head and neck emergencies. J Laryngol Otol. 2005;119(8):634–8.
13. Morris IR. Fibreoptic intubation. Can J Anaesth. 1994;41(10):996–1007.
14. Wulf H, Brinkmann G, Rautenberg M. Management of the difficult airway. A case of failed fiberoptic intubation. Acta Anaesthesiol Scand. 1997;41(8):1080–2.
15. Bramwell KJ, Davis DP, Cardall TV, Yoshida E, Vilke GM, Rosen P. Use of the Trousseau dilator in cricothyrotomy. J Emerg Med. 1999;17(3):433–6.
16. McGrath BA, Bates L, Atkinson D, Moore JA, National Tracheostomy Safety Project. Multidisciplinary guidelines for the management of tracheostomy and laryngectomy airway emergencies. Anaesthesia. 2012;67(9):1025–41.
17. Roh JL, Suh DC, Kim MR, Lee JH, Choi JW, Choi SH, et al. Endovascular management of carotid blowout syndrome in patients with head and neck cancers. Oral Oncol. 2008;44(9):844–50.
18. Tunkel DE, Anne S, Payne SC, Ishman SL, Rosenfeld RM, Abramson PJ, et al. Clinical practice guideline: nosebleed (epistaxis). Otolaryngol Head Neck Surg. 2020;162(1_suppl):S1–38.
19. Corbridge RJ, Djazaeri B, Hellier WP, Hadley J. A prospective randomized controlled trial comparing the use of Merocel nasal tampons and BIPP in the control of acute epistaxis. Clin Otolaryngol Allied Sci. 1995;20(4):305–7.
20. Holland NJ, Sandhu GS, Ghufoor K, Frosh A. The Foley catheter in the management of epistaxis. Int J Clin Pract. 2001;55(1):14–5.
21. Alshehri WM, Alwehaibi WM, Ahmed MW, Albathi A, Alqahtani B. Merocel surgicel wrap technique to manage diffuse epistaxis in patients with comorbidities. Int J Otolaryngol. 2020;2020:8272914.
22. Smyth C, Hanna B, Scally C. Rapid rhino nasal packs: demonstration of depressurisation but not deflation. J Laryngol Otol. 2009;123(5):522–7.
23. Hiro-oki O, Kamiyama R, Takiguchi Y, Kimizuka K, Ishikawa N, Kishimoto S. Histopathological examination of ruptured carotid artery after irradiation. ORL J Otorhinolaryngol Relat Spec. 2002;64(3):226–8.
24. Mazumdar A, Derdeyn CP, Holloway W, Moran CJ, Cross DT. Update on endovascular management of the carotid blowout syndrome. Neuroimaging Clin N Am. 2009;19(2):271–81.
25. Imai S, Kajihara Y, Kamei T, Komaki K, Tamada T, Shirai H, et al. Arterial embolization for control of bleeding in advanced head and neck malignancy. Int J Clin Oncol. 1998;3(4):228–32.

26. Sittel C, Gossmann A, Jungehülsing M, Zähringer M. Superselective embolization as palliative treatment of recurrent hemorrhage in advanced carcinoma of the head and neck. Ann Otol Rhinol Laryngol. 2001;110(12):1126–8.
27. Kakizawa H, Toyota N, Naito A, Ito K. Endovascular therapy for management of oral hemorrhage in malignant head and neck tumors. Cardiovasc Intervent Radiol. 2005;28(6):722–9.
28. Mok JS, Marshall JN, Chan M, van Hasselt CA. Percutaneous embolization to control intractable epistaxis in nasopharyngeal carcinoma. Head Neck. 1999;21(3):211–6.
29. Remonda L, Schroth G, Caversaccio M, Lädrach K, Lövblad KO, Zbären P, et al. Endovascular treatment of acute and subacute hemorrhage in the head and neck. Arch Otolaryngol Head Neck Surg. 2000;126(10):1255–62.
30. Morrissey DD, Andersen PE, Nesbit GM, Barnwell SL, Everts EC, Cohen JI. Endovascular management of hemorrhage in patients with head and neck cancer. Arch Otolaryngol Head Neck Surg. 1997;123(1):15–9.
31. Wilner HI, Lazo A, Metes JJ, Beil KA, Nowack P, Jacobs J. Embolization in cataclysmal hemorrhage caused by squamous cell carcinomas of the head and neck. Radiology. 1987;163(3):759–62.
32. Zimmerman RA, McLean G, Freiman D, Golestaneh Z, Perez M. The diagnostic and therapeutic role of angiography in lingual arterial bleeding. Radiology. 1979;133(3 Pt 1):639–43.
33. Earnest F, Forbes G, Sandok BA, Piepgras DG, Faust RJ, Ilstrup DM, et al. Complications of cerebral angiography: prospective assessment of risk. AJR Am J Roentgenol. 1984;142(2):247–53.
34. Greve J, Bas M, Schuler P, Turowski B, Scheckenbach K, Budach W, et al. Acute arterial hemorrhage following radiotherapy of oropharyngeal squamous cell carcinoma. Strahlenther Onkol Organ Dtsch Rontgengesellschaft Al. 2010;186(5):269–73.
35. Risley J, Mann K, Jones NS. The role of embolisation in ENT: an update. J Laryngol Otol. 2012;126(3):228–35.
36. Jones JW, Reynolds M, Hewitt RL, Drapanas T. Tracheo-innominate artery erosion: successful surgical management of a devastating complication. Ann Surg. 1976;184(2):194–204.
37. Byard RW, Gilbert JD. Potentially lethal complications of tracheostomy: autopsy considerations. Am J Forensic Med Pathol. 2011;32(4):352–4.
38. Miyake N, Ueno H, Kitano H. Pathological consideration of tracheo-innominate artery fistula with a case report. Int J Pediatr Otorhinolaryngol. 2013;77(8):1322–4.
39. Epstein SK. Late complications of tracheostomy. Respir Care. 2005;50(4):542–9.
40. Kuhn JG. Chemotherapy-associated hematopoietic toxicity. Am J Health Syst Pharm AJHP. 2002;59(15 Suppl 4):S4–7.
41. Estrera AS, Landay MJ, Grisham JM, Sinn DP, Platt MR. Descending necrotizing mediastinitis. Surg Gynecol Obstet. 1983;157(6):545–52.
42. Beck HJ, Salassa JR, McCaffrey TV, Hermans PE. Life-threatening soft-tissue infections of the neck. Laryngoscope. 1984;94(3):354–62.
43. Chen MK, Wen YS, Chang CC, Huang MT, Hsiao HC. Predisposing factors of life-threatening deep neck infection: logistic regression analysis of 214 cases. J Otolaryngol. 1998;27(3):141–4.
44. Mettias B, Robertson S, Buchanan MA. Retropharyngeal abscess after chemotherapy. BMJ Case Rep. 2018;2018:bcr-2017-222610.
45. Huang TT, Liu TC, Chen PR, Tseng FY, Yeh TH, Chen YS. Deep neck infection: analysis of 185 cases. Head Neck. 2004;26(10):854–60.
46. Bakir S, Tanriverdi MH, Gün R, Yorgancilar AE, Yildirim M, Tekbaş G, et al. Deep neck space infections: a retrospective review of 173 cases. Am J Otolaryngol. 2012;33(1):56–63.
47. Rolston KVI, Bodey GP. Factors responsible for increased susceptibility to infections. In: Kufe DW, Pollock RE, Weichselbaum RR, et al., editors. Holland-Frei cancer medicine. 6th ed. Hamilton: BC Decker; 2003.
48. Magrini SM, Pasinetti N, Belgioia L, Triggiani L, Levis M, Ricardi U, et al. Applying radiation protection and safety in radiotherapy. Radiol Med (Torino). 2019;124(8):777–82.

49. Wang CP, Ko JY, Lou PJ. Deep neck infection as the main initial presentation of primary head and neck cancer. J Laryngol Otol. 2006;120(4):305–9.
50. Lin YY, Hsu CH, Lee JC, Wang HW, Lin YS, Wang CH, et al. Head and neck cancers manifested as deep neck infection. Eur Arch Otorhinolaryngol. 2012;269(2):585–90.
51. Daramola OO, Flanagan CE, Maisel RH, Odland RM. Diagnosis and treatment of deep neck space abscesses. Otolaryngol Head Neck Surg. 2009;141(1):123–30.
52. Wang LF, Tai CF, Kuo WR, Chien CY. Predisposing factors of complicated deep neck infections: 12-year experience at a single institution. J Otolaryngol Head Neck Surg. 2010;39(4):335–41.
53. Soon SR, Kanagalingam J, Johari S, Yuen HW. Head and neck cancers masquerading as deep neck abscesses. Singap Med J. 2012;53(12):840–2.

Adrenal Emergencies in the Acute Care Setting

2

Molly Oberdoerster, Patrick Shahan, and Dawn Elfenbein

2.1 Introduction

Adrenal emergencies occur in both the traumatic and nontraumatic settings. Adrenal gland hemorrhage may be a direct result of blunt or penetrating trauma, whereas nontraumatic hemorrhage may occur from spontaneous rupture of an adrenal gland tumor or in the setting of acute illness or coagulopathy. Additionally, patients with known tumor pathology such as a pheochromocytoma or Cushing's syndrome are at risk for developing rare but life-threatening adrenal crises. The clinical manifestations and the degree of hemodynamic stability are key factors in determining the appropriate evaluation and intervention.

2.2 Adrenal Hemorrhage

Adrenal hemorrhage occurs in the traumatic and nontraumatic setting. Traumatic adrenal hemorrhage is usually discovered on computed tomography (CT) imaging during routine trauma workup and is very rarely an isolated finding. Traumatic adrenal hemorrhage is present in approximately 0.5% of blunt trauma cases and very rarely occurs in penetrating trauma. Recent studies have demonstrated that the presence of blunt adrenal gland injury is not a marker of severe injury or associated with increased mortality rate [1]. Blunt adrenal trauma is usually seen in high-impact mechanisms and is typically associated with other intra-abdominal injuries. Patient presentation may vary widely from hemodynamically stable to critically ill depending on other associated injuries.

M. Oberdoerster · P. Shahan · D. Elfenbein (✉)
University of Wisconsin School of Medicine and Public Health, Madison, WI, USA
e-mail: Shahan@surgery.wisc.edu; elfenbein@surgery.wisc.edu

A. Tarasconi et al. (eds.), *Oncologic Surgical Emergencies*, Hot Topics in Acute Care Surgery and Trauma, https://doi.org/10.1007/978-3-031-36860-8_2

Nontraumatic adrenal hemorrhage may present in the setting of ruptured adrenal tumor, illness, and coagulopathies including antiphospholipid antibody syndrome. Tumors associated with spontaneous hemorrhage include pheochromocytoma, myelolipoma, metastasis, carcinoma, and adenoma. Patients may present in hemorrhagic shock associated with flank pain and fever. Typically, unilateral hemorrhage is seen in tumors and blunt trauma, whereas bilateral hemorrhage may be seen in the setting of acute illness and coagulopathies. The evaluation and management of adrenal hemorrhage are based on the clinical presentation and stability of the patient.

Adrenal hemorrhage often presents with nonspecific symptoms including abdominal, flank, or loin pain as well as nausea, vomiting, weakness, and lethargy, making the diagnosis challenging. In cases of severe hemorrhage, symptoms of adrenal insufficiency may be present. Adrenal hemorrhage on CT scan appears as a round-to-ovoid lesion [2]. In the setting of acute adrenal hemorrhage, peri-adrenal fat stranding and bleeding into the perinephric space may be present (Fig. 2.1a). Attenuation is dependent on the age of the hematoma with acute hematomas having high attenuation. Adrenal congestion (adrenal gland thickening, peri-adrenal fat stranding) on CT may indicate impending adrenal hemorrhage [3]. Laboratory evaluation ranges from patients with normal laboratory parameters to those with leukocytosis and anemia as well as evidence of adrenal insufficiency including hyponatremia and hyperkalemia. Derangements in levels of cortisol, ACTH, and catecholamine levels may be present and aid in identifying the extent of gland destruction/involvement.

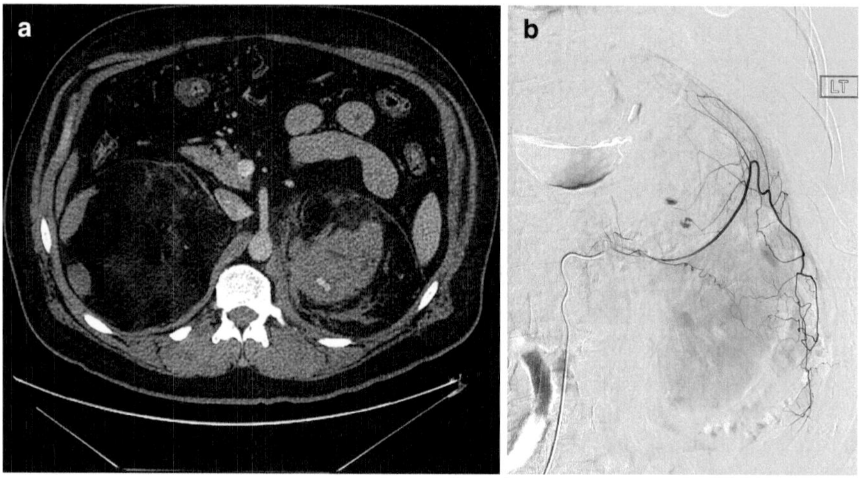

Fig. 2.1 (**a**) CT images of bilateral adrenal myelolipomas; the left has fat stranding and active extravasation of contrast suggestive of acute hemorrhage. (**b**) Angiography of the same adrenal tumor showing two areas of active hemorrhage

In a hemodynamically unstable patient with concerns for acute blood loss anemia and expanding hemorrhage, it is advisable for admission to an intensive care unit for close hemodynamic monitoring, blood product resuscitation, serial labs, and arterial embolization by interventional radiology. Angioembolization with interventional radiology is first-line therapy [4] (Fig. 2.1b). However, if angioembolization is not feasible or fails, proceeding to the operating room for an emergent adrenalectomy is the next best course of action.

For adrenal hemorrhage in the clinically stable patient (regardless of traumatic vs. nontraumatic etiology) identified on imaging, conservative management with admission for observation, IV fluid resuscitation, monitoring labs, and serial abdominal exams is advisable. Patients who have had a nontraumatic hemorrhage should ultimately be referred to an experienced adrenal surgeon for elective adrenalectomy, particularly in large tumors at risk for rebleeding (Fig. 2.2a, b).

In the setting of trauma, when emergent exploratory laparotomy is indicated for other reasons and an adrenal injury is incidentally discovered during surgical exploration, the decision of whether to repair versus proceed with resection should be based on the clinical status of the patient, viability of the adrenal tissue, and presence of a contralateral gland [5].

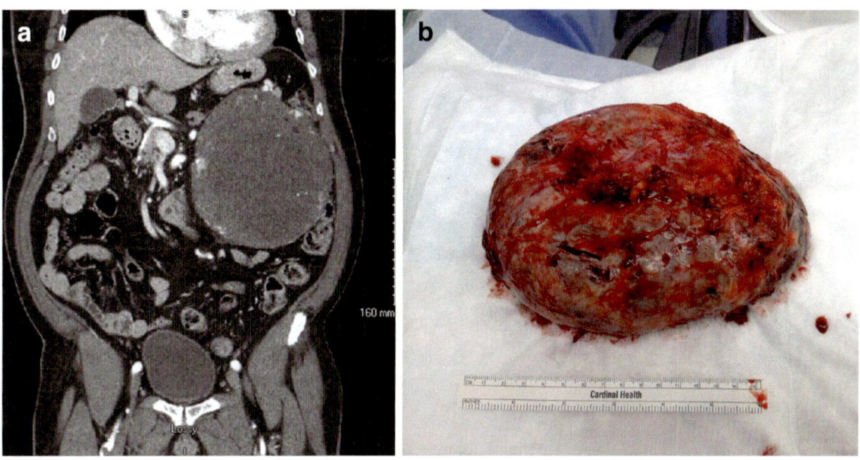

Fig. 2.2 (**a**) CT image of a giant left adrenal myelolipoma that had bled about 6 months prior to obtaining this CT. (**b**) Giant left adrenal myelolipoma surgical specimen

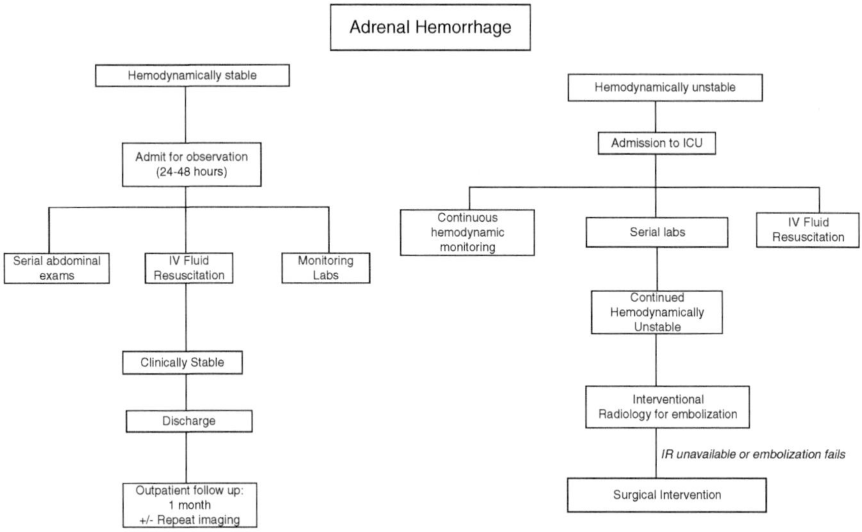

2.3 Pheochromocytoma

Pheochromocytoma is a rare catecholamine-secreting tumor of the adrenal gland, and symptoms manifest due to excessive catecholamine release. Symptoms may occur at any age, although the sporadic form is most common in the fourth and fifth decades. However, hereditary pheochromocytoma may present in younger patients with persistently elevated blood pressure despite maximal medical therapy. This may be seen in the setting of associated genetic syndromes such as multiple endocrine neoplasia (MEN) type 2, neurofibromatosis type 1, tuberous sclerosis, and ataxia telangiectasia. The classic triad of symptoms associated with a pheochromocytoma consists of episodic headache, sweating, and tachycardia, whereas sustained or paroxysmal hypertension is the most common sign of a pheochromocytoma. Patients with pheochromocytomas are at risk for developing a pheochromocytoma crisis or pheochromocytoma multisystem crisis. Crises typically present as a hypertensive emergency and may be associated with multiorgan failure and cardiopulmonary collapse. It is important to recognize that while the classic presentation is a hypertensive emergency, patients may also present with severe hypotension. Other manifestations include metabolic derangements, encephalopathy, and hyperthermia. Pheochromocytoma crisis may be triggered by acute stress (mechanical or psychological) or may be drug induced (glucocorticoids, dopamine receptor antagonist, opioids, norepinephrine reuptake inhibitors, neuromuscular blocking agents) [6]. Moreover, patients with a known pheochromocytoma are at risk for tumor rupture resulting in potential life-threatening adrenal hemorrhage and subsequent transient hypocortisolism.

Pheochromocytoma crisis should be considered in patients who present in a hypertensive crisis with associated relatively vague complaints of abdominal pain, headache, and tachycardia, and suspicion should be raised in those with laboratory values demonstrating end-organ damage. While 24-h urine metanephrine and plasma metanephrines are diagnostic for a pheochromocytoma and should be collected in the emergent setting, treatment of a presumed pheochromocytoma crisis should not be delayed for diagnostic confirmation. Imaging evaluation with CT abdomen and pelvis may demonstrate a large heterogeneous mass on the adrenal gland, and the gland itself may have evidence of hemorrhagic changes (Fig. 2.3a). Pertinent relevant history including refractory blood pressure control despite optimal medical management in conjunction with imaging findings concerning for an adrenal mass raises suspicion for a pheochromocytoma crisis. In the inpatient setting, it is important to consider a pheochromocytoma multisystem crisis (hypertension, hypothermia, and encephalopathy) in critically ill patients with concomitant comorbidities, evidence of end-organ damage, and hypertension refractory to typical medical management [7].

Pheochromocytoma crisis may result in severe cardiovascular collapse, pulmonary edema, and acute respiratory failure. Unfortunately, laboratory confirmation requires an extended period of time, and no rapid testing has yet to be established. In patients with a high index of suspicion for pheochromocytoma crisis, immediate and rapid treatment of blood pressure control should be initiated with a combination of alpha-blockade (phentolamine), calcium channel blockade (nicardipine), and direct vasodilators (nitroprusside). Beta-blockade may be initiated for residual/refractory tachycardia only once adequate alpha-blockade has been achieved as unopposed alpha-adrenergic activity can lead to cardiovascular collapse.

Despite maximal medical intervention, patients may continue to clinically deteriorate. In hemodynamically unstable patients who continue to deteriorate clinically, despite maximal medical treatment, consideration should be given to proceeding to the operating room for an emergent adrenalectomy [8] (Fig. 2.3b). Postoperatively, patients should be carefully monitored for transient hypocortisolism and subsequently treated with intravenous hydrocortisone as needed, and medical endocrinology consult is advised.

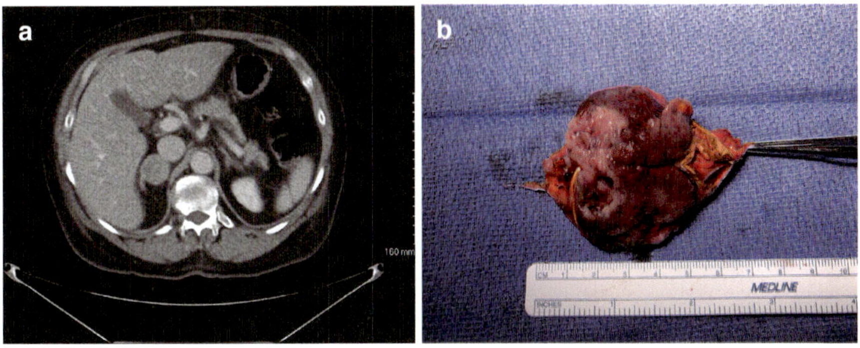

Fig. 2.3 (**a**) CT scan showing right adrenal mass that was a pheochromocytoma. (**b**) Surgical specimen of the pheochromocytoma after it was removed

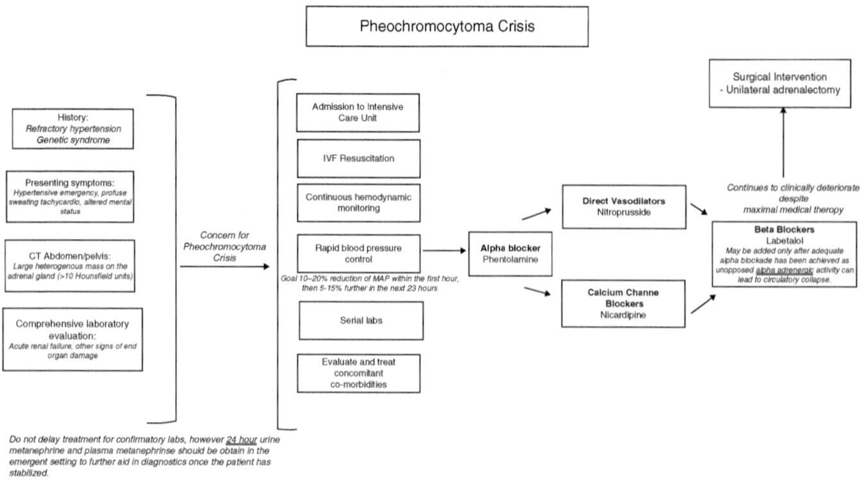

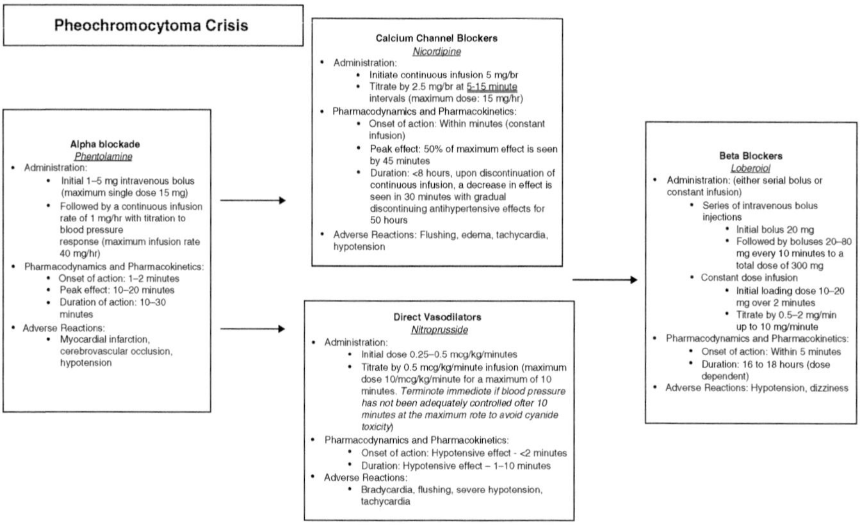

2.4 Hypercortisolism

Prolonged tissue exposure to grossly elevated concentrations of glucocorticoids, either from an endogenous or an exogenous source, may result in hypercortisolism and in severe cases constitutes an acute emergency. Exogenous sources include oral steroid medications, whereas endogenous sources may be caused by ACTH-secreting pituitary adenoma (Cushing's disease), benign adrenal lesions (adrenal adenoma, micronodular hyperplasia), malignant adrenal lesions (adrenocortical carcinoma), or ectopic ACTH secretion tumors (small-cell carcinoma). Cushing's disease is the most frequent cause of endogenous Cushing's syndrome and is characterized by secretion of cortisol secondary to an underlying pituitary adenoma. However, acute, severe clinical presentations of hypercortisolism are more typical of ectopic ACTH-secreting lesions (secretion of ACTH by a non-pituitary tumor) and account for approximately 20% of dependent Cushing's syndrome. The rapid control of severe cortisol excess is crucial and lifesaving. Patients with ectopic ACTH-secreting lesions in acute, hypercortisolism crises present with hypokalemia, hypertension, hyperglycemia, and muscle weakness.

The definition of acute, severe hypercortisolism is fluid and should be considered in the context of laboratory abnormalities, presenting symptoms, past history, and clinical exam. Severe hypercortisolism may present in conjunction with the onset of other acute morbidities including sepsis, heart failure, gastrointestinal hemorrhage, thromboembolism, myopathy, opportunistic infections, or ketoacidosis. Laboratory abnormalities of hyperglycemia, hypokalemia, and metabolic alkalosis with concomitant hypertension should raise suspicion for hypercortisolism, particularly in patients with established diagnoses known to elevate circulating glucocorticoids (i.e., *Cushing's syndrome, adrenocortical carcinoma, or ectopic paraneoplastic*). However, patients may present with no prior history and relatively vague complaints. A broad differential and workup should be initiated including comprehensive laboratory evaluation with comprehensive metabolic panel, complete blood count, serum cortisol and ACTH, as well as multiphase CT imaging. Imaging findings must be taken into consideration, particularly those with no previously established diagnoses but with other clinical evidence concerning severe hypercortisolism. Ectopic ACTH-secreting tumors may be seen as lesions in the adrenal glands, lung, or pancreas.

Severe hypercortisolism is associated with a random serum cortisol higher than 40 μg/dL (normal range 5–25 μg/dL) or a 24-h urine free cortisol more than four times the upper limit of normal (normal range 10–100 mcg/24). This is often seen in the setting of severe hypokalemia (defined as a serum potassium of <3 mmol/L) (normal range 3.6–5.2 mmol/L). In the setting of acute, severe hypercortisolism, the classic features of Cushing's syndrome are not evident; however, significant metabolic/electrolyte disturbances are apparent on laboratory analysis [9]. These laboratory abnormalities coupled with imaging findings and presenting symptoms should raise a high level of suspicion for severe hypercortisolism. Marked increase in serum cortisol and adrenocorticotropic hormone with other associated laboratory abnormalities in conjunction with concerning imaging findings should prompt rapid treatment. If the diagnosis of severe hypercortisolism is presumed, it is imperative to immediately initiate treatment and to not delay for diagnostic confirmation.

Treatment includes the rapid reduction of cortisol, correction of metabolic derangements, and management of any concomitant comorbidities. Rapid correction of cortisol should be initiated with oral ketoconazole and/or metyrapone. If enteral access is not available or if appropriate cortisol levels are not able to be achieved with oral medications, intravenous etomidate has been shown to be effective and safe in reducing elevated cortisol levels. Patients treated with etomidate should be carefully monitored in the intensive care unit with sedation scores, continuous hemodynamic monitoring, and serial serum cortisol to closely monitor levels (every 4–6 h) [10–12].

Intervention is directed at addressing the etiology of the severe hypercortisolism with optimal therapy being complete resection of the cortisol-secreting tumor or ACTH-secreting tumor. In the setting of severe hypercortisolism, admission to intensive care unit with close hemodynamic monitoring and rapid correction of elevated cortisol and electrolyte abnormalities with medical therapy should be initiated. Once the acute crisis is medically stabilized, then further treatment with either prolonged medical therapy or surgery may be initiated. Transsphenoidal surgery is the treatment of choice for ACTH-producing pituitary adenoma when a clearly circumscribed adenoma is identified. In patients with hypercortisolism secondary to ACTH secretion (pituitary adenoma or ectopic ACTH tumor) where the tumor is not resectable or non-localized, some patients may benefit from bilateral adrenalectomy, but careful patient selection and a multidisciplinary approach are required for this decision as medical management of lack of adrenal function is challenging.

In patients with primary adrenal disease, treatment is directed at removal of the adrenal gland or glands. Adrenal tumors should be removed with unilateral adrenalectomy, while bilateral adrenalectomy is indicated for bilateral micronodular and macronodular adrenal hyperplasia [13]. Unilateral tumors incidentally discovered on the adrenal gland should never be biopsied to determine etiology; rather, they should be removed with an oncologic reaction (en bloc with any nodes/invading structures) (Fig. 2.4a, b). In patients who continue to clinically deteriorate despite maximal medical therapy, emergent adrenalectomy may be considered as a lifesaving measure [14]. Finally, for tumors that are unable to be resected due to local invasion, palliative debulking may still be indicated to improve patient quality of life.

Either open or laparoscopic surgical approach is reasonable. While the laparoscopic approach is associated with less postoperative morbidity and mortality, ultimately surgical intervention should be at the discretion of the comfort level of the operative surgeon. Additionally, it is important to recognize that adrenal crisis is an emergent complication of bilateral adrenalectomy. Any patient who has bilateral adrenalectomy should wear a medic alert bracelet in case of trauma or other crises, as patients are unable to mount an acute stress response to trauma or severe illness. All patients receiving medical or surgical intervention should be monitored for adrenal insufficiency and treated accordingly with intravenous hydrocortisone with subsequent taper to oral steroids.

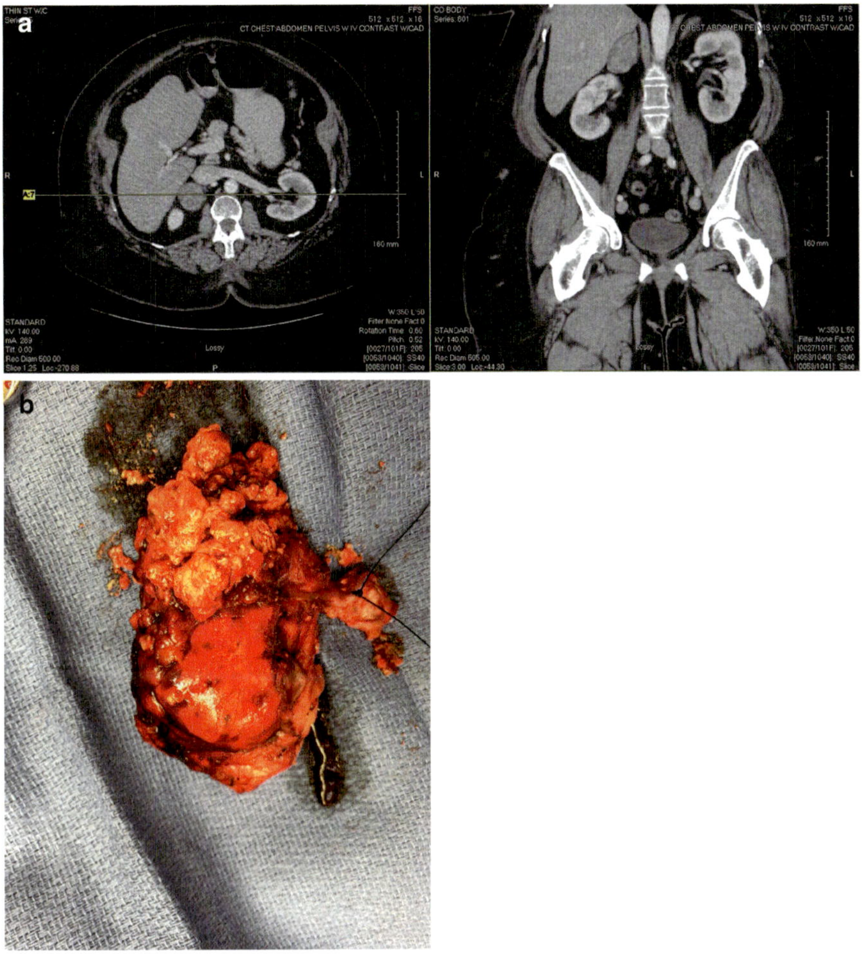

Fig. 2.4 (**a**) CT scan of a right adrenal tumor in a patient with severe Cushing's symptoms. (**b**) Surgical specimen of the same right adrenal tumor that turned out to be a low-grade adrenal cortical cancer

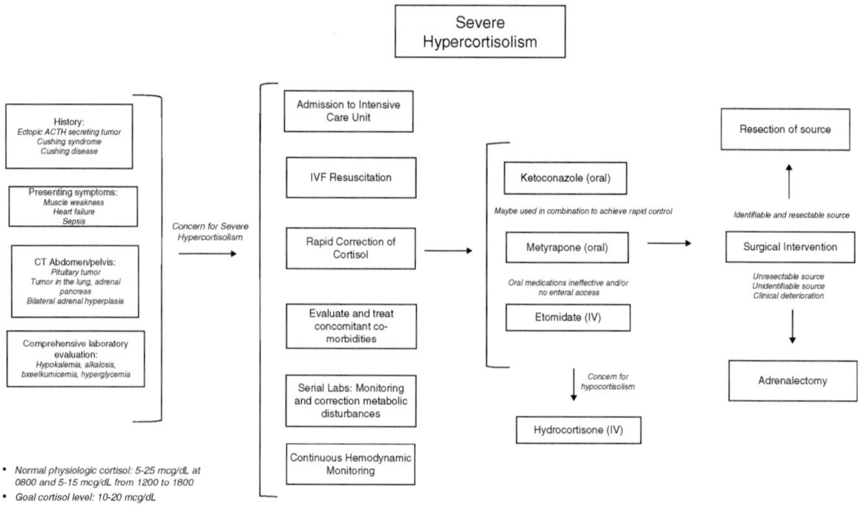

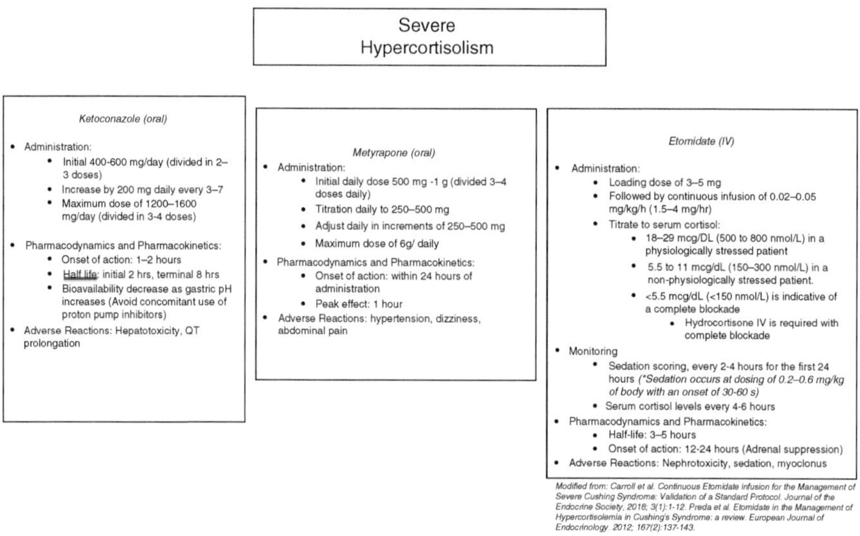

2.5 Adrenal Crisis (Acute Adrenal Insufficiency)

Adrenal insufficiency results from a deficiency of adrenal cortisol production and is categorized as primary, secondary, or tertiary adrenal insufficiency. Primary adrenal insufficiency arises from a direct insult/failure of the adrenal gland. Secondary and tertiary adrenal insufficiency are due to disorders of the pituitary or hypothalamus. Adrenal crisis (acute adrenal insufficiency) most commonly occurs in patients with primary adrenal insufficiency; however, it may also be seen in those with secondary and tertiary adrenal insufficiency [15]. Adrenal crisis is a life-threatening emergency associated with significant morbidity and mortality and requires prompt treatment.

Primary adrenal insufficiency may occur with bilateral adrenal hemorrhage, bilateral adrenalectomy, congenital hyperplasia, drug-induced adrenal enzyme inhibition (i.e., mitotane, ketoconazole, and metyrapone), etomidate when continuously infused or frequently dosed, as well as other pharmacologic agents such as carbamazepine, phenytoin, and phenobarbitone [16]. Adrenal hemorrhage may occur in the setting of trauma, or spontaneously ruptured adrenal tumor. Although less common, acute adrenal insufficiency may occur in secondary and tertiary adrenal insufficiency and is typically precipitated by acute stress, pituitary infarct, or traumatic brain injury or following surgical cure of Cushing's syndrome. Additionally, patients on exogenous steroids (prednisone 5 mg/day or equivalent for 4 weeks or longer across all routes of administration—oral, optical, inhaled, or intranasal) are at increased risk for adrenal insufficiency, and abrupt withdrawal from exogenous glucocorticoids may provoke adrenal crisis.

The clinical features of adrenal crisis include hypotension and hypovolemia with laboratory abnormalities of hyperkalemia and hyponatremia. However, patients often present with vague, nonspecific symptoms such as nausea, vomiting, fever, abdominal pain, fatigue, and altered consciousness.

In patients with a suspected adrenal crisis, prompt initiation of treatment is crucial. Serum chemistry, blood serum cortisol, ACTH, renin, and aldosterone should be collected as part of the initial evaluation; however, treatment should not be delayed for diagnostic confirmatory tests. Rapid correction of hypocortisolism can be done with bolus injection of 100 mg IV hydrocortisone (intramuscular may be substituted pending intravenous access) followed by 200 mg hydrocortisone per 24 h (continuous IV infusion or 50 mg of hydrocortisone intravenous injection every 6 h). Concurrently, rehydration should be started with isotonic saline or 5% dextrose in isotonic saline via continuous IV and titrated based on volume status/urine output. Patients should be admitted to an intensive care unit for close monitoring of vitals and serial serum chemistry laboratory tests to carefully monitor electrolyte abnormalities. Intravenous hydrocortisone replacement should continue at 50 mg every 6 h until the patient is clinically stable [16]. Following clinical stability (normalization of vitals, ability to tolerate oral intake/medication), parenteral glucocorticoid therapy may be tapered over 24–72 h and transitioned to oral stress or maintenance dose. Once the patient is clinically stable, tapering of intravenous hydrocortisone to replacement doses can be initiated within 24–72 h. Patients with primary adrenal insufficiency should additionally receive mineralocorticoid replacement when the total daily hydrocortisone dose is lower than 50 mg/24 h. Additionally, once a patient has stabilized, precipitating causes of the adrenal crisis should be investigated and appropriately treated.

It is important to note that all patients with adrenal insufficiency should take emergency precautions by wearing a medical alert bracelet/necklace as well as carry an emergency card with the diagnosis, daily medication, and doses listed. Patients and family/support members should be educated on the use of injectable glucocorticoids in the setting of an emergency and be instructed to inject the medication if symptoms of acute adrenal insufficiency occur, nausea/vomiting and inability to tolerate oral intake/medications, or if the patient is found unresponsive. Following medication administration, the family/support person(s) should seek medical help immediately [16].

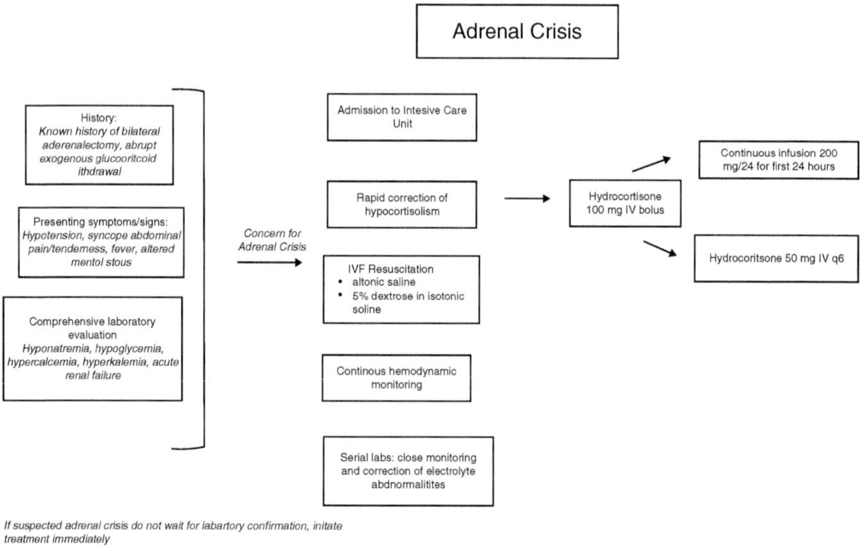

2.6 Conclusion

Adrenal emergencies are rare but potentially life-threatening diagnoses that present a challenge in the acute care setting. Due to their often vague presentation, a high index of suspicion for diagnoses is required. History, presentation, imaging, and laboratory values are helpful in aiding the clinician to ascertain the correct diagnosis. However, in the setting of a potentially life-threatening adrenal emergency, if the index of suspicion is high, initiation of treatment should not be delayed for diagnostic confirmation. Rapid intervention and treatment may be lifesaving in adrenal emergencies.

References

1. Di Gaiacomo JC, et al. Acute traumatic injuries of the adrenal gland: Pennsylvania trauma outcomes study registry. Trauma Surg Acute Care Open. 2020;15(5):e000487.
2. Bharucha T, Broderick C, Easom N, et al. Bilateral adrenal haemorrhage presenting as epigastric and back pain. JRSM Short Rep. 2012;3(3):15.
3. Godfrey RL, Clark J, Field B. Bilateral adrenal hemorrhagic infarction in patient with antiphospholipid syndrome. BMJ Case Rep. 2014;2014:bcr2014207050.

4. Madhusudhanan J, Robert JA, Sekar TV. Successful angioembolization for blunt adrenal gland trauma. Indian J Urol. 2020;36(1):59–61.
5. Gomez R, McAninch J, Carroll P. Adrenal gland trauma: diagnosis and management. J Trauma Injury Infect Crit Care. 1993;35(6):870–4.
6. Bartikoski S, Reschke D. Pheochromocytoma crisis in the emergency department. Cureus. 2021;13(3):e13683.
7. Katsura K, et al. Pheochromocytoma multisystem crisis treated with emergency surgery: a case report and literature review. BMC Res Notes. 2015;8:758.
8. Salinas C, Beltran O, Sanchez-Hidalgo J, et al. Emergency adrenalectomy due to acute heart failure secondary to complicated pheochromocytoma: a case report. World J Surg Oncol. 2011;9:49.
9. Lutgers HL, et al. Severe hypercortisolism: medical emergency requiring urgent intervention. Crit Care Med. 2010;38(7):1598–601.
10. Castinetti F, et al. Ketoconazole in Cushing's disease: is it worth a try? J Clin Endocrinol Metab. 2014;99(5):1623–30.
11. Carroll TB, et al. Continuous etomidate infusion for the management of Severe Cushing Syndrome: validation of a standard protocol. J Endocr Soc. 2018;3(1):1–12.
12. Preda et at. Etomidate in the management of hypercortisolemia in Cushing's syndrome: a review. Eur J Endocrinol. 2012;167(2):137–43.
13. Vieira Oberger Marques J, Boguszewski CL. Medical therapy in severe hypercortisolism. Best Pract Res Clin Endocrinol Metab. 2021;35(2):101487.
14. Davenport E, Lennard T. Acute hypercortisolism: what can the surgeon offer? Clin Endocrinol. 2014;81(4):498–502.
15. Huecker MR, Bhutta BS, Dominique E. Adrenal insufficiency. Treasure Island (FL): StatPearls; 2021.
16. Dineen R, Thompson C, Sherlock M. Adrenal crisis: prevention and management in adult patients. Ther Adv Endocrinol Metab. 2019;10:1–12.

Thoracic Emergencies

3

A. Hecker, J. Noll, M. A. Weigand, Markus Hirschburger, Jens G. Riedel, M. Reichert, W. Padberg, and M. Hecker

3.1 Introduction

The most frequent acute thoracic emergencies in oncologic patients include airway obstruction, endobronchial bleeding, and poststenotic complications such as development of fistula with concomitant bleeding, infection, and/or respiratory impairment. Clinical presentations in the emergency room range from slow deterioration of the general condition of the patient to acute complications with lethal outcome. Securing of the airway is the main task for both emergency and intensive care doctors. Subsequently, the treatment of the cause relies on interventional radiologists, bronchoscopy, and eventually intervention of thoracic surgeons.

Table 3.1 provides some overview on typical clinical diagnoses of lung cancer patients in the emergency room, published by Gorham et al. in 2013 [1]. Respiratory symptoms are—as expected—the most common clinical signs on admission. Of patients presenting with respiratory symptoms, 62.8% have dyspnea, 17.7% cough, 11.5% chest pain, and 8% hemoptysis as the main symptom.

A. Hecker (✉) · J. Noll · J. G. Riedel · M. Reichert · W. Padberg
Department of General and Thoracic Surgery, University Hospital of Giessen, Giessen, Germany
e-mail: Andreas.Hecker@chiru.med.uni-giessen.de; Julia.Noll@chiru.med.uni-giessen.de; Jens.G.Riedel@chiru.med.uni-giessen.de; Martin.Reichert@chiru.med.uni-giessen.de; Winfried.Padberg@chiru.med.uni-giessen.de

M. A. Weigand
Department of Anesthesiology, University Hospital of Heidelberg, Heidelberg, Germany
e-mail: Markus.Weigand@med.uni-heidelberg.de

M. Hirschburger
Department of General Surgery, Worms Hospital, Worms, Germany
e-mail: Markus.Hirschburger@klinikum-worms.de

M. Hecker
Medical Clinic II, University Hospital of Giessen, Giessen, Germany
e-mail: Matthias.Hecker@innere.med.uni-giessen.de

A. Tarasconi et al. (eds.), *Oncologic Surgical Emergencies*, Hot Topics in Acute Care Surgery and Trauma, https://doi.org/10.1007/978-3-031-36860-8_3

Table 3.1 Typical diagnoses in lung cancer patients on admission in the emergency room (ER) [1]

Infection	29.4%	Pulmonary infection, febrile neutropenia, GIT
Neoplastic progression	21.9%	Locoregional, brain metastasis
Pain	12.4%	Acute and chronic pain
Gastrointestinal complications	8.4%	Side effects of chemotherapy, constipation, GERD
Cardiovascular complications	7.1%	Pulmonary embolism, deep vein thrombosis Arrhythmias Myocardial infarction
Pulmonary complications	3.3%	Respiratory distress Hemoptysis
Others (metabolic, hematologic, urological, neurological, etc.)	17.5%	Acute renal failure, anemia, thrombocytopenia, diabetic decompensation

3.1.1 Airway Obstruction

Both extraluminal airway compression and endoluminal tumor growth can lead to airway obstruction, which bears the risk of acute dyspnea and suffocation.

Mediastinal tumor masses (e.g., lymphoma, thymoma, teratoma, bulky disease with large lymph node metastases) could lead to compression of the trachea and the main bronchi. A concomitant compression of the superior vena cava is clinically apparent as an upper venous congestion (see Sect. 3.1.2). After initial airway securing, definitive management relies on bronchoscopic implantation of self-expanding metal stents (SEMSs), silicone stents (without metal stabilization), or hybrid stents. The use of a jet ventilation system enables the endoscopist to implant the stent via rigid bronchoscopy. In case of malignancy, covered metal stents as well as silicone stents are typically used to avoid in-stent tumor growth. Tumors that are primarily located endobronchially or infiltrate the bronchial lumen could lead to endobronchial obstruction. While endobronchial tumor growth in trachea and main bronchi can be typically managed by interventional bronchoscopy, obstruction of peripheral bronchi (e.g., segmental bronchi) requires surgical tumor resection in the absence of formal inoperability criteria. If resection (e.g., by lobectomy with systemic lymphadenectomy) is functionally or technically unfeasible, radiotherapy could be an alternative (palliative) therapeutic option. In cases of tumor obstruction of the larger airways, flexible (diagnostic) bronchoscopy is the first step to evaluate the tumor size and texture; such information allows the choice of the optimal therapeutic option. Several therapeutic approaches are available including mechanical tumor removal, electrocoagulation, argon plasma coagulation, etc. In contrast to these techniques, which offer only temporary solutions for critical respiratory situations, the use of endobronchial brachytherapy has long-term efficiency. Nearly all bronchoscopic methods require both rigid bronchoscopic devices in combination with jet ventilators (caveats: risk of burning/explosion if high oxygen concentrations are required). Table 3.2 provides a short overview on some advantages and disadvantages of these different techniques.

Table 3.2 A short overview on the different endobronchial techniques for interventional tumor therapy

Therapeutic approach	Characteristics	Advantages	Disadvantages/side effects
Mechanical procedure	Tumor removal/debulking by endoscopic forceps and loops	Flexible bronchoscopy possible	Increased bleeding risk in emergency situation
Laser therapy	Tumor removal/debulking by ND-YAG laser 5–8 mm penetration depth	Lifetime prolonged about 4 months 80% success rate (trachea) 40% success rate (lobar bronchi)	Complication rate <2% (bleeding, perforation, asphyxia, burning, pneumothorax)
Electrotherapy (APC)	Argon plasma coagulation 2–3 mm penetration depth Often combined with mechanical tumor removal	Best coagulation, 80% success rate (trachea)	Argon gas emboli with cerebral and cardiac complications possible
Photodynamic therapy	i.v. Application of a sensitizer before the endoscopic intervention; radiation with red light leads to tumor necrosis	Not for emergency palliative situations, but for destruction of small tumors <1 cm (92% success rate) (>2 cm 50% only) (Low) Evidence that PDT could be superior to YAG laser therapy	CT to exclude deep tumor infiltration Increased risk for sunburn after sensitizer application
Endobronchial brachytherapy	Radioactive tracer is endoscopically and temporarily placed at the lung tumor/after loading technique (5–10 Gy) Often combined with initial tumor destruction by laser therapy	Ongoing trials in combination with percutaneous radiation therapy (boost)	In contrast to percutaneous radiation therapy, less effective

3.1.2 Superior Vena Cava Syndrome

Malignant tumor masses leading to invasion or external compression of the superior vena cava account for nearly 90% of cases of superior vena cava syndrome; nonmalignant causes include infections/inflammatory processes or thrombosis. About 3% of patients with lung cancer (10% of patients with small-cell lung cancer) suffer from symptoms of superior vena cava compression ranging from edema of the upper quadrants of the body and dysphagia to acute respiratory distress caused by laryngeal edema [2]. Diagnosis relies on CT scan, and the most effective and safe therapeutic approach relies on percutaneous endovascular stent implantation, with reported success rates of 80–100%. In patients with small-cell lung cancer, combined chemoradiation is a noninvasive alternative (success rates about 80%), but effects are delayed 7–14 days after treatment initiation.

3.1.3 Endoluminal Bleeding

Endoluminal bleeding can be caused by a wide range of benign conditions, such as tuberculosis, bronchiectasis, aspergillosis, and vasculitis. Reviews of the literature from France, the USA, and Italy reveal that about 14–25% of patients with hemoptysis presenting in the ER suffer from bronchial carcinoma, which may lead to minor (up to 20 mL per 24 h), moderate (20–500 mL per 24 h), or severe bleeding (more than 500 mL per 24 h) [3]. In contrast to other locations, even minor endobronchial bleedings bear the risk of life-threatening asphyxia. About 150 mL of blood could lead to a nearly complete obstruction of the airways with dramatic clinical consequences. It should be kept in mind that not exsanguination, but asphyxia leads to death during endobronchial bleeding. Blood loss of 200 mL per 24 h is associated with a mortality of 40%. The initial step in cases of dramatic bleeding should be airway securing, which might require single-lung ventilation, bronchial blockers, ECMO, etc. Lavage with cold saline or adrenalin solutions for vasoconstriction and argon plasma (APC) or laser coagulation through rigid bronchoscopy are the methods of choice to achieve quick bleeding cessation (see Table 3.2). Rigid bronchoscopy allows more efficient clot removal compared to flexible bronchoscopy. If hemostasis could not be achieved through bronchoscopy (e.g., in cases of peripheral bleeding of a tumor in the lung parenchyma), bronchial arterial embolization is the method of choice. Bronchial arteries originating as branches from the thoracic aorta can be occluded using interventional catheters. Success rates range between 77 and 100%, and complications such as aortic dissection, perforation, or neurologic impairments occur in 2–4% of patients. The main drawback of such techniques is the high recurrence rate (up to 53% recurrent hemoptysis within the first year) [4]. If patients fulfill operability criteria, oncologic tumor resection should be undertaken after emergency bleeding control by endoscopy or interventional radiology. Modern literature shows that mortality was dramatically increased if surgery was performed up front to obtain emergency control of endobronchial bleeding. Therapeutic algorithms should rely on first-line endoscopic or radiological bleeding control, followed by oncologic resection, if possible.

3.1.4 Pneumonia and Lung Abscess

Bronchial obstruction by malignancies is one of the most common reasons for pneumonia and has to be kept in mind by every emergency practitioner. Up to 9%

of patients with pneumonia have a poststenotic inflammation of the lung parenchyma. Due to the persisting stenosis, long-term broad-spectrum antibiotics are often necessary. If feasible, oncologic resection of the infected tumor-bearing pulmonary lobe is the gold standard. Otherwise, endoscopic treatment and recanalization are indicated.

Obstruction pneumonia can evolve to abscess formation. Tumor necrosis with concomitant infection may be another cause for abscess development. If the focus of infection gets in contact with the pleural cavity, a tumor-associated pleural empyema may develop. While a lung abscess due to tumor necrosis may be successfully treated by surgical tumor resection with curative intent, surgery is also indicated in palliative settings to achieve pulmonary/pleural source control and enable administration of systemic antitumor treatment. However, in most cases, radical surgical tumor resection is not feasible in these patients. Under such circumstances, endoscopic treatment of the tumor stenosis by stent implantation or bronchoscopy drainage of a pulmonary abscess is a possible palliative therapeutic option. Alternatively, external percutaneous transthoracic CT-guided drainage of a pulmonary abscess should be considered.

3.1.5 Tracheoesophageal Fistula (TEF)

Tracheoesophageal fistula is a life-threatening emergency in thoracic oncology. In the absence of efficient treatment, repetitive aspiration pneumonia leads to death within weeks; immediate interventional therapy is required in these patients to improve outcomes. Due to the palliative situation in most cases, surgical therapy is usually not an option. Endoscopic (bronchial and/or esophageal) stenting could bridge the TEF and avoid aspiration. Fibrin application or over-the-scope clipping (OTSC) of the fistula is a semi-experimental, individual option, which usually fails in the long-term malignant TEF. Malignant fistula between bronchi and aorta leads to fulminant hemoptysis with rapid clinical deterioration and death. Emergency concepts typically include implantations of thoracic endovascular aortic repair (TEVAR) stents.

3.1.6 Neoplastic Pleural Effusions with Trapped Lung

Pleural effusions in oncologic patients are often more complicated due to a trapped lung, which could not expand. Intrapleural instillation of cytotoxic agents has limited effects. In these cases, the use of intermittent pleural drainage, e.g., via a Denver pleuroperitoneal shunt, or an external permanent drainage (e.g., PleurX) should be considered. In rare situations, a pleurectomy can be discussed in patients with good clinical condition.

3.2 Conclusion

Cancer patients suffering from lung cancer are threatened by a variety of emergencies requiring interventional bronchoscopy or radiology in most cases. Interdisciplinary decisions from surgeons, anesthesiologists, radiologists, and pneumologists are necessary to provide best care for these complex emergency patients.

References

1. Gorham, et al. Lung cancer. Lancet. 2013;80:203–8.
2. De Potter B, et al. Imaging of urgencies and emergencies in the lung cancer patient. Insights Imaging. 2018;9:463–76.
3. Schweigert, et al. Oncologic emergencies in thoracic surgery. Onkologe. 2020;26:105–12.
4. German AWMF Guideline on Bronchial Cancer. 2018;331–322.

Oncological Emergencies: Esophageal Cancer

4

Mircea Chirica and Gaël Roth

4.1 Introduction

Esophageal cancer (EC) is the seventh most frequent cancer worldwide and is responsible for approximately 500,000 deaths yearly [1–3]. Multimodal therapies have replaced surgery alone in the curative approach of patients with advanced EC, and recent overall survival rates (currently approaching 50%) have doubled during the last decades [4, 5]. The current trend in modern oncology is offering personalized therapeutic pathways to cancer patients through a multidisciplinary decision-making process. While this process benefits a large majority of patients, it is not adapted to patients experiencing acute complications such as tumor bleeding, upper digestive tract perforation, obstruction, or airway invasion. Indeed, such oncological emergencies require quick complex decision-making, which takes into consideration the risks and chances of success of emergency therapeutic procedures as well as patients' cancer-related prognosis. Most practitioners have limited experience with the management of oncologic esophageal emergencies, and reliable management guidelines are lacking in the literature. This chapter focuses on the management of oncological emergencies in EC patients, which are

M. Chirica (✉)
Service de Chirurgie Digestive, Centre Hospitalier Universitaire Grenoble Alpes, Grenoble, France
e-mail: mchirica@chu-grenoble.fr

G. Roth
Service d'Hepatogastroenterologie, Centre Hospitalier Universitaire Grenoble Alpes, Grenoble, France

Institute for Advanced Biosciences-INSERM U1209/CNRS UMR 5309/Université Grenoble-Alpes, Grenoble, France
e-mail: groth@chu-grenoble.fr

A. Tarasconi et al. (eds.), *Oncologic Surgical Emergencies*, Hot Topics in Acute Care Surgery and Trauma, https://doi.org/10.1007/978-3-031-36860-8_4

classified according to their presentation mode in esophageal obstruction, esophageal perforation, tumor bleeding, and airway involvement. Complications of esophagectomy for cancer-requiring emergency management are beyond the scope of this chapter.

4.2 Esophageal Obstruction

Dysphagia is a predominant problem in patients with esophageal cancer and is the most frequent-onset symptom [6]. Severity of dysphagia ranges from simple discomfort to complete aphagia [7]. Management of dysphagia and particularly treatment of food impaction are an emergency in patients with EC. In patients eligible for curative treatments, the preservation of a good nutritional status is cornerstone as it allows appropriate patient conditioning for intensive chemotherapy regimens and extensive surgery. Restoring swallowing capacities is also important to improve the quality of life in patients with advanced EC undergoing palliative treatments. Complete obstruction of the esophageal lumen by EC induces regurgitation of food and saliva into the airway and can lead to aspiration pneumonia, which might compromise short-term survival. EC is a rare cause of food impaction (<2%) which requires prompt management [8].

Management of EC-related dysphagia relies mainly on endoscopic procedures (dilation, stenting), but alternatives have been described [7].

4.2.1 Endoscopic Management

Endoscopic dilation using either pneumatic balloon or wire-covered boogies is an easy and effective procedure of esophageal disobstruction in patients with EC [7]. While dilation provides quick relief of dysphagia, in the setting of malignant obstruction, long-term effects are very limited with quick symptom recurrence [7]. For this reason, dilation is usually associated with esophageal stenting for treatment of dysphagia in EC. Esophageal stenting maintains oral intake with short hospital stay and improves QOL in palliative patients [6]. Self-expanding metal stents (SEMSs) are currently the recommended up-front approach in patients with obstructive EC [9, 10]. SEMSs are efficient as up to 80% of patients experience dysphagia relief [6]. However, stenting may be complicated by retrosternal pain (9%), hemorrhage (8%), stent migration (7%), and esophageal perforation (3%) [6]. In case of food impaction, pushing the bolus beyond the obstacle is successful in 90% of cases; retrieval using a snare should be attempted in case of failure [11]. Enteral feeding should always be discussed after disobstruction as these patients are usually malnourished.

4.2.2 Alternative Techniques

Alternative techniques of esophageal disobstruction include radiotherapy, chemotherapy, endoluminal brachytherapy, photodynamic therapy, laser therapy, cryoablation, intra-tumoral injection of alcohol or chemotherapy, plasma argon coagulation, and surgery. These techniques are marginal, but in combination with endoscopy, they may prolong the duration of dysphagia-free periods and improve patient quality of life [7].

4.2.3 Surgery

Dysphagia palliation by esophagectomy or esophageal bypass procedures is no longer recommended in patients with advanced esophageal cancer. Due to high mortality and morbidity rates in patients with short life expectancy, surgery has been abandoned and replaced by local endoscopic therapies [7].

However, surgery has an important role in improving the nutritional status of patients with obstructive esophageal cancer who are eligible for either curative or palliative treatments [12]. Starting re-nutrition prior to complex multimodal therapies is an emergency in patients who had experienced severe weight loss [12]. Enteral feeding is highly preferred to intravenous nutrition due to potential infections, electrolyte abnormalities, liver tests abnormalities, and high costs associated with the use of parenteral nutrition. Parenteral nutrition should be generally limited to patients awaiting placement of an enteral delivery system [7]. In a recent study, surgical jejunostomy proved more effective and less morbid when compared to endoscopic stenting in patients with severe esophageal obstruction [13]. Placement of a feeding jejunostomy tube at the time of staging laparoscopy is a safe and reliable means of providing nutrition in patients with esophageal cancer [14, 15].

4.2.4 Endoluminal Brachytherapy

The technique relies on the endoscopic introduction of a radioactive source into the tumor, which allows delivery of high doses of radiotherapy to the tumor with a relatively small involvement of the surrounding healthy tissues [9, 16]. The treatment is performed weekly during a 3- to 8-week treatment course, and the response rate for dysphagia symptoms is up to 70%. The main drawbacks are the short duration of the symptom relief, lasting an average of 2.5 months, and the need for multiple treatments. Brachytherapy complications include esophagitis, stricture, and fistula formation [16]. Another shortcoming associated with this technique is its lack of availability: in one paper, only 6% of 59 US hospitals had access to brachytherapy [17].

4.2.5 Photodynamic Therapy

Photodynamic therapy has currently a marginal role in the palliation of dysphagia in the setting of EC [7, 18]. The technique includes parenteral administration of a systemic photosensitizer (porfimer sodium 2 mg/kg) followed (48–72 h) by the administration of locally directed light (red light of wavelengths 630 nm). The photosensitizer is preferentially taken up by tumor cells, and direct application of light through an endoscope triggers a photooxidative reaction resulting in cell death. Phototherapy was quite effective in palliating dysphagia in one study with a 90% success rate 4 weeks after the end of the treatment and a dysphagia-free period of 80 days [19]. The main drawbacks are the low efficacy rates and temporary photosensitivity with sunburns occurring in 20% of patients [18, 20].

4.2.6 Laser Therapy

Local laser therapy aims at esophageal disobstruction by tumor destruction using high-energy lasers such as the Nd:YAG laser. The laser beam is directed at the obstructing esophageal tumor through an endoscope positioned approximately 1 cm away from the tumor; the energy delivered results in tumor destruction by tissue coagulation and vaporization. Early studies have shown rapid improvement in dysphagia scores in patients undergoing laser Nd:YAG therapy with average duration of symptom improvement of about 4 weeks [7, 21].

4.2.7 Other Techniques

Other procedures have been developed with the purpose of obtaining local destruction of the tumor by chemical (intra-tumoral endoscopic injection of alcohol [21] and of chemotherapy [22]) and thermal (cryotherapy [23], argon plasma coagulation [24]) means. With the advent of endoscopic stenting, most of these techniques have been abandoned, but they can still be used in combination for the treatment of advanced esophageal cancers [25].

4.3 Esophageal Perforation

Esophageal perforation (EP) is a highly lethal condition with mortality rates of around 20% [11]. The association between EC and EP is rare, as EC represents less than 5% of causes of EP [26]. Perforation can be due to the spontaneous disruption of the esophageal wall continuity at the site of the tumor or most often the result of interventional and diagnostic endoscopic procedures [26]. Besides, some authors cautioned against liberal use of endoscopic procedures in patients with resectable EC, as EP occurring in this setting may compromise oncologic outcomes [27]. Although the incidence of iatrogenic perforation of esophageal cancer has increased in parallel with the use of esophageal dilation, perforation complicates less than 5% of endoscopic procedures [27, 28].

The management of EP in patients with EC remains controversial, with both emergency surgical resection and conservative treatment being advocated [27, 29]. The choice of treatment should be individually tailored to the mechanism of perforation (spontaneous vs. iatrogenic) as well as the patient's condition and oncological expectations.

4.3.1 Conservative Management

Criteria for nonoperative management of EP have been previously described in a series including only small numbers of patients with EC [30]. Such criteria may be suitable for select patients with perforated EC although data in the literature is scarce [27]. Nonoperative management should be considered for intraoperative EP during endoscopic maneuvers (endoscopic balloon dilation, endoscopic submucosal or mucosal dissection) [28]. Such patients usually have minimal mediastinal and pleural contamination because EP is recognized immediately and they underwent fasting before the procedure. Nonoperative management should also be discussed in patients with locally advanced, unresectable EC and patients unfit for surgery [27]. Conservative treatment requires nil per os diet, insertion of a nasogastric tube for gastric decompression, and either enteral (jejunostomy, nasojejunal tube) or parenteral nutrition [11]. Large-specter antibiotic therapy is usually recommended. First-line attempts at perforation closure rely on endoscopic clipping; use of over-the-scope clips and self-expanding metal stents should be considered in case of failure. Mediastinal and pleural collections should be drained radiologically and closely monitored by endoscopy and/or contrast radiology to assess healing [29].

4.3.2 Surgical Management

In patients with delayed presentation and massive mediastinal/pleural contamination and in patients with large perforations, surgery is often required, assuming that this is within the patient's goals of care [27]. The delay in diagnosis is the main prognostic determinant in patients with EP with mortality rates increasing significantly if management is started more than 24 h after EP [11, 26]. The clinical presentation may be atypical, especially in patients without a previous diagnosis of EC; a high grade of suspicion is required to establish the diagnosis of EP and start prompt treatment [26]. Emergency surgery for EP in patients without cancer relies on suture closure of the esophageal defect associated with pleural debridement, wide drainage, and jejunostomy construction [11]. As cancer tissues do not heal, esophageal resection is probably the only lifesaving treatment option of EP in patients with large defects of EC [31]; this option should be discussed even if R0 resections cannot be achieved as some patients may obtain prolonged survival (Fig. 4.1). In critically ill patients with massive mediastinal and pleural

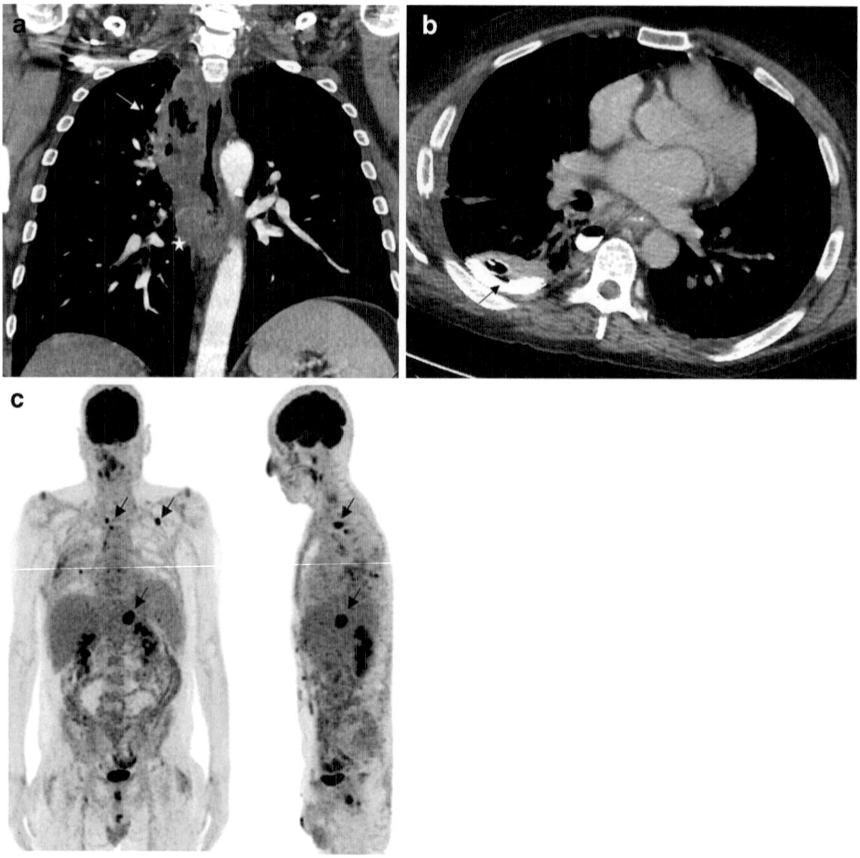

Fig. 4.1 A 63-year-old man with no previous medical history was seen in the emergency department for brutal thoracic pain, dyspnea, and hyperthermia. (**a**) Emergency CT evaluation showed extraluminal air and fluid contained to the mediastinum (arrow) and a tumor of the middle third of the thoracic esophagus. The patient underwent emergency suture repair of the esophageal defect through right thoracotomy and laparoscopic construction of a feeding jejunostomy. (**b**) Postoperative day (POD) 4 CT showed contrast leak into the pleura in a patient with persistent sepsis. Transthoracic esophagectomy with cervical esophagostoma was undertaken. The operative course was uneventful, and the patient was discharged from the hospital on POD20. (**c**) At 3 months, PET-CT showed carcinosis and bone and lymphatic metastases (arrows). Esophageal reconstruction was contraindicated, and the patient died of recurrence 3 years later

contamination, a damage control strategy including esophageal exclusion, pleural decortication, and thoracic drainage should be considered; esophagectomy, cervical esophagostoma, decompression gastrostomy, and feeding jejunostomy are then performed at the time of second-look operation. Esophageal reconstruction with the stomach may be considered in fit patients with minimal pleural contamination and resectable tumors [27]. However, if these conditions are not met, reconstruction should be delayed. Under such circumstances, gastroplasty or coloplasty is usually performed using the retrosternal route after a recurrence-free interval of 3–6 months [32]. In a recent paper focusing on esophagectomies after esophageal perforations, primary reconstruction was performed in 62% of patients while 38% underwent delayed reconstruction [33]. Irrespective of the emergency management method, the long-term oncological results of patients with EC who experience EP are disappointing. Di Franco et al. reported 48 iatrogenic esophageal perforations in EC patients of whom 16 patients underwent intention-to-cure esophageal resection; the remaining 32 patients either were unfit for surgery or had unresectable tumors. There was no significant survival difference between esophagectomy and nonoperative management. The median survival following esophagectomy was 11 months, and all patients died of recurrent disease [27].

4.4 Bleeding

Hemorrhage is a common and severe complication in patients with esophageal cancer. In a recent study focusing on gastrointestinal hemorrhage in patients with gastrointestinal cancer, EC came in fourth position after stomach, liver, and small bowel cancers regarding bleeding risks [34]. Overall, bleeding occurred in 9.3% of EC patients, and lower third cancers had higher bleeding risks (10.7%) than middle third (8.0%) or upper third cancers (6.2%) [34]. Patients with EC may present with either low-volume intermittent bleeding from their tumor or brisk and massive bleeding if the tumor erodes into the aorta. The etiology and the presentation of esophageal hemorrhage condition their management and outcomes.

4.4.1 Minor Bleeding

Patients with EC are at high risk of thromboembolism and bleeding. As occurrence of thromboembolic adverse events may reach 33% in this population, EC patients are often under anticoagulant therapy [35]. Thromboprophylaxis significantly reduces thromboembolic risks but increases tumor bleeding risks as well. Indeed, a study reporting hemorrhagic complications in EC patients under anticoagulation therapy showed that clinically relevant nonmajor bleeding occurred in 6% of patients with 24 months of follow-up [35]; the source of bleeding was gastrointestinal in half of the cases. Several options are available for the management of minor bleeding in patients with EC, including endoscopy, surgery, trans-arterial embolization, and radiation therapy. Interventional endoscopy is the most frequently employed procedure to stop minor bleeding at the tumor site and was associated with a substantial reduction in mortality [34]. Efficient endoscopic hemostasis may be difficult to obtain due to the rigidity of the tumor that hinders the use of hemostatic clips; contact thermal therapy using heater probe or bipolar electrocautery should be considered under these circumstances. Despite initial successful hemostasis, the rate of recurrence bleeding is high with 30-day rebleeding rates of 33% being reported, which is similar to control patients [36, 37]. Another option is the use of hemostatic powder (i.e., Hemospray®), which allows a good immediate hemostasis, but recurrence rates are also high [37, 38]. Thus, other procedures should be performed as a complement to endoscopy to consolidate hemostasis and in case of failure. Various options are available such as radiation therapy for diffuse tumor bleeding or embolization in case of brisk hemorrhage [7]. Transcatheter arterial embolization with *N*-butyl cyanoacrylate has been successfully used to control arterial esophageal bleeding in some EC patients [39]. Argon plasma coagulation, cryoablation, and Nd:YAG laser therapy have also been used for bleeding control in patients with EC, but their use remains marginal [7]. The large majority of these technique are still poorly studied in literature, with very low level of evidence of their benefit.

4.4.2 Massive Hemorrhage

The esophagus is close to the descending aorta in the middle and lower mediastinum, and therefore locally advanced esophageal tumors may occasionally invade the descending aorta. Tumor perforation into the aorta results in esophagoaortic fistula formation, which is a highly lethal condition unless an immediate and effective hemostatic procedure can be performed. Treatment of EC by radiotherapy is a major risk factor of aortoesophageal fistula, which was responsible for death in 7% of patients in one study [40]. A comprehensive review of 500 patients with aorto-esophageal fistulas revealed that 17% of them were caused by advanced EC [41]. Management of malignant aortoesophageal fistula is a difficult challenge, and mortality is very high. Surgical hemostasis is usually not feasible as most of the advanced esophageal tumors are unresectable. Thoracic endovascular aortic repair (TEVAR) is an established treatment for thoracic aortic aneurysms; recently, this technique was reported to enable effective hemostasis in patients with hemorrhage from aortoesophageal fistula in patients with esophageal cancer [42, 43]. Recent studies have reported the efficacy of prophylactic TEVAR to prevent fatal hemorrhagic events during treatment for locally advanced esophageal cancer [43, 44]. Moreover, survival was improved in patients who underwent prophylactic TEVAR when compared to patients who underwent TEVAR for bleeding [43]. Eventually, esophagectomy with curative intent could be offered following TEVAR, and some patients who achieved R0 resection obtained long-term survival [43]. Thus, prophylactic TEVAR should be seriously considered in patients with advanced esophageal cancer and aortic invasion [44].

4.5 Airway Invasion

Due to the proximity with the trachea and the main left bronchus, invasion of the airway is common in advanced esophageal cancer [45]. Airway invasion is suggested by symptoms such as coughing, dyspnea, and hemoptysis, and the diagnosis may be confirmed by bronchoscopy [45]. Fistulization into the tracheobronchial tree is a fearsome complication, which was reported in 0.9–4.5% of patients with EC [46]. Risk factors of malignant esotracheal fistula include dilation of esophageal stenosis, esophageal stent placement, and treatment of the primary esophageal tumor by chemotherapy and radiotherapy. The incidence of esotracheal fistula after radiotherapy for EC with airway invasion ranged between 33 and 79% [47]. Induction chemotherapy prior to radiotherapy reduced this incidence to 6% and is an option that deserves consideration in this setting [48].

The major consequence of esotracheal fistula is non-resolving aspiration pneumonia, from either direct food ingestion or backward flow of gastric contents into the esophagus. Pulmonary sepsis usually leads to patient death in about 6–12 weeks in the absence of effective anti-tumor treatment [45].

The management of malignant esotracheal fistulas is a difficult challenge because the underlying cancer is invariably incurable. It is thus important to evaluate the stage of the cancer and define the goals of treatment according to the expected patient survival. Immediate management relies on nasogastric insertion to decompress the stomach and minimize regurgitation. Providing best supportive care only is a reasonable option when the estimated duration of life of the patient is less than 12 weeks [45]. Several surgical procedures aiming at esophageal exclusion or bypass have been described, but their morbidity and mortality rates are excessive in patients with limited functional reserve. It is currently not recommended to perform complex surgery in palliative situations with limited life span [45]. Interventional endoscopy is the mainstay of esotracheal fistula treatment in patients who are in good clinical shape. Insertion of self-expanding esophageal metal stents (SEMSs) may provide rapid and effective temporary palliation although it is unlikely to seal completely the fistula. The use of a tracheal or bronchial stent, to cover the defect from the airway side, may also be effective for palliation. Tracheal stents may be used in conjunction with esophageal stents to increase the chances of fistula closure. It is recommended to place the airway stent first to prevent airway occlusion by the esophageal stent. Double stenting is at risk to further increase the fistula size due to tissue necrosis from compression of the tracheal and esophageal walls between the two stents. Use of Y-type silicone stents placed across the tracheal carina was effective in reducing the spillage and contamination of the lungs; the median duration of such stents was 4.5 months, which was consistent with the life expectancy of patients [49].

4.6 Conclusion

Oncological emergencies are rare in patients with esophageal cancer and have a strong negative impact on both short-term survival and long-term oncological outcomes. Their management must be multidisciplinary and should take into consideration the procedure-related risks, the oncological prognosis of patients, as well as their condition and desiderata. The place of surgery is quite limited, and interventional endoscopy is currently the mainstay of treatment of esophageal oncological emergencies.

References

1. Bolger JC, Donohoe CL, Lowery M, Reynolds JV. Advances in the curative management of oesophageal cancer. Br J Cancer. 2021;2021:86.
2. Arnold M, Abnet CC, Neale RE, Vignat J, Giovannucci EL, McGlynn KA, et al. Global burden of 5 major types of gastrointestinal cancer. Gastroenterology. 2020;159(1):335–49 e15.
3. Lagergren J, Smyth E, Cunningham D, Lagergren P. Oesophageal cancer. Lancet. 2017;390(10110):2383–96.
4. Al-Batran SE, Homann N, Pauligk C, Goetze TO, Meiler J, Kasper S, et al. Perioperative chemotherapy with fluorouracil plus leucovorin, oxaliplatin, and docetaxel versus fluorouracil or capecitabine plus cisplatin and epirubicin for locally advanced, resectable gastric or gastro-oesophageal junction adenocarcinoma (FLOT4): a randomised, phase 2/3 trial. Lancet. 2019;393(10184):1948–57.
5. van Hagen P, Hulshof MC, van Lanschot JJ, Steyerberg EW, van Berge Henegouwen MI, Wijnhoven BP, et al. Preoperative chemoradiotherapy for esophageal or junctional cancer. N Engl J Med. 2012;366(22):2074–84.
6. Godin A, Liberman M. The modern approach to esophageal palliative and emergency surgery. Ann Transl Med. 2021;9(10):905.
7. Halpern AL, McCarter MD. Palliative management of gastric and esophageal cancer. Surg Clin N Am. 2019;99(3):555–69.
8. Gretarsdottir HM, Jonasson JG, Bjornsson ES. Etiology and management of esophageal food impaction: a population based study. Scand J Gastroenterol. 2015;50(5):513–8.
9. Dai Y, Li C, Xie Y, Liu X, Zhang J, Zhou J, et al. Interventions for dysphagia in oesophageal cancer. Cochrane Database Syst Rev. 2014;10:CD005048.
10. Spaander MC, Baron TH, Siersema PD, Fuccio L, Schumacher B, Escorsell A, et al. Esophageal stenting for benign and malignant disease: European Society of Gastrointestinal Endoscopy (ESGE) clinical guideline. Endoscopy. 2016;48(10):939–48.
11. Chirica M, Kelly MD, Siboni S, Aiolfi A, Riva CG, Asti E, et al. Esophageal emergencies: WSES guidelines. World J Emerg Surg WJES. 2019;14:26.
12. Huddy JR, Huddy FMS, Markar SR, Tucker O. Nutritional optimization during neoadjuvant therapy prior to surgical resection of esophageal cancer—a narrative review. Dis Esophagus. 2018;31(1):1–11.
13. Velotta JB, Dusendang JR, Kwak H, Huyser M, Patel A, Ashiku SK, et al. Outcomes following interventions to sustain body weight in esophageal cancer patients starting preoperative therapy: a retrospective cohort study. J Thorac Dis. 2021;13(9):5477–86.
14. Grondona P, Andreani SM, Barr N, Singh KK. Laparoscopic feeding jejunostomy technique as part of staging laparoscopy. Surg Laparosc Endosc Percutan Tech. 2005;15(5):263–6.
15. Mastoridis S, Bracalente G, Hanganu CB, Neccia M, Giuliani A, Gillies R, et al. Laparoscopic vs. open feeding jejunostomy insertion in oesophagogastric cancer. BMC Surg. 2021;21(1):367.
16. Homs MY, Steyerberg EW, Eijkenboom WM, Tilanus HW, Stalpers LJ, Bartelsman JF, et al. Single-dose brachytherapy versus metal stent placement for the palliation of dysphagia from oesophageal cancer: multicentre randomised trial. Lancet. 2004;364(9444):1497–504.
17. Suntharalingam M, Moughan J, Coia LR, Krasna MJ, Kachnic L, Haller DG, et al. The national practice for patients receiving radiation therapy for carcinoma of the esophagus: results of the 1996–1999 patterns of care study. Int J Radiat Oncol Biol Phys. 2003;56(4):981–7.
18. Yoon HY, Cheon YK, Choi HJ, Shim CS. Role of photodynamic therapy in the palliation of obstructing esophageal cancer. Korean J Intern Med. 2012;27(3):278–84.
19. Luketich JD, Christie NA, Buenaventura PO, Weigel TL, Keenan RJ, Nguyen NT. Endoscopic photodynamic therapy for obstructing esophageal cancer: 77 cases over a 2-year period. Surg Endosc. 2000;14(7):653–7.
20. Lightdale CJ, Heier SK, Marcon NE, McCaughan JS Jr, Gerdes H, Overholt BF, et al. Photodynamic therapy with porfimer sodium versus thermal ablation therapy with Nd:YAG

laser for palliation of esophageal cancer: a multicenter randomized trial. Gastrointest Endosc. 1995;42(6):507–12.
21. Carazzone A, Bonavina L, Segalin A, Ceriani C, Peracchia A. Endoscopic palliation of oesophageal cancer: results of a prospective comparison of Nd:YAG laser and ethanol injection. Eur J Surg Acta Chir. 1999;165(4):351–6.
22. Robles-Jara C, Robles-Medranda C. Endoscopic chemotherapy with 5-fluorouracil in advanced gastric cancer. J Gastrointest Cancer. 2010;41(1):75–8.
23. Greenwald BD, Dumot JA, Abrams JA, Lightdale CJ, David DS, Nishioka NS, et al. Endoscopic spray cryotherapy for esophageal cancer: safety and efficacy. Gastrointest Endosc. 2010;71(4):686–93.
24. Akhtar K, Byrne JP, Bancewicz J, Attwood SE. Argon beam plasma coagulation in the management of cancers of the esophagus and stomach. Surg Endosc. 2000;14(12):1127–30.
25. Goetz M, Malek NP, Kanz L, Hetzel J. Cryorecanalization for in-stent recanalization in the esophagus. Gastroenterology. 2014;146(5):1168–70.
26. Chirica M, Champault A, Dray X, Sulpice L, Munoz-Bongrand N, Sarfati E, et al. Esophageal perforations. J Visc Surg. 2010;147(3):e117–28.
27. Di Franco F, Lamb PJ, Karat D, Hayes N, Griffin SM. Iatrogenic perforation of localized oesophageal cancer. Br J Surg. 2008;95(7):837–9.
28. Yamamoto Y, Kikuchi D, Nagami Y, Nonaka K, Tsuji Y, Fujimoto A, et al. Management of adverse events related to endoscopic resection of upper gastrointestinal neoplasms: review of the literature and recommendations from experts. Dig Endosc. 2019;31(Suppl 1):4–20.
29. Vogel SB, Rout WR, Martin TD, Abbitt PL. Esophageal perforation in adults: aggressive, conservative treatment lowers morbidity and mortality. Ann Surg. 2005;241(6):1016–21.
30. Altorjay A, Kiss J, Voros A, Bohak A. Nonoperative management of esophageal perforations. Is it justified? Ann Surg. 1997;225(4):415–21.
31. Yeo CJ, Lillemoe KD, Klein AS, Zinner MJ. Treatment of instrumental perforation of esophageal malignancy by transhiatal esophagectomy. Arch Surg. 1988;123(8):1016–8.
32. Reslinger V, Tranchart H, D'Annunzio E, Poghosyan T, Quero L, Munoz-Bongrand N, et al. Esophageal reconstruction by colon interposition after esophagectomy for cancer analysis of current indications, operative outcomes, and long-term survival. J Surg Oncol. 2016;113(2):159–64.
33. Abu-Daff S, Shamji F, Ivanovic J, Villeneuve PJ, Gilbert S, Maziak DE, et al. Esophagectomy in esophageal perforations: an analysis. Dis Esophagus. 2016;29(1):34–40.
34. Minhem MA, Nakshabandi A, Mirza R, Alsamman MA, Mattar MC. Gastrointestinal hemorrhage in the setting of gastrointestinal cancer: anatomical prevalence, predictors, and interventions. World J Gastrointest Endosc. 2021;13(9):391–406.
35. Mulder FI, Hovenkamp A, van Laarhoven HWM, Buller HR, Kamphuisen PW, Hulshof M, et al. Thromboembolic and bleeding complications in patients with esophageal cancer. Br J Surg. 2020;107(10):1324–33.
36. Savides TJ, Jensen DM, Cohen J, Randall GM, Kovacs TO, Pelayo E, et al. Severe upper gastrointestinal tumor bleeding: endoscopic findings, treatment, and outcome. Endoscopy. 1996;28(2):244–8.
37. Ofosu A, Ramai D, Latson W, Adler DG. Endoscopic management of bleeding gastrointestinal tumors. Ann Gastroenterol. 2019;32(4):346–51.
38. Chen YI, Barkun AN, Soulellis C, Mayrand S, Ghali P. Use of the endoscopically applied hemostatic powder TC-325 in cancer-related upper GI hemorrhage: preliminary experience (with video). Gastrointest Endosc. 2012;75(6):1278–81.
39. Aoki M, Tokue H, Koyama Y, Tsushima Y, Oshima K. Transcatheter arterial embolization with *N*-butyl cyanoacrylate for arterial esophageal bleeding in esophageal cancer patients. World J Surg Oncol. 2016;14:54.
40. Nemoto K, Takai Y, Ogawa Y, Kakuto Y, Ariga H, Matsushita H, et al. Fatal hemorrhage in irradiated esophageal cancer patients. Acta Oncol. 1998;37(3):259–62.
41. Hollander JE, Quick G. Aortoesophageal fistula: a comprehensive review of the literature. Am J Med. 1991;91(3):279–87.

42. Matsumoto A, Kanaoka Y, Baba T, Takizawa R, Hara M, Maeda K, et al. Result of thoracic endovascular aortic repair for patients with esophageal cancer. World J Surg. 2018;42(5):1551–8.
43. Watanabe M, Nakajima M, Nishikawa K, Kato H, Matsubara H. Thoracic endovascular aortic repair for esophageal cancer invading the thoracic aorta: a questionnaire survey study. Esophagus. 2020;17(1):74–80.
44. Yamatsuji T, Naomoto Y, Shirakawa Y, Gunduz M, Hiraki T, Yasui K, et al. Intra-aortic stent graft in oesophageal carcinoma invading the aorta. Prophylaxis for fatal haemorrhage. Int J Clin Pract. 2006;60(12):1600–3.
45. Shamji FM, Inculet R. Management of malignant tracheoesophageal fistula. Thorac Surg Clin. 2018;28(3):393–402.
46. Schweigert M, Posada-Gonzalez M, Dubecz A, Ofner D, Muschweck H, Stein HJ. Recurrent oesophageal cancer complicated by tracheo-oesophageal fistula: improved palliation by means of parallel tracheal and oesophageal stenting. Interact Cardiovasc Thorac Surg. 2014;18(2):190–6.
47. Martini N, Goodner JT, D'Angio GJ, Beattie EJ Jr. Tracheoesophageal fistula due to cancer. J Thorac Cardiovasc Surg. 1970;59(3):319–24.
48. Noronha V, Joshi A, Patil VM, Purandare N, Jiwnani S, Ghosh-Laskar S, et al. Efficacy and safety of induction chemotherapy in esophageal cancer with airway involvement. J Gastrointest Cancer. 2016;47(3):294–304.
49. Dutau H, Toutblanc B, Lamb C, Seijo L. Use of the Dumon Y-stent in the management of malignant disease involving the carina: a retrospective review of 86 patients. Chest. 2004;126(3):951–8.

Stomach

5

John T. Simpson, David T. Pointer Jr., and Sharven Taghavi

Highlights

- Gastric cancer is the 6th most common cancer worldwide and the 19th most common cancer in the United States [1, 2].
- Gastric oncologic emergencies occur in 14.4–39.6% of presentations and typically include perforation, hemorrhage, and obstruction [3, 4].
- Perforated gastric cancer is rare, and the initial operation should focus on controlling contamination to relieve peritonitis.
- Emergency presentations are associated with higher morbidity and mortality [5].

5.1 Gastric Cancer

Gastric cancer is the 6th most common cancer worldwide and the 19th most common cancer in the United States [1, 2]. Incidence is highest in East Asia, Eastern Europe, and South America. As the third leading cause of cancer-related deaths, gastric cancer is a major contributor to the global healthcare burden [1]. Males are disproportionately affected with global annual incidence rates approximately twice their female counterparts [1]. Both incidence and mortality are higher among African Americans, American Indians, and Hispanics [6]. The incidence and mortality rates for gastric cancer have steadily declined, yet the 5-year survival rate in the United States is approximately 33%. Both environmental and genetic factors are implicated in the pathogenesis of gastric cancer. *Helicobacter pylori* is the most important risk factor for the development of gastric cancer with an associated six-fold increased risk of gastric cancer [7, 8]. Other environmental factors associated with the development of gastric cancer include high nitrate and salt intake, low fruit

J. T. Simpson · D. T. Pointer Jr., · S. Taghavi (✉)
Department of Surgery, Tulane University School of Medicine, New Orleans, LA, USA
e-mail: jsimpson3@tulane.edu; David.pointer@ochsner.org; staghavi@tulane.edu

A. Tarasconi et al. (eds.), *Oncologic Surgical Emergencies*, Hot Topics in Acute Care Surgery and Trauma, https://doi.org/10.1007/978-3-031-36860-8_5

and vegetable intake, obesity, and gastroesophageal reflux [9–11]. Approximately 10% of gastric cancer is aggregated in families, but germline mutations (CDH1) account for an estimated 1–3% of cases [12–14]. Emergency presentations of gastric cancer can occur in as high as 39.6% of cases and typically portend a worse prognosis [4]. The most common gastric oncologic emergencies include perforation, bleeding, and gastric outlet obstruction.

5.1.1 Anatomic Classification of Gastric Cancer

Gastric cancer can be classified according to the anatomical location into true gastric cancer and gastroesophageal junction cancer. Gastroesophageal (GE) junction cancer can be categorized according to the Siewert classification [15]. Siewert type I tumors are located between 1 and 5 cm proximal to the GE junction. Siewert type II tumors are located between 1 cm proximal and 2 cm distal to the GE junction. Siewert type III tumors are located between 2 and 5 cm distal to the GE junction. This classification directs the oncologic management of GE junction tumors according to the most recent National Comprehensive Cancer Network (NCCN) guidelines—Siewert type I and II tumors are managed according to the esophageal adenocarcinoma pathway, whereas Siewert type III tumors are considered true gastric cancer and should be managed as such.

5.1.2 Gastric Cancer: Diagnosis and Additional Evaluation in the Non-emergent Setting

Ideally, diagnosis of gastric cancer begins with a focused history and physical exam. In the non-emergent setting, diagnostic endoscopy is performed to identify the location of the neoplasm and to obtain biopsies of any potentially malignant lesions. Standard size or large endoscopy forceps should be used to obtain 6–8 biopsies. Staging generally begins with chest/abdomen/pelvis computed tomography (CT) imaging with oral and intravenous contrast. Endoscopic ultrasound should be performed to detect the depth of tumor invasion and signs of lymphatic spread. 18-Fluorodeoxyglucose positron-emission tomography (FDG-PET) should be performed in patients without radiographic evidence of metastasis. Staging laparoscopy with cytology should be considered to evaluate for peritoneal spread in patients with clinical stage T1b or higher [16].

5.2 Gastric Oncologic Emergencies

Gastric cancer is typically asymptomatic or presents with vague, nonspecific symptoms such as dyspepsia. The presence of alarm symptoms, such as abdominal pain, anorexia, or weight loss, is often associated with advanced disease [17–19]. Acute, emergent presentations of gastric cancer include perforated gastric cancer, bleeding, and obstruction. Several single-center studies have demonstrated worse outcomes following emergent complications of gastric cancer [3–5, 20]. A single-center study in Britain found that among patients requiring hospitalization for an acute gastric oncologic emergency, 61% had advanced disease with only 21% undergoing potentially curative-intent resection. Furthermore, the 5-year survival rate for patients with emergent presentations was 9% [5].

5.3 Perforated Gastric Cancer

Perforated gastric cancer is a rare complication of gastric cancer. It is estimated to occur in 0.3–4% of cases and represents less than 1% of all acute abdomen cases [21–23]. Patients with perforated gastric cancer typically present with symptoms that are indistinguishable from perforated peptic ulcer disease, including abdominal pain with generalized peritonitis [24]. As such, preoperative diagnosis of malignant disease is difficult. Perforated gastric cancer is proven to be malignant preoperatively in only one-third of cases [24–26]. One systematic review identified older age (>65 years) as a risk factor for underlying malignancy in gastric perforations [25]. Another single-center study used age greater than 60 years, ulcer diameter 6 cm or larger, prolonged symptom duration (>20 h), and a white blood cell count of less than $15 \times 10^3/\mu L$ as a possible screening tool for malignant perforation. The screening tool had a sensitivity of 53.7% and a specificity of 98.7% [27]. Intraoperative diagnosis can be impaired as inflammation due to peritonitis can mimic local tumor invasion and lymph node involvement [27]. Previous reports have estimated that approximately 10–16% of all gastric perforations harbored underlying malignancy [28]. However, a more recent study identified underlying malignancy in 8% of gastric perforations [29]. Among perforated gastric cancers, tumors are typically located in the distal, middle, and upper third of the stomach in 45%, 42.9%, and 12.1% of cases, respectively [30]. Histopathologic features of perforated gastric cancer nearly uniformly demonstrate advanced stage (stage III/IV) and higher histologic grade (G3/G4) [22, 24]. Gastric cancers with perforation of the visceral peritoneum overlying the gastric ligaments or omentum are classified as T4 according to the American Joint Committee on Cancer (AJCC) Eighth Edition TNM Staging Classification [16]. Emergent surgery for perforated gastric cancer is associated with significantly worse outcomes than elective resection [31].

5.3.1 Management of Perforated Gastric Cancer

Clinicians should take note of environmental or familial risk factors for malignancy and recall the increased risk of underlying malignancy in elderly patients. Initial management should include resuscitation with crystalloids and initiation of broad-spectrum antibiotics. Per the Infectious Diseases Society of America (IDSA) and the World Society of Emergency Surgery (WSES) guidelines, routine empiric antifungal coverage is not necessary for gastric perforations that result in community-acquired peritoneal infection. WSES guidelines suggest that antifungal coverage should be administered for patients at high risk for fungal infection, such as those that are immunocompromised, at advanced age, in prolonged intensive care unit (ICU) stay, with multiple comorbid conditions, and with unresolved intra-abdominal infections. The addition of antifungal agents to patients with positive fungal culture with community-acquired fungal infection is controversial. However, in the presence of hospital-acquired fungal infection from gastric perforation and/or in the presence of critical illness, antifungal agents should be started [32, 33]. Patients that are hemodynamically unstable with generalized peritonitis should proceed to the operating room emergently for exploratory laparotomy. Radiologic evaluation can be considered in hemodynamically normal patients with generalized peritonitis. The initial goal of any surgical intervention should be to control contamination and halt the peritonitis. When a diagnosis of cancer has not been made or is unknown, it is critical that all gastric perforations are biopsied to exclude malignancy. At laparotomy, the general surgeon must decide between performing damage control surgery and resection with reconstruction. Management of perforated gastric cancer is outlined in Fig. 5.2.

Data regarding the optimal surgical management of perforated gastric cancer is limited due to the low incidence of perforated gastric cancer, declining global incidence of gastric cancer, and low likelihood of obtaining a malignant diagnosis preoperatively [1, 6, 26]. As such, consensus guidelines for the optimal management strategy do not exist, and there is some debate regarding the most appropriate surgical intervention. Current treatment options for perforated gastric cancer include simple repair of the perforation, one-stage radical gastrectomy, and two-stage radical gastrectomy. Simple repair of the perforation includes closure of the defect with a vascularized tissue patch (Graham patch or jejunal serosal patch) or wedge resection. Pedicled omental patches are appropriate for prepyloric and duodenal perforations. Jejunal serosal patches can be used when omental patch closure is insufficient or has already failed [34]. One-stage radical gastrectomy involves a formal gastric resection with negative macroscopic margins and formal D2 lymphadenectomy. During a two-stage radical gastrectomy, the first stage controls the peritonitis via wedge resection or partial gastrectomy and the second stage includes formal oncologic resection with D2 lymphadenectomy at a later date following appropriate staging workup. D1 lymphadenectomy includes the perigastric lymph nodes—right and left cardiac, lesser and greater curvature, suprapyloric, and infrapyloric. D2 lymphadenectomy includes D1 nodes plus the nodes along the named vessels of the celiac axis—left gastric artery, common hepatic artery, celiac artery, and splenic artery.

5.3.2 Graham Patch Repair

Perforated gastric cancer was previously regarded as a terminal disease due to peritoneal dissemination of cancer cells. Thus, simple closure of perforated gastric cancer was historically the treatment of choice, but it was associated with poor outcomes

[22]. Closure or plication alone resulted in a 50–68% mortality rate, attributed to a high rate of secondary leak and inflamed, friable, tumor-infiltrated tissue [35, 36]. It is possible that the poor outcomes associated with simple repair include a selection bias as it is more likely to be performed in frail, elderly patients in poor clinical condition. Over the last several decades, curative-intent gastrectomy replaced simple closure and mortality rates have fallen to 7–20% [24, 37, 38]. Graham patch is generally reserved for prepyloric perforations due to peptic ulcer disease. However, in the setting of perforated gastric cancer, Graham patch repair may play a role for patients with hemodynamic instability, extensive peritonitis, multiple comorbidities, or known metastatic disease. The goal of the index operation is to obtain source control of the intra-abdominal sepsis. In hemodynamically unstable patients, this may require damage control surgery in which the perforation should be biopsied and debrided, and then Graham patched. In cases where anatomy precludes wedge resection (such as in distal or proximal stomach), Graham patch may also be appropriate. Large perforations or perforations with underlying tumors may not be suitable for closure via Graham patch and gastric wedge resection or partial gastric resection is preferable. In such cases, the definitive procedure is a partial gastrectomy with either delayed or immediate reconstruction. In the hemodynamically unstable patient, the foregut may be left in discontinuity with a nasogastric tube in place for decompression, and a temporary abdominal closure can be placed enabling the patient to return to the ICU for ongoing resuscitation. A second-look laparotomy may be required, and definitive reconstruction can be performed once the patient's hemodynamic status has improved. Immediate reconstruction should be performed in low-risk patients with stable hemodynamics.

5.3.3 Wedge Resection

Wedge gastrectomy or wedge resection can be performed in patients with larger perforations outside of the prepyloric region. Generally, wedge resection is preferred over Graham patch because it affords the benefit of additional tissue for pathologic review. The goal of wedge resection is to obtain an appropriate margin of healthy tissue without significantly narrowing the stomach. Wedge resection can be performed using a handsewn or stapled technique. A linear stapling device can be used to excise a triangular "wedge" of gastric tissue that contains the perforation and underlying mass. Alternatively, the triangular wedge is excised sharply, and the stomach is closed in layers.

5.3.4 Partial Gastric Resection

Upon abdominal entry, the anterior surface of the stomach should be inspected for perforation. Failure to identify an anterior perforation should prompt entry to enter the lesser sac via the gastrocolic ligament to inspect the posterior surface of the stomach. Many advocate for examination of the posterior surface of the stomach in all gastric perforations regardless of whether anterior gastric perforation is identified. As seen in Fig. 5.1, reconstruction options following hemigastrectomy include gastroduodenostomy (Billroth I) and gastrojejunostomy (Billroth II or Roux-en-Y reconstruction). Generally, reconstruction with Billroth I avoids complications pertaining to the duodenal stump or afferent loop. For all reconstruction techniques, the stomach must be mobilized liberally with division of the gastrocolic, gastrophrenic, and gastrosplenic ligaments. The duodenum should be circumferentially dissected at least 2 cm distal to the pylorus. The stomach may be transected proximal to the ulcer or mass to obtain negative macroscopic margins using a linear stapling device. The duodenum should be transected approximately 1–2 cm distal to the pylorus using a linear stapling device. For Billroth I reconstruction, the duodenal stump is anastomosed to the remnant stomach in a primary end-to-end fashion. Billroth II reconstruction can be performed by anastomosis of the remnant stomach to the proximal jejunum in an end-to-side fashion. In Roux-en-Y reconstruction, the remnant stomach is anastomosed to an isoperistaltic jejunal Roux limb and an end-to-side anastomosis is performed between the distal Roux limb and proximal jejunum.

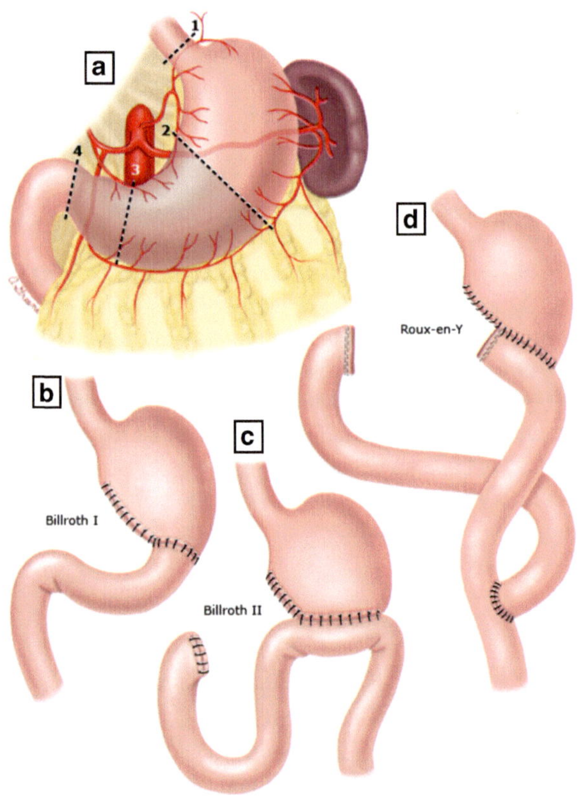

Fig. 5.1 Reconstruction options following distal (partial) gastrectomy. Intestinal continuity can be achieved via (**b**) Billroth I reconstruction, (**c**) Billroth II reconstruction, or (**d**) Roux-en-Y gastrojejunostomy. © 2022, UpToDate, Inc. and its affiliates and/or licensors. (All rights reserved. Reproduced with permission)

5.3.5 Radical Gastrectomy with Lymph Node Dissection

Formal gastric resection represents another therapeutic option for perforated gastric cancer. However, radical gastrectomy should only be performed in the rare patient where staging has been completed, is hemodynamically stable, and has minimal peritoneal contamination. There is a clear survival benefit for patients that undergo R0 resection for perforated gastric cancer, although most of this literature originates from studies in Japan, where incidence of gastric cancer is higher and routine gastric cancer screening is employed. In a Japanese retrospective cohort study of 514 cases of perforated gastric cancer, there was no significant difference in 5-year survival for one- versus two-stage gastrectomy when curative R0 resection was performed. Two-stage gastrectomy had a 78.4% rate of curative R0 resection and a hospital mortality rate of 1.9%. In contrast, the curative R0 resection rate and hospital mortality rate for one-stage gastrectomy were 50% and 11.4%, respectively. Although one- vs. two-stage gastrectomy have similar 5-year survival rates for R0 resection, one-stage gastrectomy has lower rates of curative R0 resection and higher overall hospital mortality rates. Rates of D2 lymphadenectomy were also higher for the two-stage radical gastrectomy group [39]. Other single-center studies and systematic reviews have confirmed these findings [24, 36]. In general, radical gastrectomy with lymph node dissection in the emergency setting should only be reserved for only the most exceptional cases located at tertiary academic centers where a surgical oncologist is available and the patient not only has a known diagnosis of gastric cancer but has also completed the appropriate preoperative staging. Furthermore, the patient must have limited peritonitis and exceptional performance status as measured by Eastern Cooperative Oncology Group Performance Status Scale (ECOG PS) or Karnofsky Performance Status Scale (KPS).

5.3.6 Laparoscopic vs. Open Repair

Surgical interventions can be performed open or laparoscopically. Generally, an open technique via an upper midline incision is preferred for patients with unstable hemodynamics. Like other laparoscopic surgeries, laparoscopic repair of gastric perforation may be advantageous due to smaller surgical wounds, decreased postoperative pain, and limited intestinal manipulation. Numerous studies have evaluated the outcomes following laparoscopic versus open surgical treatment for perforated peptic ulcer disease. A 2013 Cochrane review found no significant difference in postoperative mortality, abdominal septic complications, number of reoperations, operative time, or length of hospital stay when comparing laparoscopic and open surgery for perforated peptic ulcer disease [40]. Similar results were described in a 2018 meta-analysis published in *Journal of Trauma*, except for significantly less postoperative pain and fewer wound infections following laparoscopic interventions [41]. Laparoscopic intervention is at least non-inferior to open surgical repair of gastric perforations in stable patients. Further evaluation is required for certain subgroups including the elderly and patients with unstable hemodynamics (Fig. 5.2).

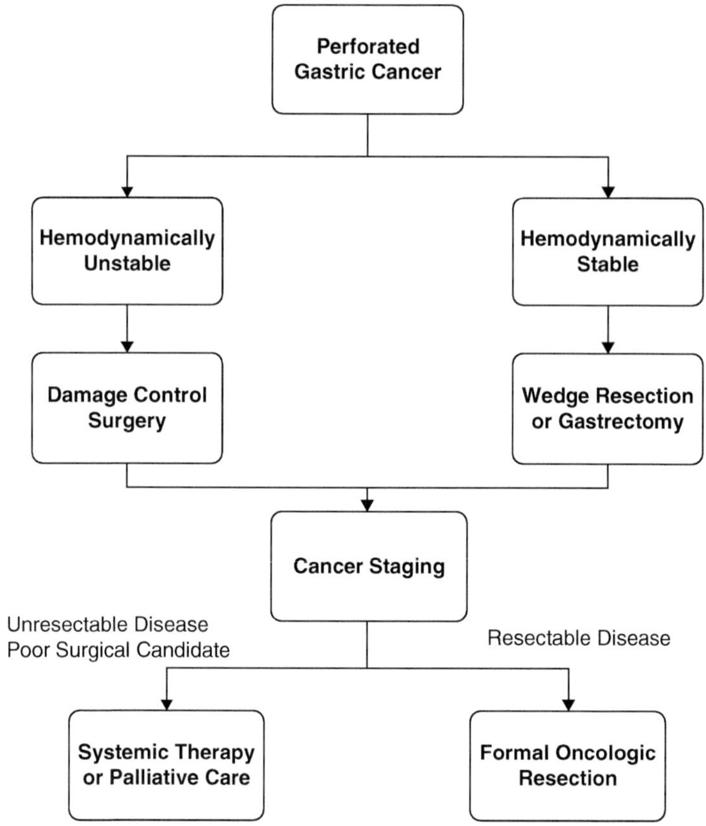

Fig. 5.2 Management of acute perforated gastric cancer

5.4 Gastrointestinal Bleeding

Acute tumor-related gastrointestinal bleeding is common in gastric cancer and occurs in up to 10% of cases [42]. Gastric cancer is the most common cause of tumor-related upper gastrointestinal (GI) bleeding and accounts for 2% of all upper GI bleeds [42, 43]. Patients will commonly present with hematemesis or melena. Initial management of bleeding gastric cancer begins with standard resuscitative practices including access with two large-bore IVs (14 or 16 gauge), nasogastric tube placement, volume resuscitation, high-dose proton pump inhibitor treatment, type and screen, and a restrictive transfusion strategy to maintain a hemoglobin level greater than 7 g/dL [44, 45]. Resuscitation with blood products should be performed using balanced component therapy consisting of packed red blood cells (PRBCs), fresh frozen plasma (FFP), and platelets administered in a 1:1:1 ratio. Functional laboratory measures of coagulation may be obtained (e.g., viscoelastic assays) to guide ongoing resuscitation [46]. Treatments for bleeding control include endoscopic therapy, transcatheter arterial embolization, radiotherapy, and surgery.

As outlined in Fig. 5.3, patients with upper GI bleeding should undergo urgent upper endoscopy (within 24 h of admission) and active bleeding should be managed with endoscopic hemostatic therapies. Recommended endoscopic hemostatic therapies include bipolar electrocoagulation, heater probes, absolute ethanol injection, clips, argon plasma coagulation, and hemostatic powder spray TC-325. The most common stigmata of recent bleeding in patients with gastric cancer is oozing hemorrhage (Forrest 1b) [43, 47]. Ablative therapies, such as argon plasma coagulation, should be considered in this setting due to likelihood of extensive superficial or diffuse lesions [47]. Recurrent bleeding following successful endoscopic management should undergo repeat endoscopy and endoscopic therapy. Failure of endoscopic

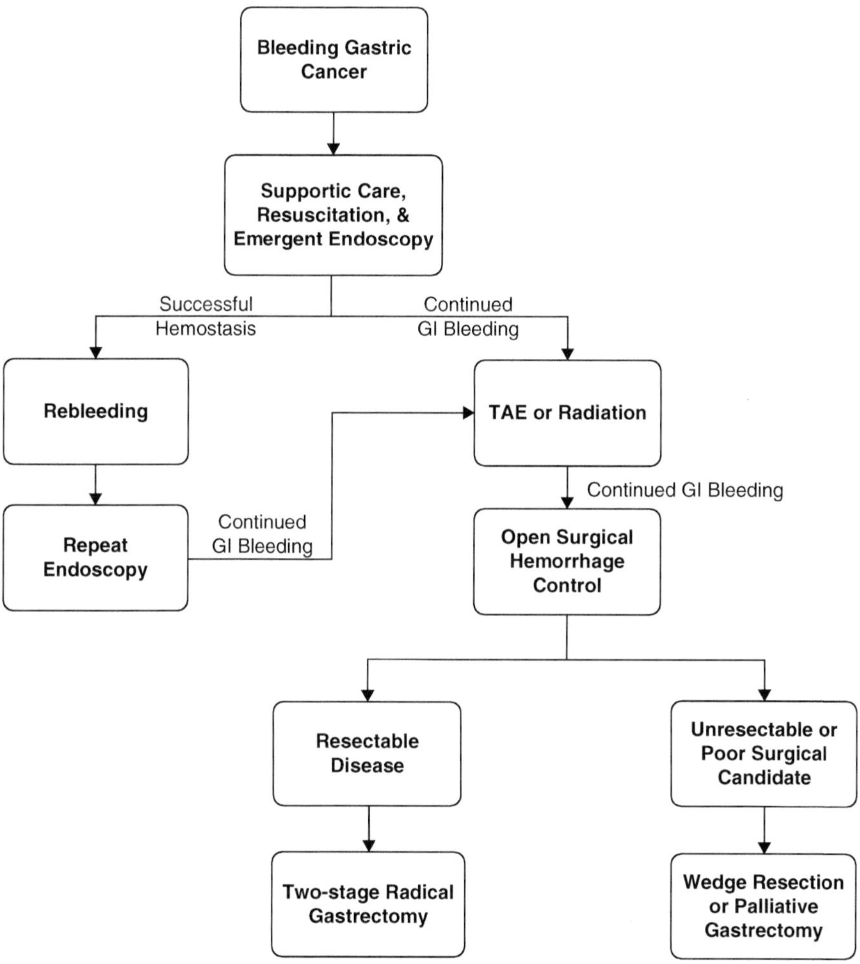

Fig. 5.3 Management of acute gastrointestinal bleeding in the setting of gastric cancer. *TAE* transcatheter arterial embolization

hemostatic therapy should be treated with transcatheter arterial embolization by interventional radiology [44].

At the time of endoscopic examination, the location of the tumor and its proximity to the gastroesophageal junction should be documented for the purposes of future surgical planning. Standard size or jumbo endoscopic forceps should be used to obtain 6–8 biopsies of the lesion. Biopsies should be obtained from both the ulcer base and margins using the strip and bite technique to ensure that adequate submucosa and muscularis propria are obtained within the histologic specimen [48]. A single biopsy is only 70% sensitive at diagnosing gastric cancer, but the sensitivity increases to 98% when seven biopsies are obtained in the fashion described above [49]. If bleeding is a concern, the endoscopist may consider using cytologic brushings in an attempt to increase the diagnostic yield, but cytologic brushings alone are rarely adequate for initial diagnosis [50]. Ultimately, the endoscopist must weigh the risks of inducing further bleeding when considering performing tissue biopsy at the time of urgent endoscopy for potential tumor-related bleeding. *H. pylori* testing should also be performed at the time of endoscopic examination via biopsy urease test or histologic diagnosis using Giemsa or immunohistochemical staining. If biopsy urease test is not performed, *H. pylori* testing should be performed using the urease breath test, stool studies, or immunoglobulin assay (although positive immunoglobulin assays indicate prior *H. pylori* infection and do not confirm current active infection) [51–53].

Endoscopic management of bleeding gastric tumors is successful in 67–100% of cases, which is comparable to the success rates of endoscopic therapy for peptic ulcer disease [54]. Rebleeding rates are higher following endoscopic treatment of bleeding gastric cancer with rates ranging from 41 to 80% compared to 8–39% for peptic ulcer bleeding [44, 54]. Factors associated with rebleeding following successful endoscopic therapy for bleeding peptic ulcer disease are extensively studied and include active bleeding on endoscopy, ulcer size >2 cm, ulcers on the lesser curvature, and posterior duodenal ulcers [55]. There is limited evidence regarding risk factors associated with gastric tumor-related rebleeding. A single-center study identified transfusion ≥5 units as an independent risk factor for tumor-related rebleeding [47]. Age ≤60 years and unstable hemodynamic status were identified in another study [43]. Finally, a third study found that a nonexposed vessel and tumor >2 cm were predictive of hemostatic failure [56]. Repeat endoscopy with endoscopic hemostatic therapy is effective in 89% of cases of rebleeding following initial successful endoscopic therapy for tumor-related bleeding [54, 57].

Transcatheter arterial embolization (TAE) should be used following failure of endoscopic hemostatic therapy. In previous studies, 22.4–50% of patients with tumor-related upper GI bleeding had negative angiography findings. Empiric embolization of the left gastric artery and other tumor-feeding vessels was performed on patients with negative angiographic finding. TAE had an overall clinical success rate of 52–74.8%. Among patients with positive angiography findings, the success rate of TAE ranged from 53.8 to 100% [58, 59].

External beam radiation therapy (EBRT) can also be considered for the management of acute and chronic gastrointestinal bleeding in the setting of advanced, unresectable gastric cancer. EBRT delivered as a total of 25–30 Gy over 5–10 fractions resulted in hemostasis of approximately 73% of tumor-related bleeding. Rebleeding occurs in approximately one-third of patients at a median of 1–3 months [60–63].

Surgery is rarely utilized as a method for achieving hemostasis for bleeding gastric cancers. Surgery should be reserved for patients that fail endoscopic hemostatic treatment and transcatheter arterial embolization or for hemodynamically unstable patients that are nonresponsive to resuscitation. Prior to any surgery, goals-of-care discussions should occur and consideration for all options including palliative care, especially in the setting of non-curable disease. Data regarding outcomes following curative- and non-curative-intent surgery in the setting of bleeding gastric cancer is extremely limited. We propose the same damage control principles as utilized in the management of perforated gastric cancer. Patients with bleeding gastric cancers that are otherwise appropriate for curative-intent surgery should undergo initial surgery aimed to halt GI bleeding by means of either oversewing bleeding vessels or partial gastrectomy. Most bleeding gastric cancers have diffuse bleeding from ulcerated and friable gastric mucosa. As such, most cases will not be amenable to ligation of a bleeding vessel. Either wedge resection or gastrectomy is the preferred method to achieve surgical hemostasis. The surgical technique is similar to that discussed previously in the management of perforated gastric cancers.

5.5 Gastric Outlet Obstruction

Gastric outlet obstruction (GOO) is a late complication of advanced gastric cancer. GOO is defined as a blockage of the distal stomach or duodenum [64]. Typical presentations of GOO include nausea, vomiting, anorexia, inability to tolerate oral intake, weight loss, dehydration, and electrolyte abnormalities [65]. It is associated with poor nutritional status, reduced quality of life, poor performance status, and decreased likelihood of receiving appropriate treatment [66]. Most patients with gastric cancer presenting with GOO have unresectable disease with over 60% of patients with metastatic disease [67]. Initial management should focus on supportive care including crystalloid resuscitation, nil per os (NPO), nasogastric tube decompression, and consideration for parenteral nutrition. Current treatment options for gastric outlet obstruction include decompressive gastrostomy tube with feeding jejunostomy tube, endoscopic self-expandable metal stent (SEMS), gastrojejunostomy, and palliative gastrectomy. The primary goal of treatment is to improve symptoms such that the patient can tolerate systemic therapy and potentially undergo surgery of curative intent.

The optimal management strategy for GOO is controversial. The patient's overall clinical condition, ability to tolerate multimodal therapy, and likelihood of undergoing future curative-intent resection should be taken into consideration when considering treatment options. Gastrojejunostomy is the traditional treatment for malignant gastric outlet obstruction. Gastrojejunostomy is associated with good functional outcomes and relief of obstructive symptoms in 72% of cases [36,

68–70]. However, other reports have shown that gastrojejunostomy can be associated with morbidity rates of up to 55% [71]. SEMS insertion is being used increasingly and has been shown to be a safe and effective modality for the management of GOO [72–74]. Comparative studies evaluating gastrojejunostomy versus SEMS for malignant GOO found that there was no significant difference in either the technical success rates, clinical improvement, or incidence of early adverse events between the two treatments. SEMS is associated with more rapid improvement of oral intake, but long-term relief is greater for gastrojejunostomy. Similarly, recurrent symptoms and recurrent intervention are more likely following SEMS [66–71, 75–77]. Figure 5.4 represents a contrast radiograph of a GOO alleviated with SEMS. In patients with a good performance status (ECOG 0–1), gastrojejunostomy is associated with lower adverse events and extended survival [71]. Therefore, most experts recommend gastrojejunostomy and reserve SEMS for poor surgical candidates with limited life expectancy. Following gastrojejunostomy, completion of staging workup and consideration for formal oncologic resection should commence.

In advanced cases, malignant GOO cannot be alleviated or bypassed. Management strategies should focus on symptomatic improvement by relieving the obstruction and ensuring adequate nutrition. Venting gastrostomy tube placement can also be considered via previously described percutaneous, endoscopic, and interventional

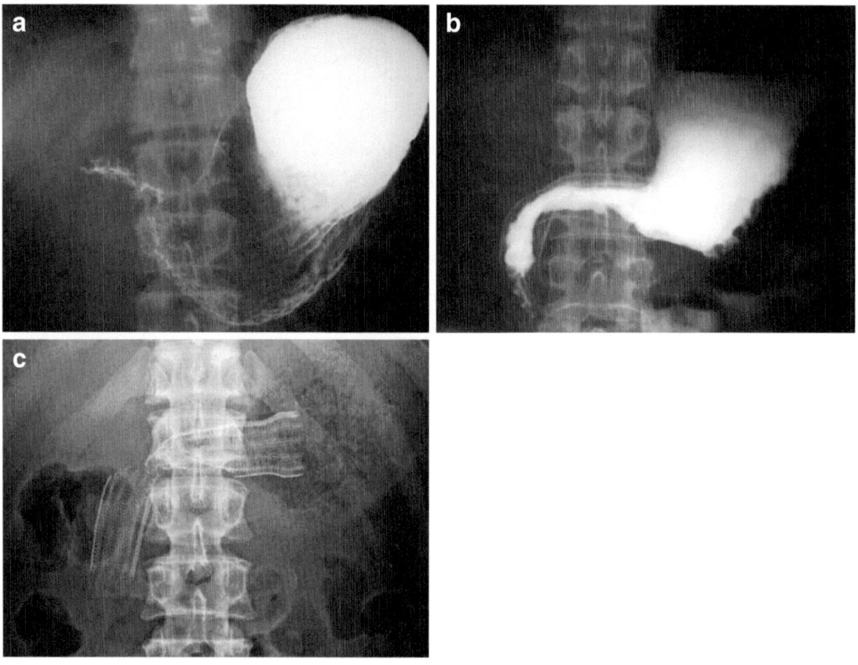

Fig. 5.4 (**a**) Contrast radiograph demonstrating gastric outlet obstruction. (**b**) SEMS placed to alleviate obstruction. (**c**) Subsequent SEMS fracture leading to recurrent symptoms

radiology or open surgical methods [78–80]. Ascites should be drained prior to venting gastrostomy tube placement to reduce the risk of infection [80, 81].

5.6 Palliative Surgery for Gastric Oncologic Emergencies

In patients that cannot undergo curative-intent radical gastrectomy, palliative care should be initiated early during the hospital course. Early consultation with a multidisciplinary palliative care team can improve quality of life and enable treatment in some patients [82]. The need for palliative care is even more important as 5-year survival for gastric cancer is increasing, in part due to advancements in chemotherapy, immunotherapy, and monoclonal antibodies [83–85]. Palliative management includes chemoradiation, systemic therapy, and palliative procedures. Indications for palliative care of gastric cancer include patients with unresectable, locally advanced, recurrent, or metastatic disease. Options for palliative surgery include palliative gastrectomy, gastrojejunostomy, bypass, and venting gastrostomy tube. Radiotherapy and endoscopic self-expandable metal stent (SEMS) are palliative procedures that can also be used in the setting of advanced gastric cancer. Palliative surgery for gastric cancer should be considered in patients with perforation, malignant gastric outlet obstruction, and gastrointestinal bleeding.

There is current debate regarding the role of palliative gastrectomy for advanced gastric cancer. Historical reports suggested that palliative gastrectomy was associated with a 40% mortality rate with limited survival benefits [86]. Some recent studies have demonstrated immediate perioperative mortality rates of 4% following palliative gastrectomy [87]. Several systematic reviews and meta-analyses have reported significantly prolonged 1-year survival following palliative gastrectomy for advanced stage IV gastric cancers [88–90]. Another 2007 retrospective review concluded that palliative gastrectomy may be associated with improved survival in patients <60 years and Asian race [91]. More recently, the REGATTA trial randomized patients with advanced, non-curable gastric cancer to receive either chemotherapy alone or gastrectomy followed by chemotherapy. Gastrectomy followed by chemotherapy offered no survival benefit when compared to chemotherapy alone [92]. The role of palliative gastrectomy to improve survival remains unclear as many early studies did not include modern chemotherapy regimens or staging modalities as standard treatment. Generally, palliative gastrectomy should be reserved for select patients presenting with significant complications of gastric cancer, including perforation, bleeding, or obstruction. However, there may be a role for palliative gastrectomy in select young patients with good performance status and limited comorbid conditions, although this should occur in the setting of a multidisciplinary team (e.g., tumor board), with shared patient decision-making.

References

1. Sung H, Ferlay J, Siegel RL, Laversanne M, Soerjomataram I, Jemal A, Bray F. Global Cancer Statistics 2020: GLOBOCAN estimates of incidence and mortality worldwide for 36 cancers in 185 countries. CA Cancer J Clin. 2021;71:209–49.
2. Siegel RL, Miller KD, Fuchs HE, Jemal A. Cancer Statistics, 2021. CA Cancer J Clin. 2021;71:7–33.
3. Vasas P, Wiggins T, Chaudry A, Bryant C, Hughes FS. Emergency presentation of the gastric cancer; prognosis and implications for service planning. World J Emerg Surg. 2012;7:31.
4. Markar SR, Mackenzie H, Jemal S, Faiz O, Cunningham D, Hanna GB. Emergency presentation of esophagogastric cancer. Ann Surg. 2018;267:711–5.
5. Blackshaw GRJC, Stephens MR, Lewis WG, Paris HJ, Barry JD, Edwards P, Allison MC. Prognostic significance of acute presentation with emergency complications of gastric cancer. Gastric Cancer. 2004;7:91–6.
6. Islami F, Ward EM, Sung H, et al. Annual Report to the Nation on the Status of Cancer, Part 1: National Cancer Statistics. J Natl Cancer Inst. 2021;113(12):1648–69.
7. Bornschein J, Selgrad M, Warnecke M, Kuester D, Wex T, Malfertheiner P. *H. pylori* infection is a key risk factor for proximal gastric cancer. Digest Dis Sci. 2010;55:3124–31.
8. Wroblewski LE, Peek RM, Wilson KT. *Helicobacter pylori* and gastric cancer: factors that modulate disease risk. Clin Microbiol Rev. 2010;23:713–39.
9. Lunet N, Valbuena C, Vieira AL, Lopes C, Lopes C, David L, Carneiro F, Barros H. Fruit and vegetable consumption and gastric cancer by location and histological type: case–control and meta-analysis. Eur J Cancer Prev. 2007;16:312–27.
10. Ladeiras-Lopes R, Pereira AK, Nogueira A, Pinheiro-Torres T, Pinto I, Santos-Pereira R, Lunet N. Smoking and gastric cancer: systematic review and meta-analysis of cohort studies. Cancer Cause Control. 2008;19:689–701.
11. Smyth EC, Nilsson M, Grabsch HI, van Grieken NC, Lordick F. Gastric cancer. Lancet. 2020;396:635–48.
12. Oliveira C, Pinheiro H, Figueiredo J, Seruca R, Carneiro F. Familial gastric cancer: genetic susceptibility, pathology, and implications for management. Lancet Oncol. 2015;16:e60–70.
13. van der Post RS, Oliveira C, Guilford P, Carneiro F. Hereditary gastric cancer: what's new? Update 2013–2018. Fam Cancer. 2019;18:363–7.
14. van der Post RS, Vogelaar IP, Carneiro F, et al. Hereditary diffuse gastric cancer: updated clinical guidelines with an emphasis on germline CDH1 mutation carriers. J Med Genet. 2015;52:361–74.
15. Siewert JR, Stein HJ. Classification of adenocarcinoma of the oesophagogastric junction. Br J Surg. 1998;85:1457–9.
16. Network NCC Gastric Cancer (Version 5.2021). https://www.nccn.org/professionals/physician_gls/pdf/gastric.pdf. Accessed 1 Nov 2021.
17. Cutsem EV, Sagaert X, Topal B, Haustermans K, Prenen H. Gastric cancer. Lancet. 2016;388:2654–64.
18. Correa P. Gastric cancer overview. Gastroenterol Clin N. 2013;42:211–7.
19. Axon A. Symptoms and diagnosis of gastric cancer at early curable stage. Best Pract Res Clin Gastroenterol. 2006;20:697–708.
20. Kasakura Y, Ajani JA, Mochizuki F, Morishita Y, Fujii M, Takayama T. Outcomes after emergency surgery for gastric perforation or severe bleeding in patients with gastric cancer. J Surg Oncol. 2002;80:181–5.
21. Kotan C, Sumer A, Baser M, Kızıltan R, Carparlar MA. An analysis of 13 patients with perforated gastric carcinoma: a surgeon's nightmare? World J Emerg Surg. 2008;3:17.
22. Gertsch P, Yip SKH, Chow LWC, Lauder IJ. Free perforation of gastric carcinoma: results of surgical treatment. Arch Surg-chicago. 1995;130:177–81.
23. Wu F-H, Chiang R-A, Tsai Y-C, Hung S-T, Huang S-S. Perforated gastric carcinoma in a young-age patient. J Cancer Res Pract. 2018;5:74–6.

24. Jwo S, Chien R, Chao T, Chen H, Lin C. Clinicopathological features, surgical management, and disease outcome of perforated gastric cancer. J Surg Oncol. 2005;91:219–25.
25. Roviello F, Rossi S, Marrelli D, Manzoni GD, Pedrazzani C, Morgagni P, Corso G, Pinto E. Perforated gastric carcinoma: a report of 10 cases and review of the literature. World J Surg Oncol. 2006;4:19.
26. Adachi Y, Mori M, Maehara Y, Matsumata T, Okudaira Y, Sugimachi K. Surgical results of perforated gastric carcinoma: an analysis of 155 Japanese patients. Am J Gastroenterol. 1997;92:516–8.
27. Ergul E, Gozetlik EO. Emergency spontaneous gastric perforations: ulcus versus cancer. Langenbecks Arch Surg. 2009;394:643–6.
28. Williams WO. Gastric carcinoma and acute perforation. Br Med J. 1952;1:164.
29. Bhaskar S, Kumari P, Sinha DK. Incidence of malignancy in gastric/antral perforation. Int Surg J. 2019;6:3347–52.
30. Melloni M, Bernardi D, Asti E, Bonavina L. Perforated gastric cancer: a systematic review. J Laparoendosc Adv Surg Tech A. 2020;30:156–62.
31. Fisher BW, Fluck M, Young K, Shabahang M, Blansfield J, Arora TK. Urgent surgery for gastric adenocarcinoma: a study of the national cancer database. J Surg Res. 2020;245:619–28.
32. Pappas PG, Kauffman CA, Andes DR, et al. Clinical practice guideline for the management of candidiasis: 2016 update by the Infectious Diseases Society of America. Clin Infect Dis. 2016;62:e1–e50.
33. Sartelli M, Chichom-Mefire A, Labricciosa FM, et al. The management of intra-abdominal infections from a global perspective: 2017 WSES guidelines for management of intra-abdominal infections. World J Emerg Surg. 2017;12:29.
34. Gupta S, Kaushik R, Sharma R, Attri A. The management of large perforations of duodenal ulcers. BMC Surg. 2005;5:15.
35. Ozmen M, Zulfikaroglu B, Kece C, Aslar A, Ozalp N, Koc M. Factors influencing mortality in spontaneous gastric tumour perforations. J Int Med Res. 2001;30:180–4.
36. Mahar AL, Brar SS, Coburn NG, Law C, Helyer LK. Surgical management of gastric perforation in the setting of gastric cancer. Gastric Cancer. 2012;15:146–52.
37. Kasakura Y, Ajani JA, Fujii M, Mochizuki F, Takayama T. Management of perforated gastric carcinoma: a report of 16 cases and review of world literature. Am Surg. 2002;68:434–40.
38. Lehnert T, Buhl K, Dueck M, Hinz U, Herfarth C. Two-stage radical gastrectomy for perforated gastric cancer. Eur J Surg Oncol. 2000;26:780–4.
39. Hata T, Sakata N, Kudoh K, Shibata C, Unno M. The best surgical approach for perforated gastric cancer: one-stage vs. two-stage gastrectomy. Gastric Cancer. 2014;17:578–87.
40. Sanabria A, Villegas MI, Uribe CHM. Laparoscopic repair for perforated peptic ulcer disease. Cochrane Database Syst Rev. 2013;2:CD004778.
41. Cirocchi R, Soreide K, Saverio SD, Rossi E, Arezzo A, Zago M, Abraha I, Vettoretto N, Chiarugi M. Meta-analysis of perioperative outcomes of acute laparoscopic versus open repair of perforated gastroduodenal ulcers. J Trauma Acute Care. 2018;85:417–25.
42. Fox JG, Hunt PS. Management of acute bleeding gastric malignancy. Aust N Z J Surg. 1993;63:462–5.
43. Sheibani S, Kim JJ, Chen B, Park S, Saberi B, Keyashian K, Buxbaum J, Laine L. Natural history of acute upper GI bleeding due to tumours: short-term success and long-term recurrence with or without endoscopic therapy. Aliment Pharmacol Ther. 2013;38:144–50.
44. Laine L, Barkun AN, Saltzman JR, Martel M, Leontiadis GI. ACG clinical guideline: upper gastrointestinal and ulcer bleeding. Am J Gastroenterol. 2021;116:899–917.
45. Odutayo A, Desborough MJR, Trivella M, et al. Restrictive versus liberal blood transfusion for gastrointestinal bleeding: a systematic review and meta-analysis of randomised controlled trials. Lancet Gastroenterol Hepatol. 2017;2:354–60.
46. Cannon JW, Khan MA, Raja AS, et al. Damage control resuscitation in patients with severe traumatic hemorrhage. J Trauma Acute Care. 2017;82:605–17.

47. Kim Y, Choi IJ, Cho S, Lee JY, Kim CG, Kim M, Ryu KW, Kim Y, Park YI. Outcome of endoscopic therapy for cancer bleeding in patients with unresectable gastric cancer. J Gastroenterol Hepatol. 2013;28:1489–95.
48. Karita M, Tada M. Endoscopic and histologic diagnosis of submucosal tumors of the gastrointestinal tract using combined strip biopsy and bite biopsy. Gastrointest Endosc. 1994;40:749–53.
49. Graham DY, Schwartz JT, Cain GD, Gyorkey F. Prospective evaluation of biopsy number in the diagnosis of esophageal and gastric carcinoma. Gastroenterology. 1982;82:228–31.
50. Wang HH, Jonasson JG, Ducatman BS. Brushing cytology of the upper gastrointestinal tract. Obsolete or not? Acta Cytol. 1991;35:195–8.
51. Chey WD, Leontiadis GI, Howden CW, Moss SF. ACG clinical guideline: treatment of *Helicobacter pylori* infection. Am J Gastroenterol. 2017;112:212–39.
52. Wang Y-K, Kuo F-C, Liu C-J, Wu M-C, Shih H-Y, Wang SS, Wu J-Y, Kuo C-H, Huang Y-K, Wu D-C. Diagnosis of *Helicobacter pylori* infection: current options and developments. World J Gastroenterol. 2015;21:11221–35.
53. Wright CL, Kelly JK. The use of routine special stains for upper gastrointestinal biopsies. Am J Surg Pathol. 2006;30:357–61.
54. Kim Y-I, Choi IJ. Endoscopic management of tumor bleeding from inoperable gastric cancer. Clin Endosc. 2015;48:121–7.
55. Elmunzer BJ, Young SD, Inadomi JM, Schoenfeld P, Laine L. Systematic review of the predictors of recurrent hemorrhage after endoscopic hemostatic therapy for bleeding peptic ulcers. Am J Gastroenterol. 2008;103:2625–32.
56. Koh KH, Kim K, Kwon DH, et al. The successful endoscopic hemostasis factors in bleeding from advanced gastric cancer. Gastric Cancer. 2013;16:397–403.
57. Tsujimoto H, Hiraki S, Sakamoto N, et al. Outcome after emergency surgery in patients with a free perforation caused by gastric cancer. Exp Ther Med. 2010;1:199–203.
58. Lee HJ, Shin JH, Yoon H-K, Ko G-Y, Gwon D-I, Song H-Y, Sung K-B. Transcatheter arterial embolization in gastric cancer patients with acute bleeding. Eur Radiol. 2009;19:960–5.
59. Cho SB, Hur S, Kim H-C, Jae HJ, Lee M, Kim M, Kim J-E, Lee JH, Chung JW. Transcatheter arterial embolization for advanced gastric cancer bleeding: a single-center experience with 58 patients. Medicine. 2020;99:e19630.
60. Kondoh C, Shitara K, Nomura M, Takahari D, Ura T, Tachibana H, Tomita N, Kodaira T, Muro K. Efficacy of palliative radiotherapy for gastric bleeding in patients with unresectable advanced gastric cancer: a retrospective cohort study. BMC Palliat Care. 2015;14:37.
61. Lee J, Byun HK, Koom WS, Lee YC, Seong J. Efficacy of radiotherapy for gastric bleeding associated with advanced gastric cancer. Radiat Oncol. 2021;16:161.
62. Kim MM, Rana V, Janjan NA, Das P, Phan AT, Delclos ME, Mansfield PF, Ajani JA, Crane CH, Krishnan S. Clinical benefit of palliative radiation therapy in advanced gastric cancer. Acta Oncol. 2009;47:421–7.
63. Asakura H, Hashimoto T, Harada H, Mizumoto M, Furutani K, Hasuike N, Matsuoka M, Ono H, Boku N, Nishimura T. Palliative radiotherapy for bleeding from advanced gastric cancer: is a schedule of 30 Gy in 10 fractions adequate? J Cancer Res Clin. 2011;137:125–30.
64. Blumenthaler AN, Ikoma N, Blum M, Das P, Minsky BD, Mansfield PF, Ajani JA, Badgwell BD. Relationship between initial management strategy and survival in patients with gastric outlet obstruction due to gastric cancer. J Surg Oncol. 2020;122:1373–82.
65. Chen X-J, Chen G-M, Wei Y-C, Yu H, Wang X-C, Zhao Z-K, Luo T-Q, Nie R-C, Zhou Z-W. Palliative gastrectomy versus gastrojejunostomy for advanced gastric cancer with outlet obstruction: a propensity score matching analysis. BMC Cancer. 2021;21:188.
66. Haga Y, Hiki N, Kinoshita T, et al. Treatment option of endoscopic stent insertion or gastrojejunostomy for gastric outlet obstruction due to gastric cancer: a propensity score-matched analysis. Gastric Cancer. 2020;23:667–76.
67. Keränen I, Kylänpää L, Udd M, Louhimo J, Lepistö A, Halttunen J, Kokkola A. Gastric outlet obstruction in gastric cancer: a comparison of three palliative methods. J Surg Oncol. 2013;108:537–41.

68. Maetani I, Tada T, Ukita T, Inoue H, Sakai Y, Nagao J. Comparison of duodenal stent placement with surgical gastrojejunostomy for palliation in patients with duodenal obstructions caused by pancreaticobiliary malignancies. Endoscopy. 2004;36:73–8.
69. Jeurnink SM, van Eijck CH, Steyerberg EW, Kuipers EJ, Siersema PD. Stent versus gastrojejunostomy for the palliation of gastric outlet obstruction: a systematic review. BMC Gastroenterol. 2007;7:18.
70. Jeurnink SM, Steyerberg EW, van Hooft JE, van Eijck CHJ, Schwartz MP, Vleggaar FP, Kuipers EJ, Siersema PD, Group for the DSS. Surgical gastrojejunostomy or endoscopic stent placement for the palliation of malignant gastric outlet obstruction (SUSTENT study): a multicenter randomized trial. Gastrointest Endosc. 2010;71:490–9.
71. No JH, Kim SW, Lim C-H, Kim JS, Cho YK, Park JM, Lee IS, Choi M-G, Choi KY. Long-term outcome of palliative therapy for gastric outlet obstruction caused by unresectable gastric cancer in patients with good performance status: endoscopic stenting versus surgery. Gastrointest Endosc. 2013;78:55–62.
72. Fujitani K, Yamada M, Hirao M, Kurokawa Y, Tsujinaka T. Optimal indications of surgical palliation for incurable advanced gastric cancer presenting with malignant gastrointestinal obstruction. Gastric Cancer. 2011;14:353–9.
73. Bessoud B, de Baere T, Denys A, Kuoch V, Ducreux M, Precetti S, Roche A, Menu Y. Malignant gastroduodenal obstruction: palliation with self-expanding metallic stents. J Vasc Interv Radiol. 2005;16:247–53.
74. van Hooft J, van Montfoort M, Jeurnink S, Bruno M, Dijkgraaf M, Siersema P, Fockens P. Safety and efficacy of a new non-foreshortening nitinol stent in malignant gastric outlet obstruction (DUONITI study): a prospective, multicenter study. Endoscopy. 2011;43:671–5.
75. Huggett MT, Ghaneh P, Pereira SP. Drainage and bypass procedures for palliation of malignant diseases of the upper gastrointestinal tract. Clin Oncol. 2010;22:755–63.
76. Jeurnink SM, Steyerberg EW, van Hof GT, van Eijck CHJ, Kuipers EJ, Siersema PD. Gastrojejunostomy versus stent placement in patients with malignant gastric outlet obstruction: a comparison in 95 patients. J Surg Oncol. 2007;96:389–96.
77. Jang SH, Lee H, Min B-H, Kim SM, Kim HS, Carriere KC, Min YW, Lee JH, Kim JJ. Palliative gastrojejunostomy versus endoscopic stent placement for gastric outlet obstruction in patients with unresectable gastric cancer: a propensity score-matched analysis. Surg Endosc. 2017;31:4217–23.
78. Issaka RB, Shapiro DM, Parikh ND, Mulcahy MF, Komanduri S, Martin JA, Keswani RN. Palliative venting percutaneous endoscopic gastrostomy tube is safe and effective in patients with malignant obstruction. Surg Endosc. 2014;28:1668–73.
79. Wollman B, D'Agostino HB. Percutaneous radiologic and endoscopic gastrostomy: a 3-year institutional analysis of procedure performance. Am J Roentgenol. 1997;169:1551–3.
80. Yuan Y, Zhao Y, Xie T, Hu Y. Percutaneous endoscopic gastrostomy versus percutaneous radiological gastrostomy for swallowing disturbances. Cochrane Database Syst Rev. 2016;2016:CD009198.
81. Lee MJ, Saini S, Brink JA, Morrison MC, Hahn PF, Mueller PR. Malignant small bowel obstruction and ascites: not a contraindication to percutaneous gastrostomy. Clin Radiol. 1991;44:332–4.
82. Harada K, Zhao M, Shanbhag N, Baba H, Ajani JA. Palliative care for advanced gastric cancer. Expert Rev Anticancer. 2020;20:575–80.
83. Fuchs CS, Tomasek J, Yong CJ, et al. Ramucirumab monotherapy for previously treated advanced gastric or gastro-oesophageal junction adenocarcinoma (REGARD): an international, randomised, multicentre, placebo-controlled, phase 3 trial. Lancet. 2014;383:31–9.
84. Kang JH, Lee SI, Lim DH, et al. Salvage chemotherapy for pretreated gastric cancer: a randomized phase III trial comparing chemotherapy plus best supportive care with best supportive care alone. J Clin Oncol. 2012;30:1513–8.
85. Thuss-Patience PC, Kretzschmar A, Bichev D, Deist T, Hinke A, Breithaupt K, Dogan Y, Gebauer B, Schumacher G, Reichardt P. Survival advantage for irinotecan versus best

supportive care as second-line chemotherapy in gastric cancer—a randomised phase III study of the Arbeitsgemeinschaft Internistische Onkologie (AIO). Eur J Cancer. 2011;47:2306–14.
86. Hallissey MT, Allum WH, Fielding JWL, Roginski C. Palliative surgery for gastric cancer. Cancer. 1988;62:440–4.
87. Dittmar Y, Rauchfuss F, Goetz M, Jandt K, Scheuerlein H, Heise M, Settmacher U. Non-curative gastric resection for patients with stage 4 gastric cancer—a single center experience and current review of literature. Langenbecks Arch Surg. 2012;397:745–53.
88. Kim DY, Joo JK, Park YK, Ryu SY, Kim YJ, Kim SK, Lee JH. Is palliative resection necessary for gastric carcinoma patients? Langenbecks Arch Surg. 2008;393:31–5.
89. Lasithiotakis K, Antoniou SA, Antoniou GA, Kaklamanos I, Zoras O. Gastrectomy for stage IV gastric cancer. a systematic review and meta-analysis. Anticancer Res. 2014;34:2079–85.
90. Sun J, Song Y, Wang Z, Chen X, Gao P, Xu Y, Zhou B, Xu H. Clinical significance of palliative gastrectomy on the survival of patients with incurable advanced gastric cancer: a systematic review and meta-analysis. BMC Cancer. 2013;13:577.
91. Lim S, Muhs BE, Marcus SG, Newman E, Berman RS, Hiotis SP. Results following resection for stage IV gastric cancer; are better outcomes observed in selected patient subgroups? J Surg Oncol. 2007;95:118–22.
92. Fujitani K, Yang H-K, Mizusawa J, et al. Gastrectomy plus chemotherapy versus chemotherapy alone for advanced gastric cancer with a single non-curable factor (REGATTA): a phase 3, randomised controlled trial. Lancet Oncol. 2016;17:309–18.

Duodenum

6

Justin S. Hatchimonji, Robert E. Roses, and Jose L. Pascual

6.1 Introduction

Surgical emergencies associated with duodenal neoplasms pose a substantial challenge. In this chapter, we present an overview of common duodenal neoplasms, followed by a discussion of the presentation and management of three primary surgical emergencies: obstruction, perforation, and bleeding.

6.2 Neoplasms of the Duodenum

6.2.1 Primary Duodenal Malignancies

Small bowel cancers are rare, contributing to an estimated 0.6% of all new cancer cases and 0.3% of all cancer deaths in the United States in 2021 [1]. The distribution of these lesions across the small intestine varies widely by histologic subtype; over 50% of small bowel adenocarcinomas arise in the duodenum, while neuroendocrine tumors (NETs), lymphomas, and gastrointestinal stromal tumors (GISTs) occur less frequently in this location (15–20%, respectively). In contrast, most NETs arise in the ileum [2, 3]. Incidence of these tumors has not changed significantly over time [4], with the exception of a marked increase in the diagnosis of NETs over the last 2–3 decades [3]. Overall, duodenal malignancies comprise about 25% of all small

J. S. Hatchimonji · J. L. Pascual (✉)
Division of Traumatology, Surgical Critical Care, and Emergency Surgery, Department of Surgery, Perelman School of Medicine, University of Pennsylvania, Philadelphia, PA, USA
e-mail: justin.hatchimonji@pennmedicine.upenn.edu; Jose.Pascual@pennmedicine.upenn.edu

R. E. Roses
Division of Endocrine and Oncologic Surgery, Perelman School of Medicine, University of Pennsylvania, Philadelphia, PA, USA
e-mail: robert.roses@pennmedicine.upenn.edu

A. Tarasconi et al. (eds.), *Oncologic Surgical Emergencies*, Hot Topics in Acute Care Surgery and Trauma, https://doi.org/10.1007/978-3-031-36860-8_6

bowel cancers [5]. Duodenal neoplasms may be difficult to diagnose, as they are not screened for routinely and often only present with nonspecific symptoms such as abdominal pain, nausea, vomiting, and/or indolent weight loss [6, 7]. In the emergent setting, histologic subtypes may present in any fashion, but GISTs most often manifest with bleeding, lymphomas most commonly with perforation, and adenocarcinomas most often with obstruction [6].

6.2.1.1 Adenocarcinoma

The duodenum is the site of more than half of all intestinal adenocarcinomas accounting for nearly 60% of all duodenal malignancies [2]. A single-center series by Halfdanarson et al. suggested that duodenal tumors present at an earlier stage than jejunal or ileal tumors, likely owing to earlier onset of symptoms from higher flow obstruction [8]. Risk factors for small bowel adenocarcinoma include inflammatory bowel disease, celiac disease, and familial polyposis syndromes [9]. In the absence of powerful evidence supporting systemic or regional nonsurgical therapies, surgical resection is often a treatment priority. Notwithstanding, many patients present with locally advanced or disseminated disease precluding complete resection, and a broadening experience supports first-line systemic therapy in patients with higher risk or metastatic disease [3].

6.2.1.2 Neuroendocrine Tumors (NETs)

Neuroendocrine tumors (NETs) of the small intestine were traditionally referred to as carcinoids, though the term NET is increasingly favored and encompasses both low-grade, more indolent tumors and higher grade lesions [10, 11]. These tumors account for 15–20% of primary duodenal malignancies [2, 3]. Approximately one-third of NETs are functional, the majority of which are gastrinomas or somatostatinomas [11, 12]. Risk factors for NETs include smoking, alcohol use [13], and multiple endocrine neoplasia type 1 (MEN-1) [14]. Endoscopic resection may be adequate for small nonfunctional NETs, but larger tumors and gastrinomas often require operative management, frequently including regional lymph node removal. A more permissive approach to localized NETs of the duodenum may be appropriate in patients with MEN-1 who often have multifocal disease [12]. A landmark study on the Zollinger-Ellison syndrome demonstrated that, even among the small proportion of MEN-1 patients free of disease immediately after operation, almost all recurred at 5 years, suggesting limited impact of surgery in this population other than for palliation [15].

6.2.1.3 Lymphomas

Small bowel lymphomas are rare (0.2–0.5 per 100,000 in the United States) and primarily present in the jejunum and ileum [16] (Fig. 6.1). Lymphomas comprise approximately 10% of all duodenal malignancies [2, 3]. The histologic subtypes of duodenal lymphomas vary significantly and are beyond the scope of this chapter. The mainstay of first-line treatment for all small bowel lymphomas is chemotherapy, with the notable addition of *H. pylori* treatment for mucosa-associated

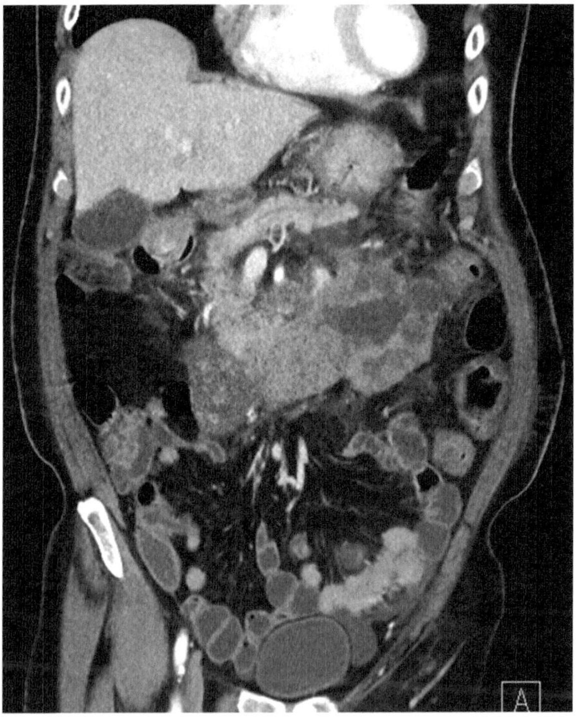

Fig. 6.1 68-Year-old male with known duodenal lymphoma. CT scan shows the distal duodenum and a proximal jejunal mass with a mesenteric calcified focus next to the duodenum. The patient ultimately underwent a pyloric exclusion and gastrojejunostomy

lymphoid tissue tumors (MALTs) [17, 18]. There is a role, in selected cases, for surgical palliation of symptoms or to improve candidacy for systemic therapy [6].

6.2.1.4 Gastrointestinal Stromal Tumors (GISTs)

GISTs are the most common GI sarcoma and are more commonly diagnosed through increased recognition over the past two decades [19]. Approximately 28% of all GISTs are located in the small intestine; a quarter of these arise in the duodenum. Six percent of duodenal malignancies are GISTs [2, 19]. Surgical resection is the treatment of choice for localized disease; negative margin resection is the goal. Lymphadenectomy is unnecessary as GISTs rarely metastasize to lymph nodes, and this may allow for more conservative surgical approaches. The tyrosine kinase inhibitor imatinib is active against the majority of GISTs and may be indicated in the adjuvant and/or neoadjuvant setting [20].

6.2.2 Benign Duodenal Neoplasms

Benign neoplasms including lipomas, adenomas, leiomyomas, and other entities are relatively uncommon in the duodenum. They are often incidental findings or present with nonspecific symptoms of abdominal pain, nausea, and/or vomiting. Adenomas are the most common of benign lesions. While periampullary location may complicate treatment approaches, many of these tumors can be managed with endoscopic or limited operative resection [21, 22].

6.2.3 Extension of a Pancreatic Malignancy

Pancreatic malignancies may infiltrate or compress the duodenum. Pancreatic cancer accounts for 3% of all new cancer cases and 8% of cancer deaths [1]. Up to 80% of patients with pancreatic cancer present with metastatic or locally advanced disease; 10–25% of patients develop symptoms of duodenal or gastric outlet obstruction at some point in their course [23]. The treatment for duodenal obstruction traditionally included operative gastrojejunostomy [24], but advances in endoscopic approaches have afforded alternatives including plastic or self-expanding metal stents [25] (Fig. 6.2). Decompressive gastrostomy tubes placed in surgery, by endoscopy, or by interventional radiology may also provide palliation in patients with particularly poor prognoses [23].

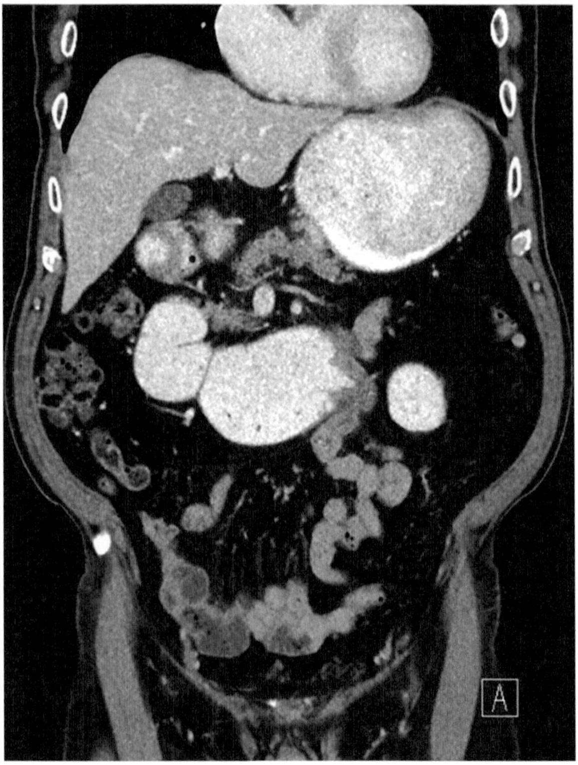

Fig. 6.2 CT scan tomogram from a 70-year-old male who presented acutely obstructed at the distal duodenum from an adenocarcinoma. Note the distended duodenum and stomach. The patient ultimately underwent resection with duodenojejunostomy anastomosis

6.2.4 Metastatic Disease to the Duodenum

Metastatic disease to the small bowel is relatively rare. Melanoma is the most common malignancy to metastasize to the gastrointestinal tract; the stomach or duodenum is involved in 5–50% of these cases [26, 27]. Other potential primary cancers to metastasize to the duodenum include colon, lobular breast, pancreatic, lung, and renal cell carcinomas [7]. Similarly to primary duodenal tumors, metastases may present with obstruction or bleeding, though the latter is uncommon [28, 29].

6.3 Surgical Emergencies

6.3.1 Intestinal Obstruction

6.3.1.1 Presentation

Patients presenting with an obstructing mass in the duodenum may manifest a combination of abdominal pain, bloating, and vomiting [30]. The likelihood of an obstructive presentation is dependent on the type and location of malignancy; for example, about 25% of duodenal adenocarcinomas present with obstruction, but this is less common if the tumor is located near the ampulla [31]. Vomiting is a hallmark of obstructive presentations, occurring in up to 80% of patients [32], and may be large volume and projectile in nature [33]. A shorter duration and rapid progression of abdominal pain may indicate a benign etiology rather than malignancy [32], and pain associated with peptic stricture may be more colicky in nature [33]. Weight loss is commonly endorsed by patients with gastroduodenal malignancy that has been present long enough to cause obstruction [32].

6.3.1.2 Physical Exam and Laboratory Findings

On examination, patients with a duodenal obstruction may display vague epigastric tenderness. A "succussion splash," or a splashing sound audible through a stethoscope when the abdomen is rocked or tapped, may be present, indicating gastroduodenal accumulation of contents. Mild diffuse abdominal distention may be present, though this is unlikely to be diffuse as the distal bowel will be decompressed. Patients may appear dehydrated or malnourished. If patients have been vomiting, laboratory examination may reflect hypokalemia and/or a hypochloremic metabolic alkalosis [34, 35].

6.3.1.3 Imaging

A variety of imaging techniques may demonstrate the gastric outlet obstruction resulting from a duodenal mass. Plain-film X-ray may reveal a "double-bubble" sign indicating a distended stomach adjacent to a distended duodenum [36]. Similarly, a fluoroscopic upper GI series may demonstrate partial or complete obstruction at some segment of the duodenum. However, most commonly, a computed tomography (CT) scan is readily available and used to make the diagnosis of an obstructive duodenal mass. Computed tomography offers several imaging characteristics that may help differentiate the various types of duodenal masses. GISTs are often relatively large, lobular, well-circumscribed, vascular masses [37], while lipomas have the appearance (density) of fat and often appear intraluminal on imaging due to their size despite their submucosal location [38]. Adenocarcinomas may have an "apple-core" appearance with associated narrowing or thickening of the duodenal wall, with or without ulceration or invasion into adjacent structures. If there is question as to the extent of local invasion of adjacent structures or encasement of vessels, or if the lesion is periampullary, an MRI can be helpful [39]. NETs tend to occur in the proximal portion of the duodenum (first or second segments) and appear as focal intraluminal masses [40]. In the setting of clinical intestinal obstruction, it may be useful to perform a CT of the abdomen with oral contrast to radiographically evaluate for complete or partial obstruction. Oral contrast should be preferentially administered via a nasogastric tube and subsequently followed with rapid evacuation to avoid high-volume emesis and aspiration.

6.3.1.4 Management

As in any case of gastrointestinal obstruction, a nasogastric tube for gastric decompression is warranted. Electrolyte abnormalities (particularly Mg^{2+}, Ca^{2+}, $PO4^{-}$, and K^{+}) as well as volume depletion should be aggressively corrected. Surgical management should focus on both decompression and restoration of gastrointestinal continuity, with or without resection of the primary lesion. If the patient's condition allows for pathologic diagnosis and oncologic staging, resection may be indicated, and if the patient is safely able to tolerate a definitive operation, an oncological operation should be performed. Otherwise, palliative surgical management with gastrojejunal bypass is often the chosen approach. If the latter is performed, it is important that the patient be maintained on acid-suppressive therapy postoperatively [30]. If bypass is not feasible, gastrostomy tube placement for drainage with or without a jejunostomy tube for feeding may be helpful. Alternatively, endoscopic stenting of the duodenal obstruction can be considered [41] (Fig. 6.3). This approach is best suited for patients with extremely poor prognosis and life expectancy (<6 months), including those with widely disseminated metastatic disease upon presentation. Duodenal stenting is not without complication risk, as stents may migrate or cause perforation or bleeding, or may also obstruct [23, 25, 42]. Depending on

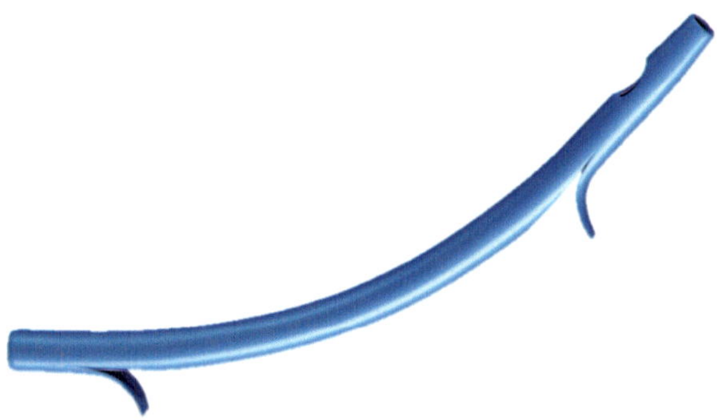

Fig. 6.3 Commercial biliary stent most often inserted endoscopically or through interventional radiology approaches. [Courtesy of Cook Medical LLC. (With permission)]

the patient and expected survival, these risks may be mitigated through the use of diverse types of stents (i.e., covered vs uncovered) [43].

A subset of patients presenting with duodenal obstruction deserve special consideration: those with some concurrent degree of biliary obstruction. These patients may additionally and/or concurrently require a biliary bypass (thus a "double bypass") with a Roux limb anastomosed to both the bile duct and the stomach [24]. Outcomes for gastrojejunostomy with or without biliary bypass are reasonable given the often debilitated and malnourished nature of this patient population; however, this procedure has definite inherent risks. An analysis of the American College of Surgeons National Surgical Quality Improvement Project (ACS NSQIP) data from 2005 to 2011 identified a 20% 30-day morbidity rate when this operation was undertaken for patients with unresectable pancreatic cancer. This was found to be higher than in patients who underwent laparotomy alone, though no difference in mortality was detected, reflecting the grave prognosis for most patients with unresectable periampullary cancer [44]. Unsurprisingly, emergent operation was associated with increased morbidity [45].

6.3.2 Duodenal Perforation

6.3.2.1 Presentation

Perforation of a duodenal malignancy may occur after an extended period of obstruction, from an aggressive necrotic tumor and/or in the context of neoadjuvant, adjuvant, or palliative therapy (i.e., radiation or chemotherapy). Patients that develop a perforation present with sudden onset of severe epigastric pain and/or diffusely throughout the abdomen, particularly if it involves the intraperitoneal portion of the duodenum. Conversely, a retroperitoneal or contained duodenal perforation may present with more indolent and subtle symptoms including malaise, nausea/vomiting, and fever. Patients with intraperitoneal perforations presenting soon after onset may have more localized pain; if later, pain may be more diffuse. The pain may radiate to the right shoulder secondary to irritation of the right diaphragm from accumulating of subdiaphragmatic succus or gastric contents [46]. In some cases, perforations may remain contained or "self-sealed," in which case the pain may actually diminish with time and be nearly resolved upon presentation. Patients may also report a history of weight loss or food intolerance leading up to the acute presentation [47]. In the case of an actively treated duodenal malignancy, perforation in this setting may result from tissue necrosis occurring secondary to treatment (i.e., following chemotherapy for lymphoma) [48].

6.3.2.2 Physical Exam and Laboratory Findings

Patients can exhibit abdominal tenderness, with or without peritonitis (including guarding and rebound tenderness). Depending on the duration of symptoms, this may be accompanied with signs of sepsis and shock, including fever, tachycardia, hypotension, and hyperlactatemia [47]. It is worth noting, however, that these are the signs and symptoms of any free intraperitoneal perforation, including that of the stomach and colon. Given that the duodenum is, in part, a retroperitoneal structure, some perforations may be contained and not cause peritonitis [49].

Laboratory workup should include a complete blood count, looking in particular for a leukocytosis, and a lactic acid elevation, particularly for patients who are clinically in shock. In those with an unidentified etiology for hollow viscus perforation, studies for other potential causes (i.e., *H. pylori*, gastrin levels) may be helpful, though these are less useful in the setting of known malignancy [47]. If malignancy is suspected based on history or imaging at the time of presentation, tumor markers such as CEA and CA 19-9 can be obtained to guide future surveillance [31].

6.3.2.3 Imaging

Upright or lateral decubitus abdominal radiographs may demonstrate pneumoperitoneum, though the sensitivity of this finding is less than 80% [46]. While in some cases such findings in themselves may be sufficient to proceed directly to laparotomy, in the absence of extreme hemodynamic instability and when at a center with rapid access to cross-sectional imaging, it is reasonable to obtain a CT scan to help rule out other sources of hollow viscus perforation and to help plan the operative intervention [50]. In the setting of perforation, a discrete tumor may not always be identifiable on CT imaging, but if a tumor is visible, adenocarcinoma will most often appear as a focal area of wall thickening. GISTs, on the other hand, will appear as exophytic masses with heterogeneous enhancement with or without ulceration, while lymphomas will appear with homogenous enhancement and may have clear lymph node involvement [50]. Even small bubbles of gas surrounding any mass suggests perforation, as does extravasation of an oral contrast agent [47]. Other findings suspicious for perforation include mesenteric fat stranding locally, bowel wall thickening, or bowel wall discontinuity [51]. Live fluoroscopic examination may be useful, but more time consuming than CT imaging, which has a sensitivity of 96% or greater for the diagnosis of hollow viscus perforation [52]. Albeit less sensitive, abdominal sonography may be useful in detecting free fluid [53].

6.3.2.4 Management

Broad-spectrum antibiotics should be administered early as mortality in septic shock rises steadily for every hour delay in antibiotic administration [54]. The patient should be resuscitated promptly while awaiting definitive management. This should continue intraoperatively and not delay surgical intervention which, if possible, should involve resection of the tumor. However, the indications to resect in the setting of perforation may be limited, particularly with a mass of unknown pathology or in the setting of extraduodenal extension or distant metastasis. Even when technically feasible, malnutrition, hemodynamic instability, and organ dysfunction (e.g., worsening acute kidney injury) represent relative contraindications to a more extensive resection [55, 56].

Intraluminal content spillage and contamination must be controlled early, even though definitive management may be delayed for a subsequent intervention ("damage control") [57]. Definitive management of duodenal perforations can be achieved by primary closure and/or omental flap or patch (Cellan-Jones or Graham patch)

[58, 59]. This is traditionally done via laparotomy but is increasingly being done laparoscopically in those familiar with the technique and in stable patients [60]. When the tumor itself perforates, these approaches often fail as the tissue is tenuous and will not hold stitches. In this case, alternative surgical management is required, and exclusion and bypass may be necessary. Pyloric exclusion involves closing the pylorus (either internally through a gastrotomy or by stapling externally across) and restoring bowel continuity with a gastrojejunal bypass [58, 61]. There is little data supporting this technique in the setting of perforated malignancy, and the benefit of pyloric exclusion in traumatic injury has also been called into question [62]. Notwithstanding, the significant challenges associated with a perforated duodenal tumor sometimes necessitate creative solutions including closure, reinforcement with vascularized tissue, exclusion, bypass, or duodenal drainage [63]. The latter can sometimes be accomplished with placement of a distal jejunostomy tube directed retrograde accompanied by extraluminal drains around the perforated bowel segment. Additionally, in the setting of failed attempt at closure or patch of a duodenal leak, percutaneous transhepatic biliary drainage may be helpful to divert bile.

6.3.3 Duodenal Bleeding

6.3.3.1 Presentation

Patients presenting with bleeding duodenal lesions may manifest similar signs and symptoms as those with any upper gastrointestinal bleed including those of simple peptic ulcers. They may present with a primary complaint of hematemesis and/or melena or experience symptoms of hypovolemia, such as lightheadedness. Most often, bleeding is slow, and occult and microcytic anemia is the only indication [64]. Melena is a somewhat sensitive sign, as it may reflect as little as 100 mL of luminal bleeding. Hematochezia may also be present, particularly if the bleed is brisk [53]. Importantly, patients may suffer an intraperitoneal or retroperitoneal duodenal bleed and never display findings of intraluminal blood [48]. Bleeding is a more common presenting symptom in patients with GISTs, as compared with other tumors [6].

6.3.3.2 Physical Exam and Laboratory Findings

On examination, patients will often have painless bleeding with hematemesis, melena, or hematochezia per rectum as described above. If the hemorrhage is brisk, the patient will also demonstrate signs of hemorrhagic shock with signs of volume depletion, such as pallor and cool, clammy extremities [65]. Vital signs may reveal tachycardia with or without hypotension, depending on the class of shock [66, 67]. It is important to realize that hypotension may not manifest until 30% of the patient's blood volume has been lost, otherwise termed class III or IV hemorrhagic shock [67]. Urine output may be decreased [68]. Laboratory examination is likely to show a low hemoglobin, though it may be normal initially. Other laboratory evidence of ongoing bleeding may include acute kidney injury with increased creatinine and electrolyte derangements [65]. In the setting of an acute bleed, anemia will more likely be normocytic, while in the setting of chronic low-grade bleeding, the anemia will be microcytic as with iron deficiency [68]. Additional laboratory abnormalities may include elevations in lactate, secondary to tissue hypoperfusion [67].

6.3.3.3 Imaging

As in the case of any upper gastrointestinal bleed, diagnosis and management mostly occur in parallel. Often, the preferred initial maneuver (after resuscitation) is upper endoscopy, as this can be both diagnostic and therapeutic [53]. Alternatively when endoscopy is not available or bleeding is too profuse to allow proper endoscopic visualization, CT angiography (CTA) is a rapid and often very accessible option. Though not the traditional first-line investigative option, CTA sensitivity and positive predictive value have improved, and this may be a reasonable place to start in the absence of other options [53]. In this context, oral contrast (i.e., Gastrografin) should be avoided in favor of intravenous contrast alone [69]. The sensitivity of CTA in gastrointestinal bleeds is about 50%, with a slightly greater sensitivity for acute as opposed to chronic bleeds [70]. Data on tumor hemorrhage in particular is sparse, but for all GI bleeds, a minimum hemorrhage rate of 0.3–0.5 cc/min is required for CTA detection [71]. Other modalities for detection of upper GI bleeding include visceral angiography, which also detects bleeding at the same rates [72], and nuclear scintigraphy, which is significantly more sensitive (minimum bleeding rate detection at 0.02–0.05 cc/min) but not offering much utility in the setting of a bleeding duodenal mass that is likely visible on endoscopy [73].

6.3.3.4 Management

As with any GI bleed, the first priority is prompt evaluation of hemodynamic status, remembering that the airway may be in jeopardy in the patient with active hematemesis and may need to be secured prior to further management. Particularly in the setting of acute hemorrhage and significant volume loss, ensuring adequate intravenous access is essential to allow for resuscitation [53, 64]. Importantly, there is some evidence that a restrictive transfusion strategy (transfusion trigger 7 g/dL) is associated with better outcomes than a liberal transfusion strategy (9 g/dL), even in upper GI bleeding patients [74]. Another randomized study demonstrated similar outcomes between transfusion thresholds of 8 g/dL and 10 g/dL, suggesting that at a minimum, a restrictive strategy may be safe [75]. For patients in acute hemorrhagic shock, permissive hypotension may result in less blood products transfused and may confer a survival benefit [76]. Coagulopathy should be corrected promptly. There is controversy regarding the use of tranexamic acid (TXA) in the setting of upper GI bleeding. Though there have been meta-analyses suggesting some benefit for GI bleeding in general (upper and lower, primarily upper in the included studies) [77, 78], the HALT-IT trial, an international, randomized, placebo-controlled trial in upper GI bleeds, found no benefit [79].

After stabilization, the primary goal should be nonoperative management of acute bleeding, in an attempt to temporize and ultimately plan an elective definitive operation (if indicated) [61]. As noted above, the first step in this process should be an upper endoscopy, not only to identify the site of bleeding but also to attempt to achieve hemostasis through the use of endoscopic clipping, submucosal epinephrine injection, cautery, or application of topical hemostatic agents [61, 80].

Endoscopic management of recurrent duodenal tumor hemorrhage can be entertained, but no data exists to support or recommend it. One might, however, extrapolate from bleeding ulcer data, which suggests that repeated attempts at endoscopic management may be beneficial [81]. When the bleeding surface has high-risk features (i.e., exposed vessel) or when there is a diffuse area of devitalized necrotic tissue, trans-arterial embolization may be the more ideal method for definitive bleeding control [61, 82, 83]. It is worth noting that, although rebleeding rates are high, in the short term, bleeding often either stops with endoscopic intervention or is self-limited [84]. This gives providers time to develop more appropriate long-term strategies, which may include up-front surgical resection in oncologic fashion or neoadjuvant treatment, which may in itself help ameliorate bleeding [85]. In the case of unresectable tumors, nonoperative management strategies may help with both tumor shrinkage and palliation of bleeding. These may include imatinib for GISTs [86] or radiation for other malignancies [87].

6.4 Special Considerations

6.4.1 Metastatic Disease

In certain cases, the surgical emergency may be the index presentation of the patient's malignancy. In some, gross metastatic disease may be readily apparent, either on preoperative imaging or intraoperatively. Surgical management of the acute issue should not deviate from the approaches described above in the face of metastatic disease. Bleeding must be controlled, perforation must be managed, and obstruction must be relieved. However, the presence of metastatic disease warrants an up-front goal-of-care discussion and might favor less invasive modalities for definitive management. For example, an obstruction that might have been manageable with a distal gastrectomy might be better managed with a gastrojejunostomy or a duodenal stent [25, 42, 43]. As discussed above, bleeding may better be managed directly with angioembolization [82, 83]. Perforation, in many cases, will mandate operation regardless of cancer stage; however, every attempt should be made to limit intervention in cases when operation is not expected to prolong life [61].

6.5 Anatomic Considerations

6.5.1 Involvement of the Ampulla

Surgical emergencies of the duodenum may be complicated by involvement of the ampulla of Vater. In cases of tumor bleeding or perforation involving the ampulla or periampullary duodenum, the approach should be the same as for metastatic disease. Less invasive or complex options are preferred, as outcomes from emergent pancreaticoduodenectomy are poor, with perioperative mortality that varies by indication but may be as high as 20% and a complication rate of 90% [88, 89]. In the case of bleeding, endoscopic or interventional radiology management should be used, and in the case of perforation, exclusion and bypass should be favored over oncologic resection [61].

Decision-making may be slightly more complex in the case of an obstructing ampullary tumor, mandating some attention to the bile duct. Indeed, as described earlier, biliary obstruction is a common presentation of duodenal and pancreatic head malignancies, with 70% of pancreatic cancers presenting with jaundice [90, 91]. As noted above, both duodenal stents [92] and biliary stents [91] are well-accepted options if the tumor is unresectable (Fig. 6.4).

6.5.2 Enteric Access

If in the operating room for one of the above surgical emergencies, one should consider placing enteral access (i.e., jejunostomy tube) prior to closing the laparotomy. This is particularly true for the patient undergoing operation for duodenal obstruction as there is a significant incidence of delayed gastric emptying after palliative gastrojejunostomy [93]. This evidence has been used by some to advocate the use of stenting over gastrojejunostomy [94, 95], but in cases where the decision has already been made to perform an operation, a jejunostomy tube may make sense. On the other hand, more recent literature suggests important morbidity from prophylactic jejunostomy tube placement [96], both following pancreaticoduodenectomy [97, 98] and after resection for gastric cancer [99]. It is unclear, however, whether these data make a legitimate argument against jejunostomy tube placement once already in surgery, as there may be confounding by indication in that surgeons may opt to place a tube in sicker and more frail patients. The issue remains controversial, but there is likely a population of patients for whom a feeding jejunostomy should be considered.

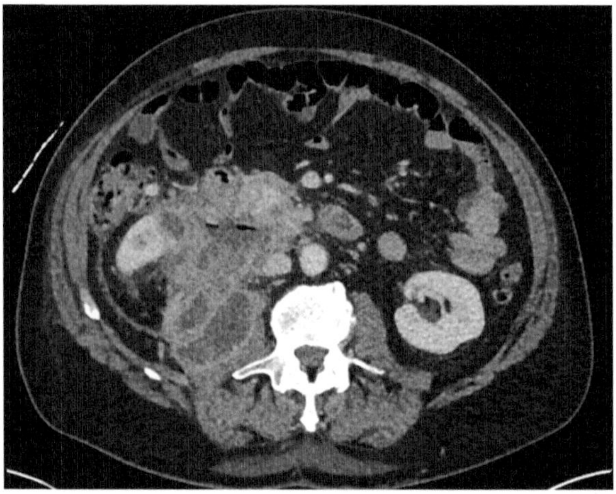

Fig. 6.4 64-Year-old male with duodenal GIST encasing the kidney and inferior vena cava who subsequently underwent gastrojejunostomy and pyloric exclusion

6.5.3 Goals of Care

Patients presenting with duodenal surgical emergencies are at high perioperative risk and are often found to have advanced disease. In general, emergency surgery carries a significantly greater mortality (12.5% vs. 2.7%) and morbidity (32.8% vs. 12.7%) risk than elective general surgery [100]. Data on oncologic surgical emergencies is limited, but these risks are likely even higher in patients with malignancies [101]. Beyond the perioperative phase, one must also consider the patient's long- and short-term prognosis prior to undertaking surgical intervention. Adequate communication regarding goals of care with the patient and his/her loved ones prior to major surgery has long been problematic [102], particularly in emergency surgery [103], but is of utmost importance [104]. A frank preoperative discussion should occur between the surgeon, patient, oncologist when possible, and family where the risks, prognosis, and goals of care are explicitly stated and all questions answered.

6.6 Conclusion

A variety of duodenal malignancies may present with obstruction, perforation, or bleeding, requiring prompt resuscitation and consideration of operative or nonoperative interventions. While general principles are largely similar to those applicable in non-oncologic emergency surgery, the extent of disease, prognosis, preexisting conditions and nutritional status, long-term treatment plan, and the patient's goals of care may complicate decision-making. Careful consideration will be needed to proceed to optimal surgical care individualized to the patient, the tumor, and the complication.

References

1. Siegel RL, Miller KD, Fuchs HE, Jemal A. Cancer statistics, 2021. CA Cancer J Clin. 2021;71(1):7–33.
2. Raghav K, Overman MJ. Small bowel adenocarcinomas—existing evidence and evolving paradigms. Nat Rev Clin Oncol. 2013;10(9):534–44.
3. Bilimoria KY, Bentrem DJ, Wayne JD, Ko CY, Bennett CL, Talamonti MS. Small bowel cancer in the United States: changes in epidemiology, treatment, and survival over the last 20 years. Ann Surg. 2009;249(1):63–71.
4. Kerremans RP, Lerut J, Penninckx FM. Primary malignant duodenal tumors. Ann Surg. 1979;190(2):179.
5. Hatzaras I, Palesty JA, Abir F, et al. Small-bowel tumors: epidemiologic and clinical characteristics of 1260 cases from the Connecticut tumor registry. Arch Surg. 2007;142(3):229–35.
6. Catena F, Ansaloni L, Gazzotti F, et al. Small bowel tumours in emergency surgery: specificity of clinical presentation. ANZ J Surg. 2005;75(11):997–9.
7. Minardi AJ Jr, Zibari GB, Aultman DF, McMillan RW, McDonald JC. Small-bowel tumors. J Am Coll Surg. 1998;186(6):664–8.
8. Halfdanarson TR, McWilliams RR, Donohue JH, Quevedo JF. A single-institution experience with 491 cases of small bowel adenocarcinoma. Am J Surg. 2010;199(6):797–803.

9. Aparicio T, Zaanan A, Svrcek M, et al. Small bowel adenocarcinoma: epidemiology, risk factors, diagnosis and treatment. Dig Liver Dis. 2014;46(2):97–104.
10. Mullen JT, Wang H, Yao JC, et al. Carcinoid tumors of the duodenum. Surgery. 2005;138(6):971–8.
11. Massironi S, Campana D, Partelli S, et al. Heterogeneity of duodenal neuroendocrine tumors: an Italian multi-center experience. Ann Surg Oncol. 2018;25(11):3200–6.
12. Sato Y, Hashimoto S, Mizuno K-I, Takeuchi M, Terai S. Management of gastric and duodenal neuroendocrine tumors. World J Gastroenterol. 2016;22(30):6817–28.
13. Chen CC, Neugut AI, Rotterdam H. Risk factors for adenocarcinomas and malignant carcinoids of the small intestine: preliminary findings. Cancer Epidemiol Biomark Prevent. 1994;3(3):205–7.
14. Hoffmann KM, Furukawa M, Jensen RT. Duodenal neuroendocrine tumors: classification, functional syndromes, diagnosis and medical treatment. Best Pract Res Clin Gastroenterol. 2005;19(5):675–97.
15. Norton JA, Fraker DL, Alexander HR, et al. Surgery to cure the Zollinger–Ellison syndrome. N Engl J Med. 1999;341(9):635–44.
16. Pan SY, Morrison H. Epidemiology of cancer of the small intestine. World J Gastrointest Oncol. 2011;3(3):33.
17. Na HK, Won SH, Ahn JY, et al. Clinical course of duodenal mucosa-associated lymphoid tissue lymphoma: comparison with gastric mucosa-associated lymphoid tissue lymphoma. J Gastroenterol Hepatol. 2021;36(2):406–12.
18. Lu PW, Fields AC, Yoo J, et al. Surgical management of small bowel lymphoma. J Gastrointest Surg. 2021;25(3):757–65.
19. Lee N, Tang D, Jayaraman S. Penetrating cardiac trauma and the use of emergent extracorporeal membrane oxygenation and therapeutic hypothermia: when cooler heads prevail. Trauma Case Rep. 2015;1(9–12):95–8.
20. Colombo C, Ronellenfitsch U, Yuxin Z, et al. Clinical, pathological and surgical characteristics of duodenal gastrointestinal stromal tumor and their influence on survival: a multi-center study. Ann Surg Oncol. 2012;19(11):3361–7.
21. Perez A, Saltzman JR, Carr-Locke DL, et al. Benign nonampullary duodenal neoplasms. J Gastrointest Surg. 2003;7(4):536–41.
22. Kemp CD, Russell RT, Sharp KW. Resection of benign duodenal neoplasms. Am Surg. 2007;73(11):1086–91.
23. Perone JA, Riall TS, Olino K. Palliative care for pancreatic and periampullary cancer. Surg Clin N Am. 2016;96(6):1415.
24. Singh SM, Longmire WP Jr, Reber HA. Surgical palliation for pancreatic cancer. The UCLA experience. Ann Surg. 1990;212(2):132–9.
25. Jeurnink SM, Steyerberg EW, van Hooft JE, et al. Surgical gastrojejunostomy or endoscopic stent placement for the palliation of malignant gastric outlet obstruction (SUSTENT study): a multicenter randomized trial. Gastrointest Endosc. 2010;71(3):490–9.
26. Liang KV, Sanderson SO, Nowakowski GS, Arora AS. Metastatic malignant melanoma of the gastrointestinal tract. Mayo Clin Proc. 2006;81(4):511–6.
27. Benedeto-Stojanov D, Nagorni A, Živković V, Milanović J, Stojanov D. Metastatic melanoma of the stomach and the duodenum. Arch Oncol. 2006;14(1–2):60–1.
28. Adamo R, Greaney PJ, Witkiewicz A, Kennedy EP, Yeo CJ. Renal cell carcinoma metastatic to the duodenum: treatment by classic pancreaticoduodenectomy and review of the literature. J Gastrointest Surg. 2008;12(8):1465–8.
29. Nazareno J, Taves D, Preiksaitis H-G. Metastatic breast cancer to the gastrointestinal tract: a case series and review of the literature. World J Gastroenterol. 2006;12(38):6219–24.
30. Dempsey DT. Pyloroplasty and gastrojejunostomy. In: Fischer JE, editor. Fischer's mastery of surgery. 6th ed. Philadelphia: Lippincott Williams & Wilkins; 2012.
31. Grandhi MS, Schulick RD. Duodenal cancer (including intestinal type ampullary cancer). In: Morita SY, Balch CM, Klimberg VS, Pawlik TM, Posner MC, Tanabe KK, editors. Textbook of complex general surgical oncology. New York: McGraw-Hill Education; 2018.

32. Khullar SK, DiSario JA. Gastric outlet obstruction. Gastrointest Endosc Clin N Am. 1996;6(3):585–603.
33. Soybel DI, Landman WB. Ileus and bowel obstruction. In: Mulholland MW, Lillemoe KD, editors. Greenfield's surgery: scientific principles and practice. 5th ed. Philadelphia: Lippincott Williams & Wilkins; 2011.
34. Gan S-I. Gastric outlet obstruction in adults. Waltham: UpToDate; 2020.
35. McQuaid KR. Complications of peptic ulcer disease. In: Papadakis MA, McPhee SJ, Rabow MW, editors. Current medical diagnosis treatment 2021. New York: McGraw-Hill Education; 2021.
36. Shen Y-C, Lin Y-S. Double-bubble sign in an adult patient. Gastroenterology. 2017;153(5):1191–2.
37. Cai P-Q, Lv X-F, Tian L, et al. CT characterization of duodenal gastrointestinal stromal tumors. Am J Roentgenol. 2015;204(5):988–93.
38. Thompson WM. Imaging and findings of lipomas of the gastrointestinal tract. Am J Roentgenol. 2005;184(4):1163–71.
39. Suh CH, Tirumani SH, Shinagare AB, et al. Diagnosis and management of duodenal adenocarcinomas: a comprehensive review for the radiologist. Abdom Imaging. 2015;40(5):1110–20.
40. Levy AD, Taylor LD, Abbott RM, Sobin LH. Duodenal carcinoids: imaging features with clinical-pathologic comparison. Radiology. 2005;237(3):967–72.
41. Roses RE, Folkert IW, Krouse RS. Malignant bowel obstruction: reappraising the value of surgery. Surg Oncol Clin N Am. 2018;27(4):705–15.
42. Dormann A, Meisner S, Verin N, Wenk LA. Self-expanding metal stents for gastroduodenal malignancies: systematic review of their clinical effectiveness. Endoscopy. 2004;36(06):543–50.
43. Woo SM, Kim DH, Lee WJ, et al. Comparison of uncovered and covered stents for the treatment of malignant duodenal obstruction caused by pancreaticobiliary cancer. Surg Endosc. 2013;27(6):2031–9.
44. Roses RE, Tzeng C-WD, Ross MI, Fournier KF, Abbott DE, You YN. The palliative index: predicting outcomes of emergent surgery in patients with cancer. J Palliat Med. 2014;17(1):37–42.
45. Bartlett EK, Wachtel H, Fraker DL, et al. Surgical palliation for pancreatic malignancy: practice patterns and predictors of morbidity and mortality. J Gastrointest Surg. 2014;18(7):1292–8.
46. Mulholland MW. Gastroduodenal ulceration. In: Mulholland MW, Lillemoe KD, Doherty GM, Maier RV, Simeone DM, Upchurch Jr GR, editors. Greenfield's surgery: scientific principles and practice. 5th ed. Philadelphia: Lippincott Wlliams & Wilkins; 2011.
47. Chikunguwo SM, Maher JW. Perforated duodenal ulcer. In: Fischer JE, editor. Fischer's mastery of surgery. 6th ed. Philadelphia: Lippincott Williams & Wilkins; 2012.
48. Bosscher MRF, van Leeuwen BL, Hoekstra HJ. Surgical emergencies in oncology. Cancer Treat Rev. 2014;40(8):1028–36.
49. Wong C-H, Chow PKH, Ong H-S, Chan W-H, Khin L-W, Soo K-C. Posterior perforation of peptic ulcers: presentation and outcome of an uncommon surgical emergency. Surgery. 2004;135(3):321–5.
50. Gosangi B, Rocha TC, Duran-Mendicuti A. Imaging spectrum of duodenal emergencies. Radiographics. 2020;40(5):1441–57.
51. Borofsky S, Taffel M, Khati N, Zeman R, Hill M. The emergency room diagnosis of gastrointestinal tract perforation: the role of CT. Emerg Radiol. 2015;22(3):315–27.
52. Reich H, Chou D, Melo N. Perforated hollow viscus. In: Butler KL, Harisinghani M, editors. Acute care surgery: imaging essentials for rapid diagnosis. New York: McGraw-Hill Education; 2015.
53. Britt LD, Peitzman A, Barie P, Peitzman A. Acute care surgery. Philadelphia: Wolters Kluwer Health; 2012.
54. Rivers E, Nguyen B, Havstad S, et al. Early goal-directed therapy in the treatment of severe sepsis and septic shock. N Engl J Med. 2001;345(19):1368–77.

55. Pidhorecky I, Cheney RT, Kraybill WG, Gibbs JF. Gastrointestinal stromal tumors: current diagnosis, biologic behavior, and management. Ann Surg Oncol. 2000;7(9):705–12.
56. Dorcaratto D, Heneghan H, Fiore B, et al. Segmental duodenal resection: indications, surgical techniques and postoperative outcomes. J Gastrointest Surg. 2015;19(4):736–42.
57. Rotondo MF, Schwab CW, McGonigal MD, et al. 'Damage control': an approach for improved survival in exsanguinating penetrating abdominal injury. J Trauma. 1993;35(3):375–82.
58. Ansari D, Torén W, Lindberg S, Pyrhönen H-S, Andersson R. Diagnosis and management of duodenal perforations: a narrative review. Scand J Gastroenterol. 2019;54(8):939–44.
59. Ricci JL, Turnbull ADM. Spontaneous gastroduodenal perforation in cancer patients receiving cytotoxic therapy. J Surg Oncol. 1989;41(4):219–21.
60. Sanabria A, Villegas MI, Morales Uribe CH. Laparoscopic repair for perforated peptic ulcer disease. Cochrane Database Syst Rev. 2013;2:CD004778.
61. Folkert IW, Roses RE. Value in palliative cancer surgery: a critical assessment. J Surg Oncol. 2016;114(3):311–5.
62. Seamon MJ, Pieri PG, Fisher CA, et al. A 10-year retrospective review: does pyloric exclusion improve clinical outcome after penetrating duodenal and combined pancreaticoduodenal injuries? J Trauma Acute Care Surg. 2007;62(4):829–33.
63. Berne TV, Donovan AJ. Nonoperative treatment of perforated duodenal ulcer. Arch Surg. 1989;124(7):830–2.
64. Schirmer BD. Bleeding duodenal ulcer. In: Fischer JE, editor. Fischer's mastery of surgery. 6th ed. Philadelphia: Lippincott Williams & Wilkins; 2012.
65. Feinman M, Haut ER. Upper gastrointestinal bleeding. Surg Clin N Am. 2014;94(1):43–53.
66. Gutierrez G, Reines H, Wulf-Gutierrez ME. Clinical review: hemorrhagic shock. Crit Care. 2004;8(5):373.
67. Cannon JW. Hemorrhagic shock. N Engl J Med. 2018;378(4):370–9.
68. Kamboj AK, Hoversten P, Leggett CL. Upper gastrointestinal bleeding: etiologies and management. Mayo Clin Proc. 2019;94(4):697–703.
69. Polotsky M, Vadvala HV, Fishman EK, Johnson PT. Duodenal emergencies: utility of multidetector CT with 2D multiplanar reconstructions for challenging but critical diagnoses. Emerg Radiol. 2020;27(2):195–203.
70. Amarteifio E, Sohns C, Heuser M, Püsken M, Lange B, Obenauer S. Detection of gastrointestinal bleeding by using multislice computed tomography acute and chronic hemorrhages. Clin Imaging. 2008;32(1):1–5.
71. Wells ML, Hansel SL, Bruining DH, et al. CT for evaluation of acute gastrointestinal bleeding. Radiographics. 2018;38(4):1089–107.
72. Walker TG, Salazar GM, Waltman AC. Angiographic evaluation and management of acute gastrointestinal hemorrhage. World J Gastroenterol. 2012;18(11):1191–201.
73. Soto JA, Park SH, Fletcher JG, Fidler JL. Gastrointestinal hemorrhage: evaluation with MDCT. Abdom Imaging. 2015;40(5):993–1009.
74. Villanueva C, Colomo A, Bosch A, et al. Transfusion strategies for acute upper gastrointestinal bleeding. N Engl J Med. 2013;368(1):11–21.
75. Jairath V, Kahan BC, Gray A, et al. Restrictive versus liberal blood transfusion for acute upper gastrointestinal bleeding (TRIGGER): a pragmatic, open-label, cluster randomised feasibility trial. Lancet. 2015;386(9989):137–44.
76. Tran A, Yates J, Lau A, Lampron J, Matar M. Permissive hypotension versus conventional resuscitation strategies in adult trauma patients with hemorrhagic shock: a systematic review and meta-analysis of randomized controlled trials. J Trauma Acute Care Surg. 2018;84(5):802–8.
77. Lee P-L, Yang K-S, Tsai H-W, Hou S-K, Kang Y-N, Chang C-C. Tranexamic acid for gastrointestinal bleeding: a systematic review with meta-analysis of randomized clinical trials. Am J Emerg Med. 2021;45:269–79.
78. Dionne JC, Oczkowski SJW, Hunt BJ, et al. Tranexamic acid in gastrointestinal bleeding: a systematic review and meta-analysis. Crit Care Med. 2022;50(3):e313–9.

79. Roberts I, Shakur-Still H, Afolabi A, et al. Effects of a high-dose 24-h infusion of tranexamic acid on death and thromboembolic events in patients with acute gastrointestinal bleeding (HALT-IT): an international randomised, double-blind, placebo-controlled trial. Lancet. 2020;395(10241):1927–36.
80. Hwang JH, Fisher DA, Ben-Menachem T, et al. The role of endoscopy in the management of acute non-variceal upper GI bleeding. Gastrointest Endosc. 2012;75(6):1132–8.
81. Lau JYW, Sung JJY, Lam Y-h, et al. Endoscopic retreatment compared with surgery in patients with recurrent bleeding after initial endoscopic control of bleeding ulcers. N Engl J Med. 1999;340(10):751–6.
82. Koo HJ, Shin JH, Shin S, Yoon H-K, Ko G-Y, Gwon DI. Efficacy and clinical outcomes of transcatheter arterial embolization for gastrointestinal bleeding from gastrointestinal stromal tumor. J Vasc Interv Radiol. 2015;26(9):1297–304.
83. Loffroy R, Rao P, Ota S, De Lin M, Kwak B-K, Geschwind J-F. Embolization of acute non-variceal upper gastrointestinal hemorrhage resistant to endoscopic treatment: results and predictors of recurrent bleeding. Cardiovasc Intervent Radiol. 2010;33(6):1088–100.
84. Ofosu A, Ramai D, Latson W, Adler DG. Endoscopic management of bleeding gastrointestinal tumors. Ann Gastroenterol. 2019;32(4):346–51.
85. Krishnamurthy G, Singh H, Sharma V, Savlania A, Vasishta RK. Therapeutic challenges in the management of bleeding duodenal gastrointestinal stromal tumor: a case report and review of literature. J Gastrointest Cancer. 2019;50(1):170–4.
86. Liu Q, Kong F, Zhou J, Dong M, Dong Q. Management of hemorrhage in gastrointestinal stromal tumors: a review. Cancer Manag Res. 2018;10:735–43.
87. Kondoh C, Shitara K, Nomura M, et al. Efficacy of palliative radiotherapy for gastric bleeding in patients with unresectable advanced gastric cancer: a retrospective cohort study. BMC Palliat Care. 2015;14(1):37.
88. Tsai C-Y, Lai B-R, Wang S-Y, et al. The impact of preoperative etiology on emergent pancreaticoduodenectomy for non-traumatic patients. World J Emerg Surg. 2017;12(1):21.
89. Gulla A, Tan WP, Pucci MJ, et al. Emergent pancreaticoduodenectomy: a dual institution experience and review of the literature. J Surg Res. 2014;186(1):1–6.
90. Lillemoe KD, Pitt HA. Palliation: surgical and otherwise. Cancer. 1996;78(3):605–14.
91. Kruse EJ. Palliation in pancreatic cancer. Surg Clin N Am. 2010;90(2):355–64.
92. Oh SY, Edwards A, Mandelson M, et al. Survival and clinical outcome after endoscopic duodenal stent placement for malignant gastric outlet obstruction: comparison of pancreatic cancer and nonpancreatic cancer. Gastrointest Endosc. 2015;82(3):460–8.
93. Doberneck RC, Berndt GA. Delayed gastric emptying after palliative gastrojejunostomy for carcinoma of the pancreas. Arch Surg. 1987;122(7):827–9.
94. Jeurnink SM, Steyerberg EW, van't Hof G, van Eijck CHJ, Kuipers EJ, Siersema PD. Gastrojejunostomy versus stent placement in patients with malignant gastric outlet obstruction: a comparison in 95 patients. J Surg Oncol. 2007;96(5):389–96.
95. Chandrasegaram MD, Eslick GD, Mansfield CO, et al. Endoscopic stenting versus operative gastrojejunostomy for malignant gastric outlet obstruction. Surg Endosc. 2012;26(2):323–9.
96. Zapas JL, Karakozis S, Kirkpatrick JR. Prophylactic jejunostomy: a reappraisal. Surgery. 1998;124(4):715–20.
97. Padussis JC, Zani S, Blazer DG, Tyler DS, Pappas TN, Scarborough JE. Feeding jejunostomy during Whipple is associated with increased morbidity. J Surg Res. 2014;187(2):361–6.
98. Nussbaum DP, Zani S, Penne K, et al. Feeding jejunostomy tube placement in patients undergoing pancreaticoduodenectomy: an ongoing dilemma. J Gastrointest Surg. 2014;18(10):1752–9.
99. Patel SH, Kooby DA, Staley CA III, Maithel SK. An assessment of feeding jejunostomy tube placement at the time of resection for gastric adenocarcinoma. J Surg Oncol. 2013;107(7):728–34.
100. Havens JM, Peetz AB, Do WS, et al. The excess morbidity and mortality of emergency general surgery. J Trauma Acute Care Surg. 2015;78(2):306–11.

Table 7.1 Tumour subtypes

Histological subtype	Portion of cases	Portion of cases by site
Neuroendocrine tumour	37.4%	Duodenum 16% Jejunum 15% Ileum 57%
Adenocarcinoma	36.9%	Duodenum 59% Jejunum 42% Ileum 15%
Lymphoma	17.3%	Duodenum 10% Jejunum 22% Ileum 17%
Gastrointestinal stromal tumour	8.4%	Duodenum 6% Jejunum 16% Ileum 4%
Other		Duodenum 9% Jejunum 5% Ileum 4%

predisposition syndromes such as Lynch syndrome, familial adenomatous polyposis, and Peutz-Jeghers syndrome [4]. Coeliac disease confers an increased risk, with absolute risk estimated at 0.06 [5] to 0.65% [6] for affected individuals. Likewise, Crohn's disease demonstrates an increased incidence, estimated at 0.2 per 1000 patient years with both site and duration of disease affecting risk [7]. Predisposing risk tends to result in lower age of presentation, with most cases arising in 50–70-year-olds.

Increasing incidence of midgut small bowel (jejunal and ileal) neuroendocrine tumours (NETs) has led to them overtaking adenocarcinoma as the most common subtype of small bowel tumour in the USA, accounting for 37% of cases [3]. Small bowel NETs are epithelium tumours characterised by neuroendocrine differentiation, which can secrete functional amines or neuroendocrine hormones. In over 20–56% of cases, they are multifocal [8, 9].

The gastrointestinal tract is the most common site of extranodal presentation of non-Hodgkin's lymphoma (NHL), accounting for 4–12% of NHL cases in the UK and 18–24% of small bowel malignancy. Diffuse large B cell lymphoma is the most common subtype, ahead of extranodal marginal zone B cell lymphoma of mucosa-associated lymphoid tissue (MALT) [10].

Gastrointestinal stromal tumours (GISTs) arise from the interstitial cells of Cajal, which act as smooth muscle pacemaker cells, controlling gut peristalsis. They classically develop due to gain-of-function mutations in the tyrosine kinase receptor c-KIT (80%) or PDGFRα genes [11]. They account for 8.4% of small intestinal tumours, most commonly arising in the jejunum and ileum [3].

The small intestine may be involved as a metastatic site of primary malignancies, either with extraluminal involvement such as with peritoneal carcinomatous or by haematogenous spread from melanoma, sarcoma, breast, or colon cancer.

7.2 Emergency Presentation

Small bowel tumours have an indolent onset, often resulting in late presentation. Symptoms are non-specific and include abdominal pain, nausea and vomiting, anaemia, and weight loss. However, they can present acutely with obstruction, perforation, and gastrointestinal bleeding [12, 13]. Historically, small bowel obstruction in the virgin abdomen raised concern of small bowel tumours; they are in fact identified in only 4% of such cases, with adhesions accounting for 62% [14].

Data on the percentage of small bowel tumours that present as emergencies is limited. Most case series or cohorts examine a histological subset or emergency presentation as an isolated entity. Tumours present most commonly with acute haemorrhage, and obstruction occurs more commonly than perforation [15–17]. The exact patterns of presentation depend on underlying histopathology. In a case series of 34 patients presenting as acute emergencies across a 10-year period, 44% of patients presented with obstruction, 32% with perforation, and 24% with bleeding. All the patients with acute haemorrhages had underlying stromal tumours, most perforations were lymphomas (88%), and all carcinoid tumours presented with obstruction [12].

Up to 35% of small bowel NETs present acutely: 80% of these present with obstruction, 3% with ischaemia, 3% with intussusception, and 9% with pain. Compared to other small bowel tumours, they rarely present with acute haemorrhage [18]. An estimated 20–56% of small bowel NETs are multifocal at presentation [9]. Carcinoid syndrome is a unique feature of NETs. It is characterised by flushing, diarrhoea, and bronchospasm. It is typically a late feature, suggestive of metastatic disease.

Outside of limited case reports and small patient series, there is a lack of data surrounding the acute presentation of adenocarcinoma. Between 52 and 64.7% of small bowel adenocarcinomas occur in the duodenum and can present with a broader symptom complex including gastric outlet obstruction and biliary obstruction as well as perforation, bleeding, and obstruction seen with jejunal and ileal tumours [19, 20]. Duodenal and periampullary tumours are complex, often requiring specialist endoscopic and/or interventional radiology interventions, which in many countries are not located outside of specialist centres.

A report on the Dutch GIST registry reports 19% of small bowel GISTs having required emergency surgery for ileus, perforation, or gastrointestinal haemorrhage. When operated on emergently, 23% of patients had R1 or R2 resection [11]. A further case series investigating emergency presentation of GISTs—of which the primary site was stomach in over 50%—reported GI bleeding as the most common reason for emergency presentation (48.9%). Interestingly, of this cohort, 15.2% presented with intraperitoneal haemorrhage as opposed to intraluminal, 28.3% presented with intestinal obstruction, and 7.6% with perforation and peritonitis [21]. When compared to non-bleeding GISTs, bleeding appears to be a protective factor for GIST recurrence, as well as a predictor for smaller tumours and longer relapse-free survival [22].

Contemporaneous review suggests that emergency surgical intervention is required in 11–64% of primary intestinal lymphomas, with rates of perforation of 1–25% and gastrointestinal bleeding a feature in 2.2–22%. Obstruction was estimated to occur in 5–39% of intestinal NHL [10] cases. A further case series of 82 patients across 15 years at a single centre reported tumour complications as the indication for surgery in 38 cases with 18 operated on for perforation, 14 for obstruction, and 6 for bleeding [23]. See Table 7.2.

Metastatic small bowel tumours or extraluminal peritoneal carcinomatous may also present as an emergency. Classically, gastrointestinal metastases from cutaneous melanoma present with acute haemorrhage; however, they may also present with abdominal pain and obstruction [24].

For patients presenting with acute haemorrhage or peritonism due to obstruction, ischaemia, or perforation, definitive histological diagnosis will often follow surgical intervention. Despite this, understanding the patterns associated with each pathology is important to the diagnostic and surgical approach. The non-specificity and vagueness of symptoms at early stages warrant consideration of axial imaging for patients even without overt signs, especially in high-risk patient cohorts such as coeliacs, Crohn's disease, cancer predisposition syndromes, and those with previous carcinoma. Identification of a small bowel tumour on axial imaging should prompt a skin survey and a carefully considered history of risk factors, carcinoid symptoms, and B symptoms.

Table 7.2 Presentation patterns

Histological subtype	Emergency presentation	Pattern of presentation
Overall		Haemorrhage 23–41% Obstruction 22–26% Perforation 6–9%
Neuroendocrine tumour	35%	Obstruction 80% Pain 9% Ischaemia 3% Intussusception 3%
Adenocarcinoma	Limited data	Biliary obstruction (duodenal) Gastric outlet obstruction (duodenal) Perforation Haemorrhage Obstruction Intussusception
Lymphoma	11–64%	Perforation 1–25% Obstruction 5–39% Bleeding 2.2–22%
Gastrointestinal stromal tumour	19%	Gastrointestinal bleeding 48.9% Intraperitoneal haemorrhage 15.2% Obstruction 28.3% Perforation 7.6%

7.3 Initial Management and Diagnosis

Initial patient management in the emergency department should focus on resuscitation, analgesia, and early identification and treatment of sepsis with appropriate broad-spectrum antibiotics. For bleeding patients and those with obstructive symptoms, early transfusion of blood products and insertion of a nasogastric tube for decompression, respectively, should be considered.

In rare occasions, patients may not respond to resuscitation due to ongoing acute haemorrhage or established peritonism with septic shock and multiorgan failure. For these cases, prompt involvement of anaesthesia and critical care is essential. With due consideration for patient factors including age, comorbidity, and frailty, a diagnostic laparotomy for haemorrhage or source control may be warranted in those patients that cannot be stabilised. In the responsive patient, choice of axial imaging should be guided by the clinical picture.

7.3.1 Radiology

In a patient with haematemesis, melaena, or fresh blood per rectum when gastroscopy either has been completed or is not indicated, plain abdominal X-ray offers little, and computer tomography angiography (CTA) of the abdomen and pelvis should be undertaken with IV contrast. On probability, the colon and stomach are the more likely source sites than small intestine. In the 5–10% of cases whereby a bleeding point in the stomach or colon is not identified on bleeding study, or first-line endoscopic investigations (gastroscopy, sigmoidoscopy, or colonoscopy), and the patient has been stabilised, consideration can be given to radionuclide scanning with technetium sulphur colloid or 99mTc pertechnetate-labelled red cells, though they add little in the initial acute emergent setting. These scans require a minimum rate of 0.1–0.5 mL/min to detect bleeding. The usefulness of these investigations has been questioned by several studies, which have shown a trend towards high incorrect positive rates (10%) or incorrect identification of bleeding site [25–28]. Similarly, small bowel capsule endoscopy and/or double-balloon enteroscopy are usually not suitable in the acute situation, but can be useful in the stable patient with persistent, unexplained anaemia and occult bleeding.

For responders with peritonism and/or obstruction, CT abdomen and pelvis with contrast should be performed to guide further management. CT is estimated to detect 73% of small bowel tumours. Thickening of the small bowel wall of greater than 1.5 cm is highly suspicious for neoplasia. Associated luminal narrowing, obstruction, perforation, or ischaemia may be seen. Adenocarcinoma classically appears as an annular or ulcerated lesion or a discrete tumour mass. Lymphoma may appear as a lead point of intussusception, a nodular filling defect, or an ill-defined infiltrating lesion with or without involvement of adjacent tissues, often associated with bulky lymphadenopathy. NETs are associated with a desmoplastic reaction seen as stellate stranding of soft tissues and mesenteric calcification (Fig. 7.1).

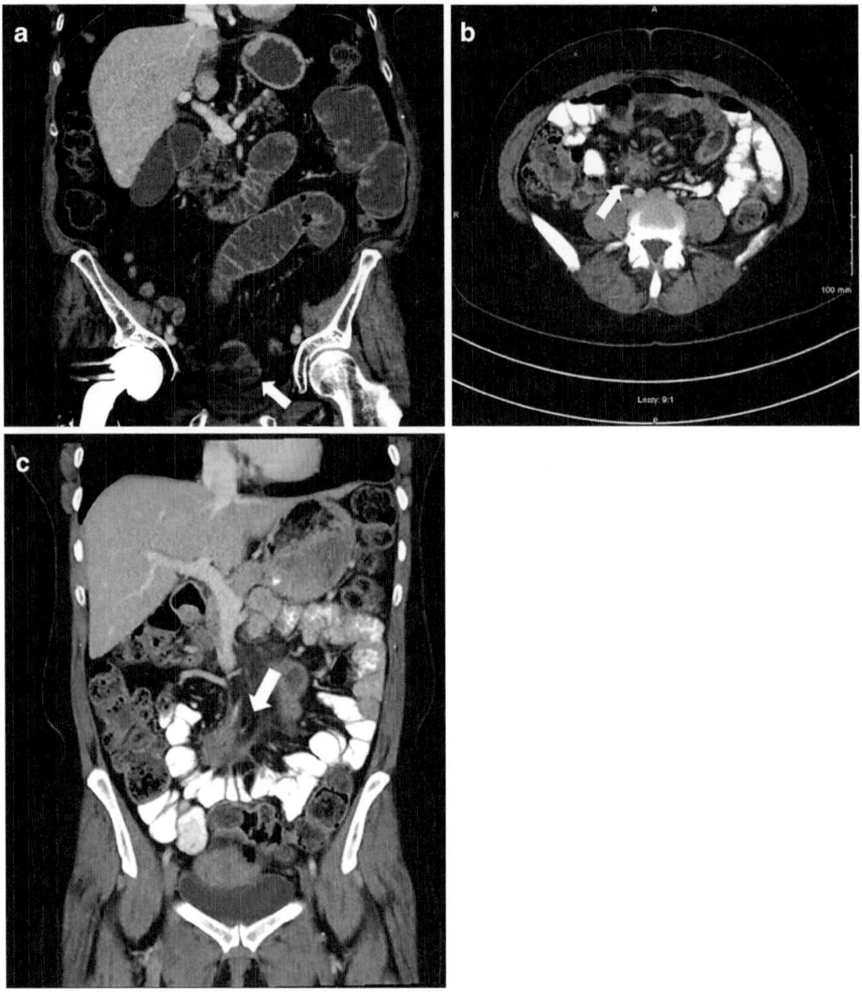

Fig. 7.1 Radiological examples of small bowel tumours. (**a**) Coronal image showing thickened small bowel wall, interpretation of images limited by artefact from hip prosthesis. Post-operative histology showed a stenotic, annular adenocarcinoma of the small intestine. (**b**) Axial and (**c**) coronal images desmoplastic stellate reaction in mesentery associated with primary small bowel neuroendocrine tumour. The primary lesion was not identifiable at CT

These features may be more readily identified than the primary tumour. GISTs are typically submucosal, solitary masses, but may appear subserosal or intraluminal. Features suggestive of malignancy are central liquefication due to necrosis, calcification, and irregularity [29]. CT will determine, in cases with associated obstruction, not only the site and nature of the obstruction but also whether it is complete or incomplete, the presence of complications such as ischaemia, or loco-regional nodal involvement or metastases.

CT enteroclysis is highly sensitive (92.8%) and specific (99.2%) for diagnosis of small bowel tumours, but it is not useful in the emergency setting, as both perforation and obstruction are absolute contraindications [30, 31]. Contrast media is delivered directly to the small intestine via nasoenteric tube, to distend the lumen and aid in the identification of luminal pathology. Exact protocols and media used vary between institutes. Enterography by comparison involves ingestion of contrast per os. Enteroclysis is thought to be marginally more sensitive (94% vs. 93%) and more specific (100% vs. 94%) than enterography for identification of small bowel pathology, but enterography is more readily accepted and tolerated by patients, with a lower dose of radiation [32].

Similar techniques of magnetic resonance (MR) enteroclysis and enterography provide radiation-free alternatives to CT. MR enteroclysis has a diagnostic accuracy of up to 96.6% for small bowel tumours, with excellent interobserver agreement. MRI provides enhanced soft tissue characterisation when compared to CT, which can provide more information regarding histological subtype [33]. MR enterography has demonstrated to have accuracy (96%) comparable to enteroclysis for 7–70 mm small bowel tumours [34]. Ongoing advances in MR and CT technology are continuing to produce new accurate approaches to diagnostic imaging for small bowel pathology. Again, MRI is difficult in the acute presentations as there is a requirement for significant breath holding. Its use should be limited largely to elective and urgent workup.

For completion of staging, thoracic axial imaging in the form of CT should be performed perioperatively, with timing dictated by the clinical scenario.

7.3.2 Endoscopy

Standard gastroscopy and colonoscopy do not evaluate the small intestine, except the proximal duodenum and terminal ileum. Modern and emerging technologies such as small bowel capsule endoscopy and double-balloon enteroscopy provide a means of visualising small bowel mucosa and, in the latter, the potential for tissue harvesting and/or therapeutic intervention. In the setting of acute GI haemorrhage, gastroscopy and/or colonoscopy provide an opportunity for definitive diagnosis and therapy. In the small number of cases whereby the bleeding source is the small intestine, advanced endoscopic techniques can be employed with the important caveat that obstruction and perforation are contraindications warranting primary surgical intervention.

Small bowel capsule endoscopy (SBCE) entails the ingestion of a small capsule containing a camera, which continually images the lumen of the small intestine as it travels through it. Capsule retention occurs in 1–2% of cases; this increases to 3.6–13% in Crohn's disease (Fig. 7.2) [35]. Dissolvable capsules have been developed to try tackle this, but retention at 30 h remains high [36]. The yield for small bowel lesions on capsule endoscopy is estimated at 60–78%, with a better yield than CT angiography. It should be reserved for stable patients without any evidence of obstruction and for that reason has limited use in emergency presentations [37].

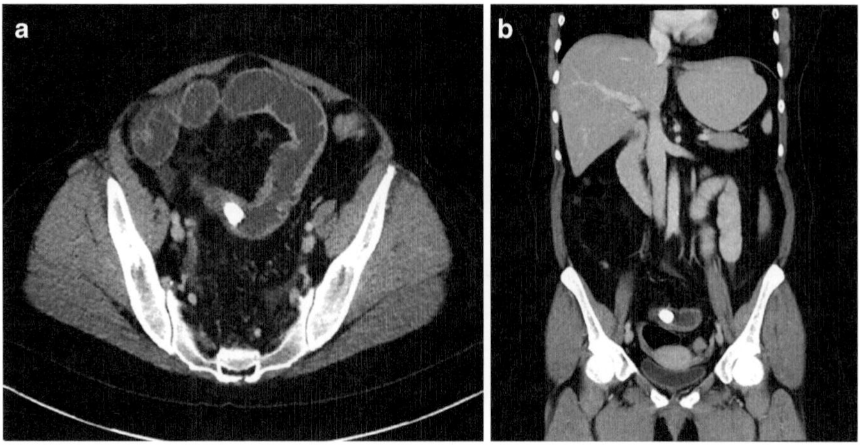

Fig. 7.2 Complications of capsule endoscopy. (**a**) Axial and (**b**) coronal images showing small bowel capsule endoscope impacted in a fibrostenotic segment of terminal ileal Crohn's disease with resultant small bowel obstruction. While useful in routine and urgent workup of small bowel pathology and occult bleeding, its role in the emergency setting is limited

Double-balloon enteroscopy (DBE) can provide histological diagnosis prior to resection. A retrospective study of 627 patients undergoing 880 DBE identified 28 patients with small bowel tumours. Of these, initial histological diagnosis was made at DBE for 64.3% compared to 25% at surgery. In 25% of cases, DBE modified outcome by delaying or avoiding emergency surgery in three, prompting emergent resection in two, and modifying approach in three [38]. The diagnostic yield ranges from 12 to 17% for small bowel tumours on DBE [35]. DBE has also provided therapeutic options such as argon plasma coagulation, polypectomy, and balloon dilatation. As with capsule endoscopy, use of DBE may not be appropriate in the acute setting, dependent on the clinical scenario and patient factors.

7.4 Operative Approach

The clinical history supplemented by physical examination will help decide if the acute presentation is complicated or simple. Generally, complicated presentation will have perforated with signs of peritonism and absent bowel sounds.

Elevated inflammatory markers may also be a guide to early surgery, and the trend analysis of the white cell count and C-reactive protein is important. The use of a wound bundle will improve outcomes [39], and this should be combined with a laparotomy closure bundle to reduce fascial dehiscence, surgical site infection, seroma, and dehiscence.

The first inflection point is whether, or not, to operate. Preoperative histological diagnosis broadens options when it can be safely obtained; however, in the emergent case, this is often not possible. In some cases, patients may already have a known small bowel GIST, neuroendocrine tumour, or lymphoma and be actively undergoing neoadjuvant, medical, conservative, or palliative treatment at presentation [40].

The approach to surgery will be dictated by patient characteristics, outcomes of perioperative investigations, and urgency of the case. In the critically unwell, undifferentiated case in extremis whereby a diagnostic laparotomy is performed, a methodical approach must be employed. Rarely, in the unstable bleeding patient, the source will be a small bowel tumour, typically a GIST which may bleed into the lumen of the GI tract or intraperitoneally.

Identification of a small bowel tumour at laparotomy should prompt a full assessment of the stomach, small intestine, large intestine, peritoneal surfaces, and liver (all of which should be performed routinely at diagnostic laparotomy); up to 50% of small bowel NETs have multifocal disease at presentation. Presentation with perforation and obstruction suggests advanced disease in the setting of adenocarcinoma and lymphoma, and metastatic disease may be present at surgery. Synchronous tumours in bowel are very hard to detect at laparotomy and can be easily missed.

Laparoscopy, while associated with reduced length of stay, has a limited role in the management of small bowel tumours outside of select cases due to the commonality of multifocal disease; however, it can be used to guide and minimise the size of open incision [41]. Surgery should be performed with curative intent, aiming to resect macroscopic disease by segmental resection of the involved portion of small intestine with its mesenteric lymph nodes followed by anastomosis or diversion (Fig. 7.3). Care should be taken when performing the anastomosis. When employing a stapled technique, it is important that the stapler be held for 30 s before firing and that the surgeon has a clear understanding of the difference between a transabdominal and linear cutter in terms of stapler ergonomics, use cases, and outcomes.

In the case of bulky terminal ileal disease, this may require ileocolic resection. Likewise, advanced disease may require multivisceral and/or extensive mesenteric resection. Depending on the surgeon's skill set and training, in these circumstances, consideration should be given to bypass or diverting surgery with a view to obtaining biopsies for tissue diagnosis and referral to specialist centre for definitive treatment; this is especially true for duodenal tumours, which may require pancreaticoduodenectomy for oncological resection.

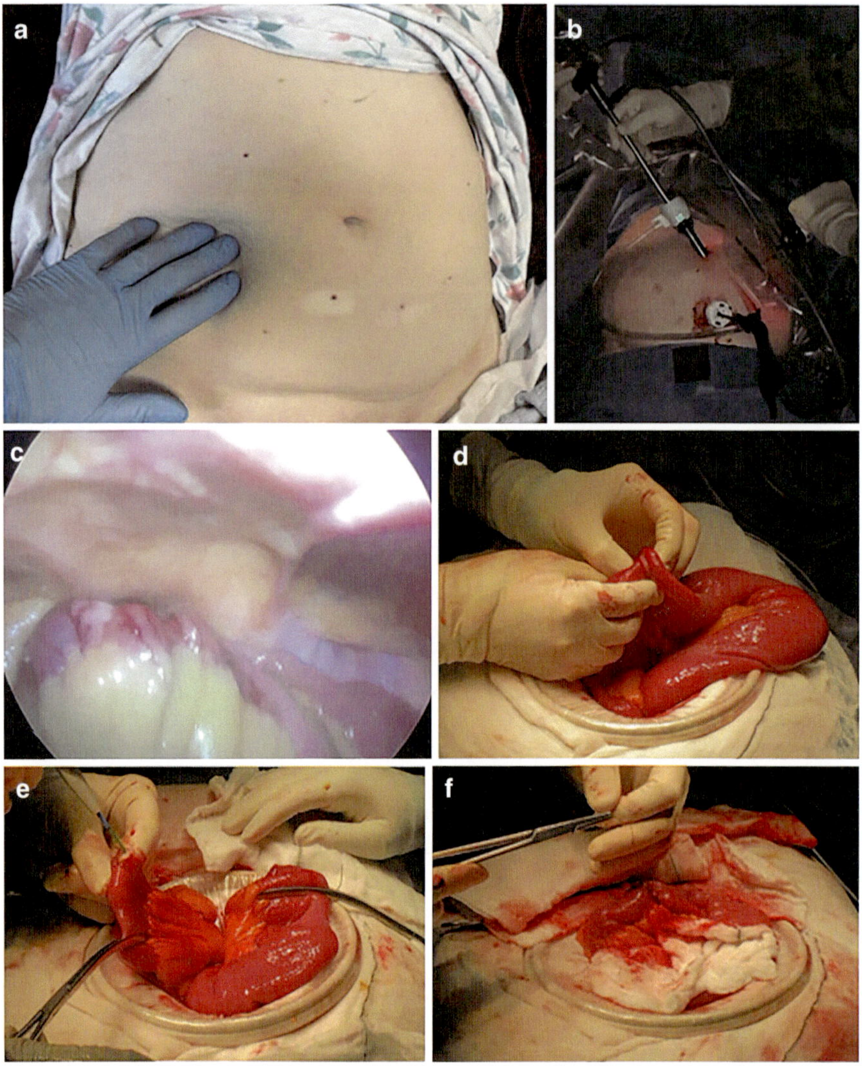

Fig. 7.3 Operative approach. Based on the (**a**) clinical assessment, a decision to begin with (**b**) laparoscopy is made. The camera and suprapubic ports are placed in the midline using longitudinal incisions. After the (**c**) the tumour is localised laparoscopically, a decision is made to convert to a small lower midline incision incorporating the port sites. (**d**) The tumour is delivered through the incision and resected along the mesenteric root. (**e**) A slit is made in the antimesenteric side of the distal limb prior to anastomosis to correct for the discrepancies in luminal diameter. (**f**) A hand-sewn anastomosis is performed with an inverting mattress suture using 3-0 PDS. The mesenteric defect is subsequently closed

7.5 Post-operative Outcomes and Complications

Emergency surgery is in and of itself a poor prognostic indicator. In-hospital mortality following surgery for an obstructing small bowel tumour is 11.3%, with reoperation and 30-day readmission rates of 4.8% and 9.7%, respectively, and a mean length of stay of 13.6 days [42]. Case series are often small, with poor outcomes. One such study investigating outcomes following emergency surgery for malignant small bowel perforation reported in-hospital mortality rates as high as 42.8% [43]. Recent systematic review of management for primary and metastatic small bowel obstruction showed 30-day mortality ranging for 13–28% in those that underwent surgery and 2–61% in those that were managed conservatively [44].

In a cohort of patients with small bowel lymphoma requiring acute surgery, 11.3% had major surgical complications including anastomotic leak and prolonged peritonitis. Early mortality was also 11.3% [23]. Emergency surgery for SB GISTs is associated with a significant rate of tumour spill [11], which in turn is associated with a recurrence rate of 49–74% at 2 years [45]. 5-Year survival rate following complete resection is 73%, but 26% after incomplete resection [21]. Interestingly, a recent large retrospective population study of patients with small bowel NETs and synchronous metastases has suggested that upfront resection of primary disease confers a survival benefit (11.6 vs. 6.2 years), reduced rate of unplanned acute care admissions (48.1% vs. 71.1% at 1 year), and less unplanned subsequent small bowel surgeries (18.5% vs. 38.9% at 3 years). It is important to note that this study included elective and emergency upfront surgery [46].

It is vitally important that we advocate for our patients by employing evidence-based approaches to minimising post-operative complications. Surgical site infections have significant implications for long-term oncological outcomes after surgery and should not be underestimated [47]. Careful attention should be paid to minimising wound infection through the use of a wound bundle (Fig. 7.4). This should include preparation of the abdomen by the removal of hair, use of alcohol-based aseptic preparations for both scrubbing and surgical site sterilisation, use of a wound protector, and a dedicated closure trolley and instruments [39]. Negative-pressure wound therapy is associated with reduced surgical site infection rates [48], and these systems are becoming more readily available and affordable. Post-operative incisional hernia rates after laparotomy range from 20 to 40% [49] and are symptomatic in up to 84% of patients [50]; use of small bite technique for abdominal closure and prophylactic mesh placement can reduce this to 3.9–16% [51, 52].

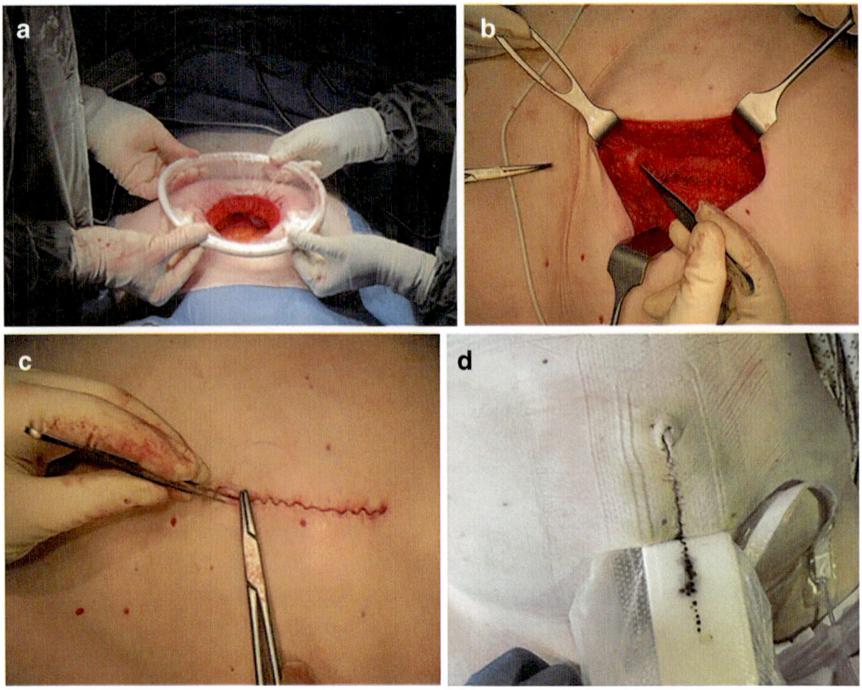

Fig. 7.4 Wound closure bound. These images demonstrate elements of a wound bundle including (**a**) use of a wound protector, (**b**) prophylactic mesh placement, (**c**) subcuticular skin closure with a self-locking stitch, and (**d**) a negative-pressure wound therapy system. Collectively, these interventions aim to reduce post-operative complications such as surgical site infection and incisional hernia

7.6 Post-operative Prognosis and Management

Definitive histological diagnosis and pathological staging will dictate prognosis and adjuvant treatment.

For adenocarcinoma, nodal involvement is the strongest indicator of long-term disease-free survival. Duodenal tumours confer significantly worse 5-year survival when compared to jejunal or ileal. Positive margins, lymphovascular invasion, T4 disease, and poorly differentiated histology are poor prognostic indicators. For duodenal adenocarcinoma, node-positive disease has a 5-year survival rate of 21%, compared to 65% for node negative [53]. Outcomes are better for jejunal disease, with 41% overall survival rate at 5 years. Limited data is available on the use of adjuvant chemotherapy in small bowel adenocarcinoma; hence, approaches are largely dictated by data from colonic adenocarcinoma. Adjuvant chemotherapy is generally advised in the setting of node-positive disease, with some advocating for chemotherapy in T3 and T4 tumours. Multivariant analysis shows that chemotherapy is associated with improved overall survival for stage II and III disease [54].

The BALLAD trial is ongoing, investigating the role of adjuvant 5-FU/leucovorin or 5-FU/LV plus oxaliplatin (FOLFOX) compared to observation alone for stage I–III small bowel adenocarcinoma [55].

5-Year survival rate for small bowel NETs is excellent, ranging from 52 to 100% dependent on stage. For NETs smaller than 1 cm, 1.1–1.9 cm, and larger than 2 cm, nodal disease is present in 12%, 70%, and 85%, respectively [56]. Even with advanced metastatic disease, 10-year survival rate can be greater than 50%. Multiple randomised control trials show improvements in progression-free survival with the use of systemic agents including octreotide (PROMID), lanreotide (CLARINET), everolimus (RADIANT4), and peptide radioreceptor therapy (NETTER-1) in the setting of metastatic well-differentiated disease [57–60]. Where curative resection is possible, resection of hepatic metastases can prolong disease-free survival [61].

Adjuvant treatment with imatinib is the standard of care for high-risk GISTs with at least one of the following features: size greater than 5 cm and a mitotic rate higher than 5 per high-power field units, size greater than 10 cm, or greater than 10 mitosis per high-power units [62]. It is also used as a first-line therapy for locally advanced and metastatic disease, as well as in the neoadjuvant setting for tumour downsizing [63]. Prognosis depends on gender, nodal disease, tumour size, site, and resection margins.

The adjuvant treatment of small bowel tumours is a complex and evolving field, limited by the rarity of small bowel neoplasia and the diversity of histological subtypes. It is a largely specialist field, with multiple strong non-surgical management options in certain patient cohorts.

7.7 Conclusion

Small bowel tumours are rare, with emergency presentation rarer yet. However, in the event of obstruction, perforation, or haemorrhage, disease is commonly advanced and urgent surgical intervention often warranted. Though the elective management of many subtypes of small bowel tumours is a specialist field, all general surgeons must have an appreciation for the common patterns of presentation and pathology, so that when faced with the acute case, they are equipped to deal with the patient appropriately and expediently when required.

Depending on the skill set and training of the surgeon, they may or may not be intimately familiar with the nuisances of management for all varieties of small bowel tumours. For those surgeons that do not manage these cases on a regular basis, a recognition that temporisation by resuscitation, diversion, or bypass as required can be an acceptable strategy for cases that are suitable for transfer to specialist centres owing to the benefits of preoperative histological diagnosis and neoadjuvant treatment options.

Acknowledgements This project was supported by the European Union's INTERREG VA Programme, managed by the Special EU Programmes Body (SEUPB) and Donegal Clinical Research Academy.

References

1. Reynolds I, Healy P, Mcnamara D. Malignant tumours of the small intestine. Surgeon. 2014;12(5):263–70.
2. Faivre J, Trama A, De Angelis R, Elferink M, Siesling S, Audisio R, et al. Incidence, prevalence and survival of patients with rare epithelial digestive cancers diagnosed in Europe in 1995–2002. Eur J Cancer. 2012;48(10):1417–24.
3. Bilimoria K, Bentrem D, Wayne J, Ko C, Bennett C, Talamonti M. Small bowel cancer in the United States: changes in epidemiology, treatment, and survival over the last 20 years. Ann Surg. 2009;249(1):63–71.
4. Aparicio T, Henriques J, Manfredi S, Tougeron D, Bouché O, Pezet D, et al. Small bowel adenocarcinoma: results from a nationwide prospective ARCAD-NADEGE cohort study of 347 patients. Int J Cancer. 2020;147(4):967–77.
5. Emilsson L, Semrad C, Lebwohl B, Green P, Ludvigsson J. Risk of small bowel adenocarcinoma, adenomas, and carcinoids in a Nationwide cohort of individuals with celiac disease. Gastroenterology. 2020;159(5):1686–94.
6. Caio G, Volta U, Ursini F, Manfredini R, De Giorgio R. Small bowel adenocarcinoma as a complication of celiac disease: clinical and diagnostic features. BMC Gastroenterol. 2019;19(1):45.
7. Elriz K, Carrat F, Carbonnel F, Marthey L, Bouvier A, Beaugerie L. Incidence, presentation, and prognosis of small bowel adenocarcinoma in patients with small bowel Crohn's disease: a prospective observational study. Inflamm Bowel Dis. 2013;19(9):1823–6.
8. Tran C, Sherman S, Howe J. The landmark series: management of small bowel neuroendocrine tumors. Ann Surg Oncol. 2021;28(5):2741–51.
9. Ethun C, Postlewait L, Baptiste G, McInnis M, Cardona K, Russell M, et al. Small bowel neuroendocrine tumors: a critical analysis of diagnostic work-up and operative approach. J Surg Oncol. 2016;114(6):671–6.
10. Abbott S, Nikolousis E, Badger I. Intestinal lymphoma—a review of the management of emergency presentations to the general surgeon. Int J Color Dis. 2015;30(2):151–7.
11. Boonstra P, Steeghs N, Farag S, van Coevorden F, Gelderblom H, Grunhagen D, et al. Surgical and medical management of small bowel gastrointestinal stromal tumors: a report of the Dutch GIST registry. Eur J Surg Oncol. 2019;45(3):410–5.
12. Catena F, Ansaloni L, Gazzotti F, Gagliardi S, Di Saverio S, De Cataldis A, et al. Small bowel tumours in emergency surgery: specificity of clinical presentation. ANZ J Surg. 2005;75(11):997–9.
13. Talamonti M, Goetz L, Rao S, Joehl R. Primary cancers of the small bowel: analysis of prognostic factors and results of surgical management. Arch Surg. 2002;137(5):564–70.
14. Ng Y, Ngu J, Wong A. Small bowel obstruction in the virgin abdomen: time to challenge surgical dogma with evidence. ANZ J Surg. 2018;88(1–2):91–4.
15. Ciresi D, Scholten D. The continuing clinical dilemma of primary tumors of the small intestine. Am Surg. 1995;61(8):698–702.
16. Minardi A, Zibari G, Aultman D, McMillan R, McDonald J. Small-bowel tumors. J Am Coll Surg. 1998;186(6):664–8.
17. Ojha A, Zacherl J, Scheuba C, Jakesz R, Wenzl E. Primary small bowel malignancies: single-center results of three decades. J Clin Gastroenterol. 2000;30(3):289–93.
18. Rajaretnam N, Meyer-Rochow G. Surgical management of primary small bowel NET presenting acutely with obstruction or perforation. World J Surg. 2021;45(1):203–7.
19. Huffman B, Jin Z, Yadav S, Patel S, Nagorney D, Truty M, et al. Novel prognostic factors in resected small bowel adenocarcinoma. Clin Colorectal Cancer. 2019;18(3):218–25.
20. Colina A, Hwang H, Wang H, Katz M, Sun R, Lee J, et al. Natural history and prognostic factors for localised small bowel adenocarcinoma. ESMO Open. 2020;5(6):e000960.
21. Sorour M, Kassem M, Ghazal Ael H, El-Riwini M, Abu NA. Gastrointestinal stromal tumors (GIST) related emergencies. Int J Surg. 2014;12(4):269–80.
22. Yin Z, Gao J, Liu W, Huang C, Shuai X, Wang G, et al. Clinicopathological and prognostic analysis of primary gastrointestinal stromal tumor presenting with gastrointestinal bleeding: a 10-year retrospective study. J Gastrointest Surg. 2017;21(5):792–800.

23. Hong Y, Kuo I, Liu Y, Yeh T. The role of surgical management in primary small bowel lymphoma: a single-center experience. Eur J Surg Oncol. 2017;43(10):1886–93.
24. Gallino G, Maurichi A, Patuzzo R, Mattavelli I, Barbieri C, Leva A, et al. Surgical treatment of melanoma metastases to the small bowel: a single cancer referral center real-life experience. Eur J Surg Oncol. 2021;47(2):409–15.
25. Tabibian J, Wong Kee Song L, Enders F, Aguet J, Tabibian N. Technetium-labeled erythrocyte scintigraphy in acute gastrointestinal bleeding. Int J Color Dis. 2013;28(8):1099–105.
26. Hunter J, Pezim M. Limited value of technetium 99m-labeled red cell scintigraphy in localization of lower gastrointestinal bleeding. Am J Surg. 1990;159(5):504–6.
27. Levy R, Barto W, Gani J. Retrospective study of the utility of nuclear scintigraphic-labelled red cell scanning for lower gastrointestinal bleeding. ANZ J Surg. 2003;73(4):205–9.
28. Olds G, Cooper G, Chak A, Sivak M, Chitale A, Wong R. The yield of bleeding scans in acute lower gastrointestinal hemorrhage. J Clin Gastroenterol. 2005;39(4):273–7.
29. Buckley J, Fishman E. CT evaluation of small bowel neoplasms: spectrum of disease. Radiographics. 1998;18(2):379–92.
30. Soyer P, Aout M, Hoeffel C, Vicaut E, Placé V, Boudiaf M. Helical CT-enteroclysis in the detection of small-bowel tumours: a meta-analysis. Eur Radiol. 2013;23(2):388–99.
31. Parrish F. Small bowel CT-enteroclysis: technique, pitfalls and pictorial review. Australas Radiol. 2006;50(4):289–97.
32. Minordi L, Vecchioli A, Mirk P, Bonomo L. CT enterography with polyethylene glycol solution vs CT enteroclysis in small bowel disease. Br J Radiol. 2011;84(998):112–9.
33. Masselli G, Gualdi G. MR imaging of the small bowel. Radiology. 2012;264(2):333–48.
34. Amzallag-Bellenger E, Soyer P, Barbe C, Diebold M, Cadiot G, Hoeffel C. Prospective evaluation of magnetic resonance enterography for the detection of mesenteric small bowel tumours. Eur Radiol. 2013;23(7):1901–10.
35. Ching H, McAlindon M, Sidhu R. An update on small bowel endoscopy. Curr Opin Gastroenterol. 2017;33(3):181–8.
36. Hosoe N, Takabayashi K, Ogata H, Kanai T. Capsule endoscopy for small-intestinal disorders: current status. Digest Endosc. 2019;31(5):498–507.
37. Chetcuti Zammit S, Sidhu R. Small bowel bleeding: cause and the role of endoscopy and medical therapy. Curr Opin Gastroenterol. 2018;34(3):165–74.
38. Robles E, Delgado P, Conesa P, Andrés B, Guggiana M, Mateos E, et al. Role of double-balloon enteroscopy in malignant small bowel tumors. World J Gastrointest Endosc. 2015;7(6):652–8.
39. McGeehan G, Edelduok I, Bucholc M, Watson A, Bodnar Z, Johnston A, et al. Systematic review and meta-analysis of wound bundles in emergency midline laparotomy identifies that it is time for improvement. Life. 2021;11(2):138.
40. Singh H, Krishnamurthy G, Kumar H, Mandavdhare H, Sharma V, Yadav T. Surgical management of jejunal tumors: experience from tertiary care centre. J Gastrointest Cancer. 2020;51(3):901–7.
41. Figueiredo M, Maggiori L, Gaujoux S, Couvelard A, Guedj N, Ruszniewski P, et al. Surgery for small-bowel neuroendocrine tumors: is there any benefit of the laparoscopic approach? Surg Endosc. 2014;28(5):1720–6.
42. Pisano M, Ceresoli M, Cimbanassi S, Gurusamy K, Coccolini F, Borzellino G, et al. 2017 WSES and SICG guidelines on acute calculous cholecystitis in elderly population. World J Emerg Surg. 2019;14:10.
43. Tan K, Bang S, Ho C. Surgery for perforated small bowel malignancy: a single institution's experience over 4 years. Surgeon. 2012;10(1):6–8.
44. Banting S, Waters P, Peacock O, Narasimhan V, Lynch A, McCormick J, et al. Management of primary and metastatic malignant small bowel obstruction, operate or palliate. A systematic review. ANZ J Surg. 2021;91(3):282–90.
45. Gaku C, Haruhiko C, Shinsuke S, Tsuyoshi T, Kazuhito N, Tsunehiko M, et al. Risk factors for gastrointestinal stromal tumors (GISTs) with suspicious/obvious tumor spillage. In: 2016 ASCO Annual Meeting I; 2016: American Society of Clinical Oncology; 2016.
46. Bennett S, Coburn N, Law C, Mahar A, Zhao H, Singh S, et al. Upfront small bowel resection for small bowel neuroendocrine tumors with synchronous metastases: a propensity-score matched comparative population-based analysis. Ann Surg. 2020;276(5):e450–8.

47. Lawler J, Choynowski M, Bailey K, Bucholc M, Johnston A, Sugrue M. Meta-analysis of the impact of postoperative infective complications on oncological outcomes in colorectal cancer surgery. BJS Open. 2020;4(5):737–47.
48. Sahebally SM, McKevitt K, Stephens I, Fitzpatrick F, Deasy J, Burke JP, et al. Negative pressure wound therapy for closed laparotomy incisions in general and colorectal surgery: a systematic review and meta-analysis. JAMA Surg. 2018;153(11):e183467.
49. Bevis PM, Windhaber RA, Lear PA, Poskitt KR, Earnshaw JJ, Mitchell DC. Randomized clinical trial of mesh versus sutured wound closure after open abdominal aortic aneurysm surgery. Br J Surg. 2010;97(10):1497–502.
50. van Ramshorst GH, Eker HH, Hop WC, Jeekel J, Lange JF. Impact of incisional hernia on health-related quality of life and body image: a prospective cohort study. Am J Surg. 2012;204(2):144–50.
51. Deerenberg EB, Harlaar JJ, Steyerberg EW, Lont HE, van Doorn HC, Heisterkamp J, et al. Small bites versus large bites for closure of abdominal midline incisions (STITCH): a double-blind, multicentre, randomised controlled trial. Lancet. 2015;386(10000):1254–60.
52. Bhangu A, Fitzgerald JE, Singh P, Battersby N, Marriott P, Pinkney T. Systematic review and meta-analysis of prophylactic mesh placement for prevention of incisional hernia following midline laparotomy. Hernia. 2013;17(4):445–55.
53. Meijer L, Alberga A, de Bakker J, van der Vliet H, Le Large T, van Grieken N, et al. Outcomes and treatment options for duodenal adenocarcinoma: a systematic review and meta-analysis. Ann Surg Oncol. 2018;25(9):2681–92.
54. Akce M, Jiang R, Zakka K, Wu C, Alese O, Shaib W, et al. Clinical outcomes of small bowel adenocarcinoma. Clin Colorectal Cancer. 2019;18(4):257–68.
55. Benson A, Venook A, Al-Hawary M, Arain M, Chen Y, Ciombor K, et al. Small bowel adenocarcinoma, Version 1.2020, NCCN clinical practice guidelines in oncology. J Natl Compr Cancer Netw. 2019;17(9):1109–33.
56. Rorstad O. Prognostic indicators for carcinoid neuroendocrine tumors of the gastrointestinal tract. J Surg Oncol. 2005;89(3):151–60.
57. Strosberg J, El-Haddad G, Wolin E, Hendifar A, Yao J, Chasen B, et al. Phase 3 trial of 177 Lu-Dotatate for midgut neuroendocrine tumors. N Engl J Med. 2017;376(2):125–35.
58. Caplin M, Pavel M, Ćwikła J, Phan A, Raderer M, Sedláčková E, et al. Lanreotide in metastatic enteropancreatic neuroendocrine tumors. N Engl J Med. 2014;371(3):224–33.
59. Yao J, Fazio N, Singh S, Buzzoni R, Carnaghi C, Wolin E, et al. Everolimus for the treatment of advanced, non-functional neuroendocrine tumours of the lung or gastrointestinal tract (RADIANT-4): a randomised, placebo-controlled, phase 3 study. Lancet. 2016;387(10022):968–77.
60. Rinke A, Müller H, Schade-Brittinger C, Klose K, Barth P, Wied M, et al. Placebo-controlled, double-blind, prospective, randomized study on the effect of octreotide LAR in the control of tumor growth in patients with metastatic neuroendocrine midgut tumors: a report from the PROMID Study Group. J Clin Oncol. 2009;27(28):4656–63.
61. Boudreaux J, Klimstra D, Hassan M, Woltering E, Jensen R, Goldsmith S, et al. The NANETS consensus guideline for the diagnosis and management of neuroendocrine tumors: well-differentiated neuroendocrine tumors of the jejunum, ileum, appendix, and cecum. Pancreas. 2010;39(6):753–66.
62. Fletcher C, Berman J, Corless C, Gorstein F, Lasota J, Longley B, et al. Diagnosis of gastrointestinal stromal tumors: a consensus approach. Int J Surg Pathol. 2002;10(2):459.
63. Casali P, Abecassis N, Aro H, Bauer S, Biagini R, Bielack S, et al. Gastrointestinal stromal tumours: ESMO-EURACAN clinical practice guidelines for diagnosis, treatment and follow-up. Ann Oncol. 2018;29(Suppl 4):468–78.

Right Colon

8

Silvia Strambi, Dario Tartaglia, Camilla Cremonini,
Serena Musetti, Massimo Chiarugi, and Federico Coccolini

About one-third of colon rectal cancer (CRC) reveals itself with obstruction, perforation, or hemorrhage, without having a prior elective diagnosis. Emergency CRC surgery is still affected by high morbidity and mortality rates, especially in elderly patients (11–35% and 9–22%, respectively) [1].

Right-sided colon cancer more often represents a surgical emergency despite CRC screening programs, due to its nonspecific and gradual symptoms (e.g., asthenia, anorexia, dyspnea, nausea, or vomiting) and the tendency to affect older patients [2]; in addition, for anatomical reasons (greater diameter of the cecum and ascendant than the left colon), right obstructive tumors have often an advanced stage at onset compared to the left ones [3].

For all these reasons, patients presenting with colorectal cancer as a surgical emergency have a poorer prognosis than elective ones. The postoperative morbidity rate after emergency surgery for obstructive right colon cancer ranges from 46 to 54%, resulting in higher than elective right hemicolectomy (30%) and also increased mortality rate (14.5% vs. 2.6% of elective cases).

The surgical treatment has two main goals: palliation of symptoms and oncological radicality. The emergency surgeon has the difficult task of deciding how to balance these two aspects of treatment to provide the patient with the most appropriate standard of care for its specific condition. For this purpose, the surgeon must take into consideration the patient's age, his/her physiological reservoir, comorbidities, medication intake, nutritional status (e.g., albuminemia), degree of autonomy in daily life activities, and his/her disposition of treatment and wills (relatives and caregivers may be involved in the decision). Moreover, a precise cancer stadiation during the diagnostic process should be pursued in order to plan the treatment.

S. Strambi (✉) · D. Tartaglia · C. Cremonini · S. Musetti · M. Chiarugi · F. Coccolini
General, Emergency and Trauma Surgery Unit, Pisa University Hospital, Pisa, Italy
e-mail: silvia.strambi@phd.unipi.it; dario.tartaglia@unipi.it; camilla.cremonini@phd.unipi.it; serena.musetti@phd.unipi.it; massimo.chiarugi@unipi.it; federico.coccolini@unipi.it

A. Tarasconi et al. (eds.), *Oncologic Surgical Emergencies*, Hot Topics in Acute Care Surgery and Trauma, https://doi.org/10.1007/978-3-031-36860-8_8

All these conditions must be weighted with the severity of disease at presentation, hemodynamical status, specific surgical and anesthesiologic risk (assessed with ASA score), and experience of the surgeon/center. When a tailored decision has been found, it must be clearly communicated to the patient, relatives, or caregivers.

Literature shows that bowel obstruction is the most frequent cause of emergency presentation (8–60% of cases) followed by perforation (2–22% of cases) and bleeding [4].

8.1 Obstructive Right Colon Cancer (ORCC)

Mege et al. in a multicenter study on 2325 patients with obstructive colon cancer (ORCC) divided into right- and left-sided, showed that patients with ORCC were older, frailer, and more associated with worse prognosis although tumor resection and anastomosis are more frequently performed than in left-sided cases [5]. Moreover, the obstructive feature of colon cancer itself is reported to have an advanced cancer stage at presentation with poor prognostic factors and to be an independent high-risk feature of recurrence [6].

Onset of right bowel obstruction can be acute, with severe abdominal pain, abdominal distension, and constipation without passing of stool and gas, or subacute with gradual development of symptoms. If the site of obstruction is proximal, pain tends to be cramping and more associated to early vomiting, miming a small bowel obstruction. Dehydration and alteration of electrolyte balance often complicate the condition; also, respiratory dynamic can be compromised by abdominal compression on the diaphragm.

Abdominal examination often shows tenderness without abdominal guarding, tympanic and distended abdomen, and excessive or absent peristalsis.

Laboratory exams can demonstrate electrolyte imbalances and metabolic alkalosis due to dehydration and vomiting, often associated with normal/high level of hemoglobin and high hematocrit as a sign of deep dehydration; low hemoglobin, instead, suggests active or recent bleeding. Leukocytosis can be a result of associated ischemia or perforation.

Obstruction can be sometimes associated with bowel perforation, either at the site of cancer or in the preceding segments, also in relation with the continence status of the ileocecal valve; the fecal contamination further increases the postoperative morbidity and mortality rates [7].

Abdominal X-ray usually demonstrates large bowel obstruction, but it cannot discriminate between mechanical obstructions, requiring surgical treatment, from pseudo-obstructions. Abdominal contrast-enhanced CT scan allows to demonstrate the exact site of the obstructive mass and the presence of tumor-related findings. In the emergency setting, however, diagnosis is often reached only during surgical exploration and validated after surgery by histopathological examination.

For resectable ORCC, primary tumor resection should be preferred. The gold standard treatment for obstructive right-sided or transverse colon lesions is a right hemicolectomy or extended right hemicolectomy with ileocolic anastomosis. It is considered safe and feasible in most cases, even though patients with right-sided colon cancer are usually aged and with advanced locoregional diseases [8] (Fig. 8.1).

Generally, oncologic principles are respected in the resection of ORCC when considering the extent of the resection, the surgical margins, and the number of dissected lymph nodes [8], also due to favorable anatomical conditions of the right colon.

In selected cases, ORCC can be treated laparoscopically also in acute settings. The safety and feasibility of laparoscopy depend on hemodynamic stability, degree of abdominal distension, resectability of the carcinoma, and laparoscopic skills of the surgeon. The advantages of a minimally invasive approach (shorter hospital stay, faster recovery of peristalsis, less intraoperative blood loss, with adequate oncological resection) should encourage the use of laparoscopy also in emergency settings [9].

The reported rate of anastomotic leakage after emergency resection is higher compared to the rate of elective right hemicolectomy (12–16.4% vs. 2.8–4.1%, respectively). Interestingly, the risk of anastomotic leakage did not increase with age in reported series [10]; therefore, very advanced age should not in itself represent a contraindication to perform an ileocolic anastomosis.

Other major postoperative complications related to abdominal surgery could be represented by evisceration (due to abdominal wall dehiscence) or wound infection, as well as septic shock.

For high-risk patients, terminal ileostomy with colonic fistula can be created after resection [11]. If the tumor is unresectable, the creation of loop ileostomy or an internal surgical bypass can be a valid palliative option to alleviate obstructive symptoms, especially in frail elderly patients [12]. Internal bypass, when feasible, should be preferred between the option above to avoid the complications of high fecal output of ileostomies [2, 7]. Decompressive cecostomy, except for some percutaneous cases in extremely frail patients, is not anymore currently supported due to its inefficacy [7].

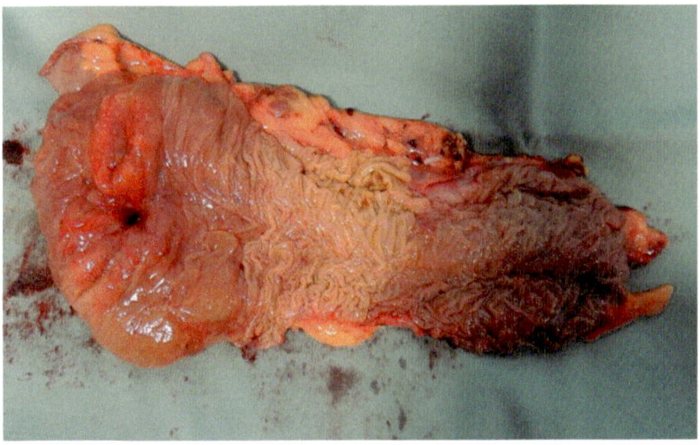

Fig. 8.1 Gross examination of right colon after right hemicolectomy for stenosing and ulcerated tumor of the cecum near the ileocecal valve

The principles of damage control surgery (DCS) may be applied in case of hemodynamic instability, with tumor resection followed by creation of open abdomen with NPWT and delayed anastomosis (after stabilization of vital parameters) [9].

The positioning of a self-expanding metallic stent (SEMS) can be an alternative to emergency surgery in high-risk patients, as it allows a prompt palliation of obstruction symptoms without the risk of postoperative complications [8]. However, since SEMS insertion is not feasible for obstructive cancer of the cecum or ileocolic valve, its use is limited in ORCC sited beyond the cecum, and it is technically challenging compared to its left-side positioning. Despite reported comparable long-term oncologic outcome after staged operation (than those of primary emergency surgery, possibly due to selection bias) [2], the insertion of SEMS as a temporary bridge to elective surgery is not recommended [8].

8.2 Perforated Right Colon Cancer

As previously stated, the site of perforation may be at the tumor itself or at the cecum, which becomes distended secondary to distal obstruction. The perforation may result in generalized fecal peritonitis leading to septic shock, even if for right-sided colon cancer, localized peritonitis with abscess formation is more common [13] (Fig. 8.2).

Right hemicolectomy with primary anastomosis, when feasible, is the procedure of choice irrespective of the degree of contamination. However, it must be kept in mind that the anastomotic leak reaches the highest rates (about 4.5%) in perforated emergency cases compared to ORCC and to 0.5–1.4% reported for elective surgery [8].

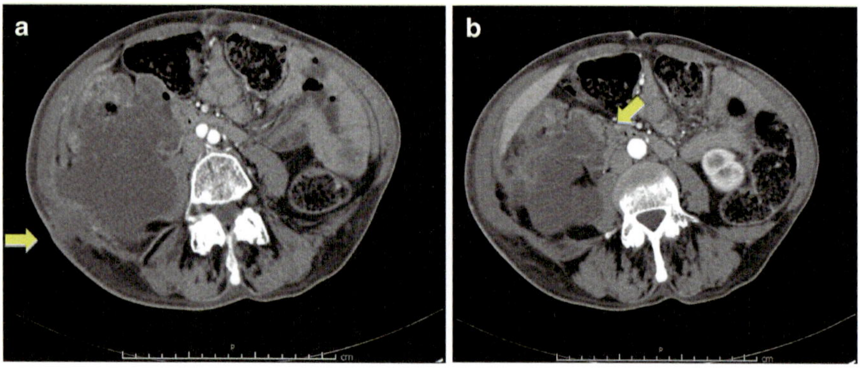

Fig. 8.2 Rough formation of about 12 cm (partially colliquated) that incorporates the right colon showing circumferential and stenosing wall thickening, the right iliopsoas muscle, the right ureter that has fistulized to the skin (**a**), and the duodenum (**b**)

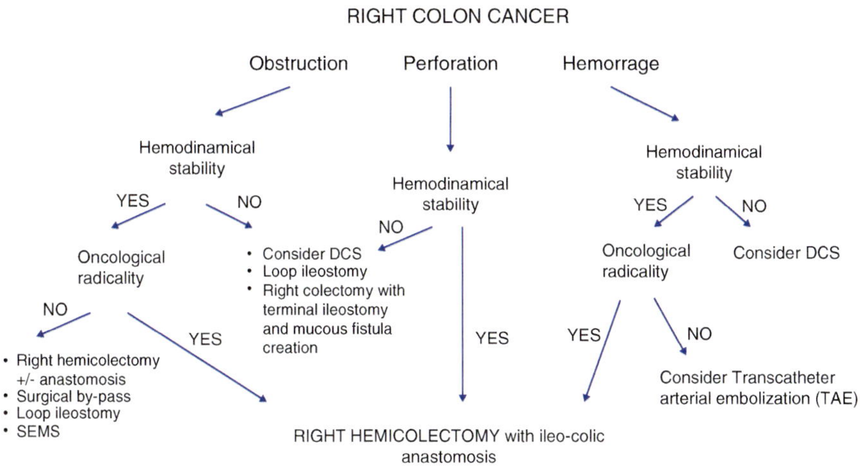

Fig. 8.3 Flowchart for the management of oncological right-sided colon emergencies

In case of hemodynamic instability, DCS with source control, bowel resection, open abdomen with NPWT, and scheduled second look (after 24/48 h, depending on the patient's stabilization) with delayed anastomosis or loop ileostomy or terminal ileostomy and mucous fistula creation may be considered [8] (Fig. 8.3).

8.3 Hemorrhagic Right Colon Cancer

Hematochezia and colonic hemorrhage are rare emergency presentation for RCC, less frequent than obstruction and perforation, that can be caused by ulcerative neoplastic lesions. In extremely rare cases, bleeding can be a consequence of the tumor's involvement of adjacent organs; Iwata et al. [14] reported a rare case of hemorrhagic shock due to a large mass in the ascending colon invading duodenum and pancreatic head and causing gastroduodenal artery bleeding into the colon, treated with en bloc pylorus-preserving pancreaticoduodenectomy and right colectomy.

In addition to fluids and blood resuscitation, emergency treatment may require investigation with angiography to detect the exact source of bleeding, followed by transcatheter arterial embolization (TAE) and/or surgical resection [8]; DCS strategy should be of choice if hemodynamic instability persists.

References

1. Costa G, Frezza B, Fransvea P, Massa G, Ferri M, Mercantini P, Balducci G, Buondonno A, Rocca A, Ceccarelli G. Clinico-pathological features of colon cancer patients undergoing emergency surgery: a comparison between elderly and non-elderly patients. Open Med (Wars). 2019;14:726–34. https://doi.org/10.1515/med-2019-0082.

2. Yoo RN, Cho HM, Kye BH. Management of obstructive colon cancer: current status, obstacles, and future directions. World J Gastrointest Oncol. 2021;13(12):1850–62. https://doi.org/10.4251/wjgo.v13.i12.1850.
3. Decker KM, Lambert P, Nugent Z, Biswanger N, Samadder J, Singh H. Time trends in the diagnosis of colorectal cancer with obstruction, perforation, and emergency admission after the introduction of population-based organized screening. JAMA Netw Open. 2020;3(5):e205741. https://doi.org/10.1001/jamanetworkopen.2020.5741.
4. Teixeira F, Akaishi EH, Ushinohama AZ, Dutra TC, Netto SD, Utiyama EM, Bernini CO, Rasslan S. Can we respect the principles of oncologic resection in an emergency surgery to treat colon cancer? World J Emerg Surg. 2015;10:5. https://doi.org/10.1186/1749-7922-10-5.
5. Mege D, Manceau G, Beyer L, Bridoux V, Lakkis Z, Venara A, Voron T, de'Angelis N, Abdalla S, Sielezneff I, Karoui M, AFC (French Surgical Association) Working Group. Right-sided vs. left-sided obstructing colonic cancer: results of a multicenter study of the French Surgical Association in 2325 patients and literature review. Int J Color Dis. 2019;34(6):1021–32. https://doi.org/10.1007/s00384-019-03286-2.
6. Cortet M, Grimault A, Cheynel N, Lepage C, Bouvier AM, Faivre J. Patterns of recurrence of obstructing colon cancers after surgery for cure: a population-based study. Color Dis. 2013;15(9):1100–6. https://doi.org/10.1111/codi.12268.
7. Otani K, Kawai K, Hata K, Tanaka T, Nishikawa T, Sasaki K, Kaneko M, Murono K, Emoto S, Nozawa H. Colon cancer with perforation. Surg Today. 2019;49(1):15–20. https://doi.org/10.1007/s00595-018-1661-8.
8. Pisano M, Zorcolo L, Merli C, Cimbanassi S, Poiasina E, Ceresoli M, Agresta F, Allievi N, Bellanova G, Coccolini F, Coy C, Fugazzola P, Martinez CA, Montori G, Paolillo C, Penachim TJ, Pereira B, Reis T, Restivo A, Rezende-Neto J, Sartelli M, Valentino M, Abu-Zidan FM, Ashkenazi I, Bala M, Chiara O, De' Angelis N, Deidda S, De Simone B, Di Saverio S, Finotti E, Kenji I, Moore E, Wexner S, Biffl W, Coimbra R, Guttadauro A, Leppäniemi A, Maier R, Magnone S, Mefire AC, Peitzmann A, Sakakushev B, Sugrue M, Viale P, Weber D, Kashuk J, Fraga GP, Kluger I, Catena F, Ansaloni L. 2017 WSES guidelines on colon and rectal cancer emergencies: obstruction and perforation. World J Emerg Surg. 2018;13:36. https://doi.org/10.1186/s13017-018-0192-3.
9. Cirocchi R, Cesare Campanile F, Di Saverio S, Popivanov G, Carlini L, Pironi D, Tabola R, Vettoretto N. Laparoscopic versus open colectomy for obstructing right colon cancer: a systematic review and meta-analysis. J Visc Surg. 2017;154(6):387–99. https://doi.org/10.1016/j.jviscsurg.2017.09.002.
10. Manceau G, Mege D, Bridoux V, Lakkis Z, Venara A, Voron T, Sielezneff I, Karoui M, French Surgical Association Working Group. Emergency surgery for obstructive colon cancer in elderly patients: results of a multicentric cohort of the French National Surgical Association. Dis Colon Rectum. 2019;62(8):941–51. https://doi.org/10.1097/DCR.0000000000001421.
11. Mege D, Manceau G, Beyer-Berjot L, Bridoux V, Lakkis Z, Venara A, Voron T, Brunetti F, Sielezneff I, Karoui M, AFC (French Surgical Association) Working Group. Surgical management of obstructive right-sided colon cancer at a national level results of a multicenter study of the French Surgical Association in 776 patients. Eur J Surg Oncol. 2018;44(10):1522–31. https://doi.org/10.1016/j.ejso.2018.06.027.
12. De Simone B, Coccolini F, Ansaloni L, Tarasconi A, Baiocchi G, Vettoretto N, Joly P, Ferron M, Pozzo A, Charre L, Di Saverio S, Napoli JA, Agresta F, Sartelli M, Catena F. Complicated colorectal cancer in nonagenarian patients: is it better not to perform anastomosis in emergency? Ulus Travma Acil Cerrahi Derg. 2017;23(1):15–22. https://doi.org/10.5505/tjtes.2016.77178.
13. Cuffy M, Abir F, Audisio RA, Longo WE. Colorectal cancer presenting as surgical emergencies. Surg Oncol. 2004;13(2–3):149–57. https://doi.org/10.1016/j.suronc.2004.08.00.
14. Iwata T, Konishi K, Yamazaki T, Kitamura K, Katagiri A, Muramoto T, Kubota Y, Yano Y, Kobayashi Y, Yamochi T, Ohike N, Murakami M, Gokan T, Yoshikawa N, Imawari M. Right colon cancer presenting as hemorrhagic shock. World J Gastrointest Pathophysiol. 2011;2(1):15–8. https://doi.org/10.4291/wjgp.v2.i1.15.

Appendiceal Tumors

9

Gaetano Gallo, Marta Goglia, Arcangelo Picciariello, Maria Chiara Ranucci, Elena Lamirata, Maria Paula Forero Rios, Franco Roviello, and Salomone Di Saverio

9.1 Introduction

Appendiceal adenocarcinoma was first described by Berger in 1882 [1], whereas a tumor arising from neuroendocrine cells [neuroendocrine tumors (NETs)] was reported by Masson in 1928 [2]. Primary appendiceal tumors (ATs) are rare entities, occurring in <2% of all appendectomies, with an age-adjusted incidence of 0.12 cases per million people per year, even if in large databases the incidence may reach

G. Gallo · F. Roviello
Unit of General Surgery and Surgical Oncology, Department of Medicine, Surgery and Neurosciences, University of Siena, Siena, Italy
e-mail: franco.roviello@unisi.it

M. Goglia
Department of General Surgery, University Hospital Sant'Andrea, La Sapienza University of Rome, Rome, Italy
e-mail: marta.goglia@uniroma1.it

A. Picciariello
Department of Emergency and Organ Transplantation, University "Aldo Moro" of Bari, Bari, Italy

M. C. Ranucci
Department of Digestive and Emergency Surgery, Hospital Saint Mary of Terni, Nutrition Science Degree, University of Perugia, Terni, Italy

E. Lamirata
University of Catania, Catania, Italy

M. P. F. Rios
Department of Medicine, Universidad el Bosque, Bogota, Colombia

S. Di Saverio (✉)
Department of General Surgery, ASUR Marche, AV5, Hospital of San Benedetto del Tronto, San Benedetto del Tronto, Italy
e-mail: salo75@inwind.it

A. Tarasconi et al. (eds.), *Oncologic Surgical Emergencies*, Hot Topics in Acute Care Surgery and Trauma, https://doi.org/10.1007/978-3-031-36860-8_9

0.97 per year [3, 4]. Thanks to the current detection methods, including both imaging and colonoscopy, there was an increased incidence and decreased age at diagnosis of AT [5].

Nevertheless, the vast majority of these tumors are not diagnosed preoperatively and are often detected as incidental findings with a still high mortality rate [6]. Interestingly, most of the tumors are located at the tip of the appendix with a maximal diameter of <1 cm [7, 8].

AT survival varies by stage at diagnosis, with an overall 5-year survival rate of 83% for all stages [6–8].

Perforated epithelial ATs are uncommon, with a reported incidence of 0.3% in appendectomy [9].

In this context, appendiceal adenocarcinoma is the most frequently perforating carcinoma of the entire gastrointestinal tract, occurring most frequently in middle-aged or older adults, with a median age at presentation of 40–50 years, while NETs or carcinoid tumors occur in younger patients in the second decade [10]. The latter are the most common primary malignant tumors arising from the appendix representing 32–85% of all ATs [11].

9.2 Clinical Presentation and Differential Diagnosis

Preoperative diagnosis of AT is challenging, due to the nonspecificity of both radiological and clinical findings [12]. Symptoms may range from vague nonspecific abdominal symptoms to gross abdominal distension and nutritional compromise [13], fever and hydronephrosis [14], and vaginal bleeding [15].

The most common presentation is acute appendicitis (AA) (54%) [16–18] and is very frequent in adenocarcinomas or goblet cell adenocarcinomas (GCCs). Advanced or metastasized tumors may present with abdominal pain or compression [19]. Appendiceal torsion is a rare manifestation and presents with symptoms similar to those of AA [20].

NETs are most commonly related to the presence of liver metastases with a carcinoid syndrome, or rather diarrhea, palpitations, high blood pressure, skin lesions, and shortness of breath, in less than 5% of AT [21, 22].

Sometimes, AT symptoms may simulate several disorders such as primary bladder cancer [23], Crohn's disease [24], or cecal intussusception [25].

Interestingly, differential diagnosis varies according to both age and sex of the patient. During childhood, intussusception, acute gastroenteritis, and Meckel's diverticulitis present with an overlapping clinical scenario.

In young adolescent male patients, differential diagnosis includes inflammatory bowel disease, sickle cell anemia, and epididymitis, while in young women, pelvic inflammatory disease, ovarian cyst or torsion, ectopic pregnancy, ovarian cancer, and urinary tract infection should always be considered. Tumors of the gastrointestinal tract and reproductive organs, diverticulitis, perforated ulcer, and cholecystitis should also always be suspected in adults and older people.

9.3 Classification and Staging

The classification of AT has always been confusing due to the rarity and the multiple nomenclatures used to describe this kind of pathology. A recent review of the literature prefers to classify AT in four broad groups: colonic-type adenocarcinomas, mucinous neoplasms, GCCs, and NETs [26]. However, we propose a whole AT classification based on the histological features, as suggested by the American Society of Colon and Rectal Surgeons (ASCRS) and the World Health Organization (WHO) guidelines on AT [27, 28].

It is mandatory to underline that embryological and histological composition of the appendix directly correlates with the development of different types of tumors (Fig. 9.1a, b). Indeed, the appendiceal epithelium is composed of enterocytes, goblet cells, and enterochromaffin cells, which may hesitate in epithelial tumors, GCCs, and NETs, respectively. On the other side, lymphomas may arise from the lymphoid tissue of the mucosal and submucosal layers, similarly to the Peyer's patches in the small intestine.

The most common ATs are of epithelial and mesenchymal origin. NETs are often discovered incidentally. On the contrary, lymphoid tumors are rare and account for 5% of all malignant lymphomas [28].

Epithelial tumors may be divided into adenomas, a benign AT representation; mucinous neoplasms, usually of low grade producing mucin that accumulates in the peritoneal cavity; non-mucinous or colonic type which is similar to their colorectal counterparts both morphologically and genetically; adenocarcinomas; and GCCs. The latter are predominantly composed of mucin-secreting cells, and in a minor percentage of neuroendocrine cells, they show a more aggressive behavior with respect to NETs.

The **nonepithelial tumors** are represented by NETs and other rarely encountered tumors such as lymphomas, mesenchymal tumors, non-carcinoid NETs, sarcomas, and neuroectodermal and nerve sheath tumors [29] (Table 9.1).

The histologic type of the tumor predicts the biological behavior and the propensity for specific patterns of disease spread and imaging features.

Indeed, epithelial neoplasms can be broadly classified into mucinous and non-mucinous based on mucin production. The mucinous group is then divided into different subgroups on the basis of their aggressiveness.

Low-grade appendiceal mucinous neoplasms (LAMNs) are characterized by well-differentiated adenomas that usually lack infiltrative invasion ability, which is instead a characteristic of mucinous adenocarcinoma. Mucinous tumor of uncertain malignant potential, mucocele, mucinous cystadenoma, and mucinous cystadenocarcinoma are terms no longer in use, but now comprehended in the LAMNs group of classification.

High-grade appendiceal mucinous neoplasms (HAMNs) are characterized by a more aggressive cytologic atypia but lack infiltrative invasion within the appendix, like LAMNs. Although extremely rare, when found, they can be associated with invasive adenocarcinoma. The eighth edition of the American Joint Committee on Cancer (AJCC) classifies HAMNs as moderately differentiated (G2) [30].

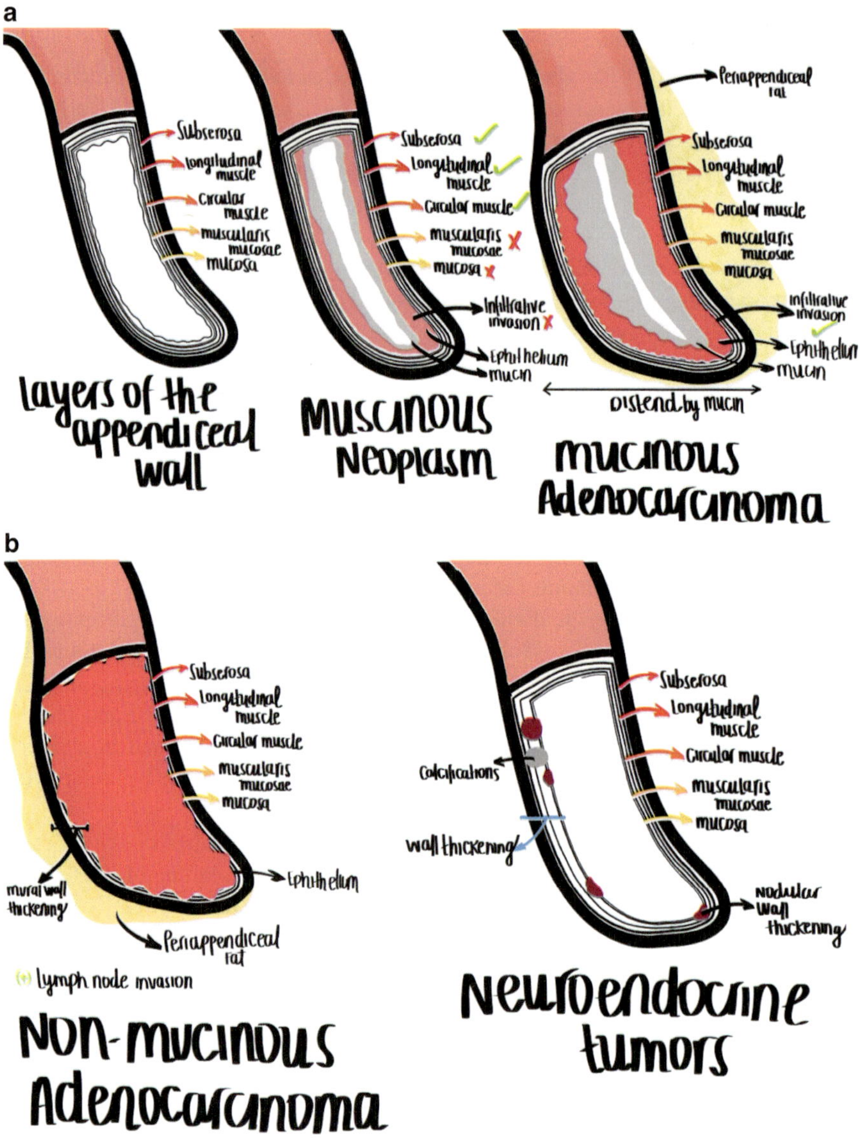

Fig. 9.1 Layers of the appendiceal wall in physiological situations and in appendiceal neoplasm. (**a**) Mucinous neoplasm and mucinous adenocarcinoma. (**b**) Non-mucinous adenocarcinoma and neuroendocrine tumors (NETs). (Illustration by Maria Paula Forero Rios)

Epithelial adenocarcinomas are the most common malignant neoplasms of the appendix considering both the mucinous and the non-mucinous histologic type (occurring in 37% and 27% of cases). GCCs are seen in 19% of all appendiceal neoplasms, while 11% of appendix malignant tumors are represented by NETs [29].

Table 9.1 Type of appendiceal tumors

Epithelial tumors	• Adenomas • Mucinous – Polyps – LAMN – HAMN – Adenocarcinomas – Adenocarcinomas with signet cells – Mucinous signet cells • Non-mucinous • Adenocarcinomas • GCCs • PMP
Nonepithelial tumors	• NETs • Mesenchymal tumors – GISTs – Desmoid – Leiomyomas – Leiomyosarcomas • Non-carcinoid NETs – Ganglioneuromas – Paragangliomas – Pheochromocytomas • Sarcomas – Desmoplastic small round cell tumor – HIV-Kaposi sarcoma • Neuroectodermal tumors – Schwannoma – Neurofibroma

Appendiceal adenocarcinomas in their mucinous subtype are characterized by invasive glands containing high-grade cytologic atypia and extracellular mucin in >50% of the lesion. They express p53, CD44, and CDX2 as their colorectal counterparts [27].

Mucinous adenocarcinomas often demonstrate signet ring cells if poorly differentiated. If the signet cells are more than 50%, then the tumor is considered mucinous signet cell adenocarcinomas, which is prone to lymphatic spread, and staged according to the TNM classification.

GCCs, also called adenoneuroendocrine carcinoma, can be considered as adenocarcinomas that show some features in common with NETs; for example, they show positive chromogranin A staining. However, their behavior is more aggressive than traditional NETs, and it is recommended to treat them as appendiceal adenocarcinomas. The term carcinoid tumor is no longer used.

Pseudomyxoma peritonei (PMP) is the term used to define a condition in which diffuse mucin deposits can be found throughout the abdomen. The most probable cause may be represented by appendiceal neoplasm perforation throughout the peritoneal cavity. It is a malignant condition, and the 10-year overall survival is estimated to be 63% after surgery [27].

PMP is classified on the basis of the degree of cellularity within the mucin in four categories: acellular, low-grade histologic features, high-grade histologic features, and PMP with signet ring cells [31].

Nonepithelial appendiceal neoplasms include **NETs**. The characteristics of this neoplasm are the same of other NETs that can be found elsewhere in the gastrointestinal tract. Appendiceal NETs follow a separate TNM staging with respect to the other appendiceal neoplasms.

Other **rare nonepithelial appendiceal neoplasms** include gastrointestinal stromal tumors (GISTs), lymphomas, and neural proliferations.

9.4 Grading

Mucinous tumors, LAMNs, HAMNs, and mucinous adenocarcinomas are graded according to a three-tiered grading system.

G1 or well-differentiated tumors are LAMNs, with low-grade cytologic atypia and no signet ring cells. Acellular mucinous tumors are with low cellularity and lack infiltration of peritoneum or other organs. G2 or moderately differentiated tumors include mucinous adenocarcinomas, low- and high-grade cytologic atypia, and no signet ring cells, and G3 or poorly differentiated tumors are non-mucinous adenocarcinomas, with high-grade cytologic atypia and signet ring cells [32].

LAMNs can be easily identified because of a broad tumor front invasion, hyalinization, and fibrosis of the underlying tissue. Since HAMNs are often focally invasive, a complete examination of the appendix specimen is strongly recommended.

Mucinous adenocarcinomas show drops of mucin with detached strips, glands, and clusters of atypical neoplastic cells inside.

GCCs are poorly differentiated with focal areas, similarly to signet ring cell adenocarcinomas.

Regarding appendiceal NETs, grading is not formally part of the staging system. However, the European Neuroendocrine Tumor Society (ENETS)/WHO grading criteria proposed another classification based on the mitotic rate [28, 33] (Table 9.2).

Table 9.2 ENETS/WHO grading system

Grade 1	Mitotic rate <2 per 10 high-power fields and Ki67 <3%
Grade 2	Mitotic rate 2–20 per 10 high-power fields or Ki67 3–20%
Grade 3	Mitotic rate >20 per 10 high-power fields or Ki67 >20%

9.5 Staging (WHO Classification of Digestive Tumor—Fifth Edition)

The TNM classification applies to adenocarcinomas of the appendix and GCCs, while NETs are classified separately. Mucinous and non-mucinous adenocarcinomas deserve different classifications.

Regarding the mucinous AT, they follow the Union for International Cancer Control (UICC) staging system (Tables 9.3 and 9.4).

Tumor is staged as a metastatic disease, when mucin and epithelial cells are found in the peritoneal surface. We can distinguish pM1a if the mucin is acellular and pM1b if mucin contains mucinous epithelial cells.

Concerning nodal metastasis, the regional lymph nodes (LNs) considered are the ileocolic ones. N1c stays for tumor deposits in the absence of nodal metastasis. Metastasis is staged as M1a for intraperitoneal acellular mucin, M1b intraperitoneal metastasis, and M1c non-peritoneal metastasis.

pT and pN are basically the same of TNM. When the LNs are negative but less than 12 (the minimum number necessary to examine lymph node metastasis), the tumor is classified as pN0 (Table 9.3).

Table 9.3 Union for International Cancer Control (UICC) staging system for mucinous appendiceal tumors

Tx	Primary tumor cannot be assessed
T0	No evidence of primary tumor
Tis	Carcinoma in situ: intraepithelial invasion of lamina propria
Tis (LAMN)	LAMN confined to the appendix
T1	Invasion of the submucosa
T2	Invasion of the muscularis propria
T3	Invasion of subserosa or mesoappendix
T4	T4a invades visceral peritoneum including mucinous peritoneal tumor or acellular mucin on the serosa of the appendix or mesoappendix T4b directly invades other organs or structures
Nx	Cannot be assessed
N0	No LN METs
N1	METs in 1–3 regional LNs N1a METs in 1 regional LN N1b METs in 2–3 regional LNs N1c tumor deposits (microscopic or macroscopic nodules)
N2	METs in 4 or more regional LNs
M0	No distant METs
M1	Distant METs M1a intraperitoneal acellular mucin only M1b intraperitoneal METs only, including mucinous epithelium M1c non-peritoneal METs

METs metastasis, *LNs* lymph nodes

Table 9.4 Mucinous appendiceal tumor staging

Stage 0	Tis	N0	M0	
Stage 0	Tis (LAMN)	N0	M0	
Stage I	T1, T2	N0	M0	
Stage IIA	T3	N0	M0	
Stage IIB	T4a	N0	M0	
Stage IIC	T4b	N0	M0	
Stage IIIA	T1, T2	N1	M0	
Stage IIIB	T3, T4	N1	M0	
Stage IIIC	Any T	N2	M1a	Any G
Stage IVA	Any T	Any N	M1b	G1
Stage IVB	Any T	Any N	M1b	G2, G3, GX
Stage IVC	Any T	Any N	M1c	Any G

Table 9.5 NET TNM

Tx	Primary tumor cannot be assessed
T0	No evidence of primary tumor
T1	Tumor 2 cm or less
T2	Tumor >2 cm but <4 cm
T3	Tumor >4 cm/with subserosal invasion/involvement of mesoappendix
T4	Peritoneum or other adjacent structures other than direct mural extension to adjacent subserosa
N0	No LN METs
N1	Regional LN METs
M0	No distant METs
M1	Distant METs M1a hepatic METs only M1b extrahepatic METs only M1c hepatic and extrahepatic METs

METs metastasis, *LNs* lymph nodes

Table 9.6 NET TNM staging

Stage I	T1	N0	M0
Stage II	T2, T3	N0	M0
Stage III	T4	N0	M0
	Any T	N1	M0
Stage IV	Any T	Any N	M1

9.6 NETs

Staging of appendiceal NETs is mainly based on tumor size and infiltration of serosa/mesoappendix. The great majority of NETs invade the subserosa or mesoappendix and are therefore classified as pT3.

pT and pN correspond to TNM categories. pN0 occurs if the LNs retrieved are less than 12 but all negative.

pM1 includes distant METs microscopically confirmed (Tables 9.5 and 9.6).

9.7 Anatomy and Imaging Features of Each Subtype

Preoperative imaging has a pivotal role both in the diagnosis and in the eventual surgery planning process. However, since the most frequent initial manifestation of these tumors is an AA, the diagnosis is often confirmed intraoperatively with a frozen section of the appendiceal specimen or later with the histopathology [4, 34, 35].

Nevertheless, morphology and type of AT can also be detected by specific radiologic examinations such as computed tomography (CT) scan when an appendiceal mass is suspected preoperatively.

Indeed, CT scan has been demonstrated as more sensitive than ultrasonography (US) and radiography in the evaluation of the anatomical relations of the tumor and other structures. Moreover, CT scan is considered more accurate than MRI in detecting calcifications inside the mass, especially in case of LAMNs [35]. However, cross-sectional imaging involving CT, US, and magnetic resonance imaging (MRI) is useful for the correct evaluation and definition of an AT [29].

9.8 Imaging Features of Epithelial Neoplasm

9.8.1 Colonic Type/Non-mucinous

These tumors are more often diagnosed after the appendectomy; therefore, little information has been reported in literature with regard to their radiologic features.

In the setting of a suspicion of acute appendicitis, on CT scan with contrast medium, they usually appear as enlarged in their size, with periappendiceal fat stranding and focal soft tissue with no evidence of LAMNs or heterogeneous masses infiltrating the entire appendix (Fig. 9.2) [29]. A dilation with diffuse mural thickening of the appendix can be associated with this type of tumor; indeed, direct invasion of the surrounding tissues and organs can be detected in some cases [29, 36].

9.8.2 Mucinous Type

Mucocele (now included in the category of LAMNs) represents the most common finding of mucinous neoplasm of the appendix that appears abnormally distended by mucin [4].

Through abdominal X-rays, mucoceles can be identified as a soft-tissue mass with peripheral calcifications usually located in the right lower quadrant of the abdomen [36]. Internal concentric echogenic layers with a typical "onionskin" appearance and curvilinear mural calcifications (in almost 50% of cases) are detected at US.

In case of evidence of mucocele on the X-ray examination, MRI usually shows characteristics of simple fluid with a variety of signal intensities depending on the protein content [37].

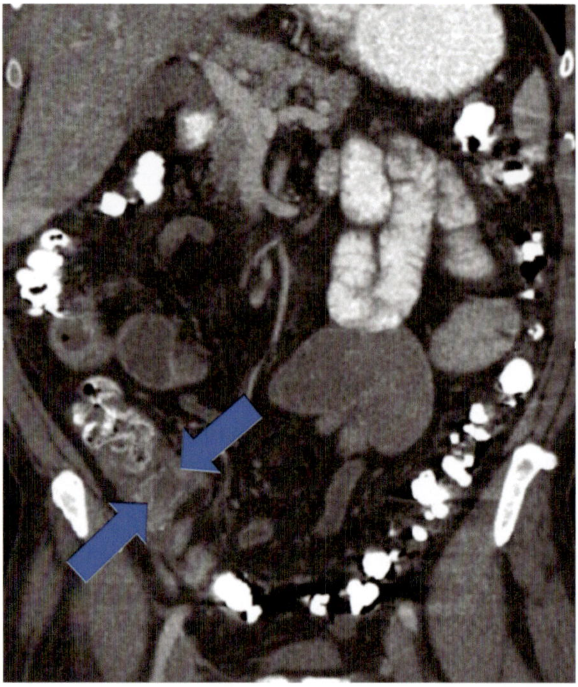

Fig. 9.2 CT scan of colonic-type neoplasm of the appendix. (Modified from Leonards et al. [29])

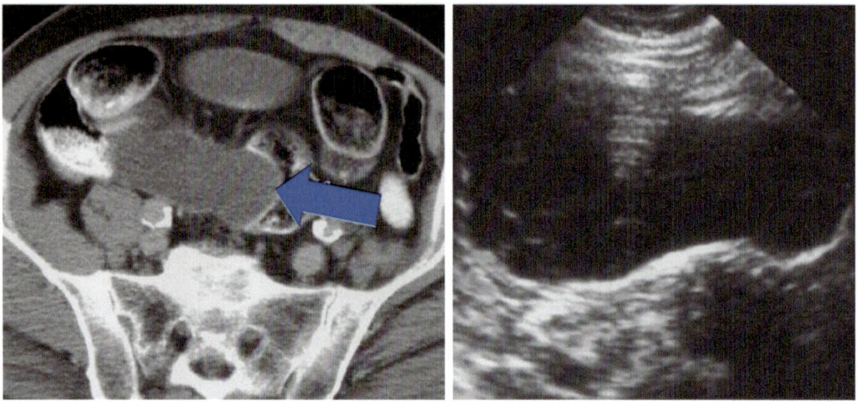

Fig. 9.3 CT scan and US of mucocele in a patient affected by mucinous-type appendiceal neoplasm. (Modified from Pickhardt et al. [36])

At CT scan, malignant mucoceles are identified due to the presence of some features such as the dilatation of the appendix with mural nodularity and an irregular wall thickening. Internal septa, wall calcifications, and straining of the periappendiceal fat are other common findings [36, 38, 39] (Fig. 9.3).

Once an appendiceal mucocele has been identified at CT, the presence of mucin within the peritoneum and pelvic organs should be carefully evaluated in order to exclude the development of a PMP [40].

9.8.3 Neuroendocrine Tumors

Although NETs may represent up to 80% of appendiceal neoplasms, their typical small size (1–2 cm) and the involvement of the distal appendix in the majority of cases (75%) make the instrumental diagnosis very rare and challenging [41].

At US, only in case of AA, appendix appears dilated and noncompressible with striated wall thickening. CT scan could identify a diffuse wall thickening of the appendix and poorly defined soft-tissue mass with a focus of calcification on the root of the mesentery [29, 42] (Fig. 9.4).

The formation of a mucocele represents a quite rare finding at imaging. ^{18}F-FDG PET and octreotide scintigraphy can be useful for the staging and follow-up after surgery or in case of NETs larger than 2 cm [43]. Moreover, CT scan and MRI should be performed to assess possible liver metastases.

9.8.4 Goblet Cell Adenocarcinoma

GCCs usually involve the entire appendix circumferentially and can be mucinous or non-mucinous [44].

A large enhancing mass with frequent aspects of infiltration of the surrounding structures and likely venous invasion with intraperitoneal spread is the most common finding at the CT scan [29, 36, 45] (Fig. 9.5). Small calcifications could be detected around the lesion.

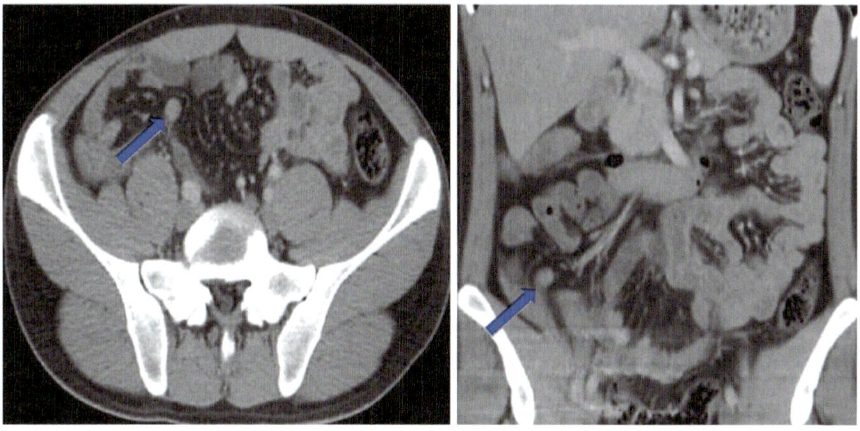

Fig. 9.4 CT scan features of a carcinoid tumor involving the appendix. (Modified from Bayhan et al. [42])

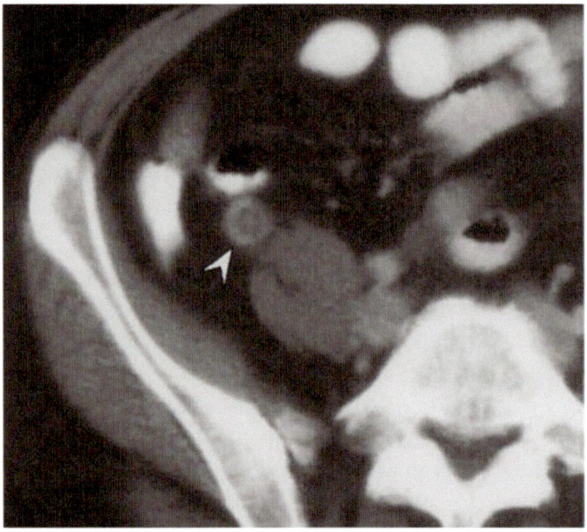

Fig. 9.5 CT scan showing a goblet cell tumor of the appendix. (From Pickhardt et al. [36])

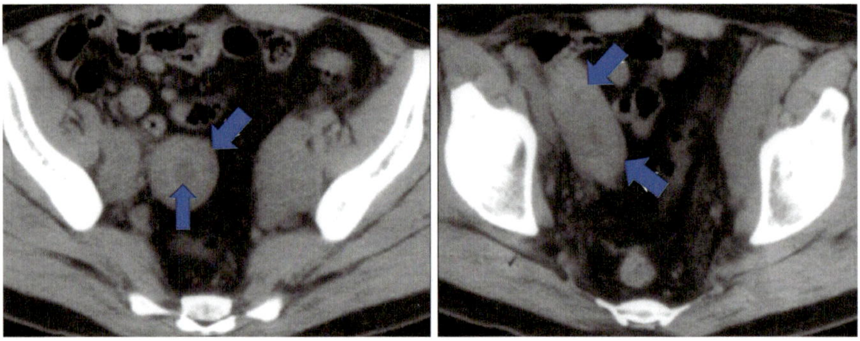

Fig. 9.6 Axial images from unenhanced CT scan showing an appendiceal non-Hodgkin's lymphoma. (Modified from Pickhardt et al. [36])

9.8.5 Lymphoma

Non-Hodgkin's lymphoma of the appendix represents an unusual entity that typically manifests with an AA in patients with no prior history of lymphoma [46].

At CT scan, lymphomatous infiltration of the appendix is shown by a diffuse mural soft-tissue thickening preserving the vermiform morphology (Fig. 9.6) [36]. Focal dilatation of the lumen, stranding of the periappendiceal fat, and abdominal lymphadenopathy could be rarely detected [47].

9.9 Treatment

There is currently no standardized treatment, and the choice of treatment depends on the tumor's subtype.

9.9.1 Adenocarcinomas

Data on the treatment of appendiceal adenocarcinomas are quite limited. Like in case of AT, colonic-type adenocarcinoma is most frequently found incidentally following appendectomy for appendicitis, and consequently, in these cases, T-stage information is immediately available and guides the treatment. Patients with **Tis** tumors resected with negative margins are treated with appendectomy alone. It is not always easy to differentiate between Tis and T1. For **T1** tumors, G1 or G2, no vascular or lymph node invasion, and negative section margins, appendectomy alone may be sufficient. Patients with unfavorable **T1** tumors (G3, vascular or lymph node invasion, and/or positive section margins) should undergo right colectomy for adequate staging and resection. For patients with **T2** or greater tumors, right colectomy is recommended. The rate of LN involvement in the colonic-type adenocarcinoma subtype was 30% in the largest population-based study of primary appendix cancer [48]. In patients with stage **T3** disease, adjuvant systemic chemotherapy is recommended, although specific studies for appendiceal adenocarcinomas are not available. As for colon adenocarcinoma, adjuvant chemotherapy should also be considered for stage II tumors with high-risk features. The rate of distant metastases at presentation is not well known but has been reported from 23 to 37%. Most often, there is peritoneal dissemination so that for these patients complete cytoreductive surgery (CRS) and hyperthermic intraperitoneal chemotherapy (HIPEC) should be considered if a complete resection can be eventually achieved. Surgical resection including metastasectomy of liver and lung lesions is reasonable for selected patients with appendix adenocarcinoma [26].

Considering the absence of high levels of evidence, experts recommended that adenocarcinomas of the appendix can be treated with systemic therapy according to the National Comprehensive Cancer Network (NCCN) guidelines for colon cancer [49].

9.9.2 Goblet Cell Adenocarcinomas

The prognosis of GCC lays intermediate between NETs and primary appendiceal adenocarcinoma, but the biological behavior of the disease is more aggressive than typical carcinoid tumor and often presents with metastatic disease. The 5-year overall survival rate based on AJCC staging system is 100% for stage I, but it becomes more severe for the other stages: 76% for stage II, 22% for stage III, and 14% for stage IV [30].

Usually, GCCs are found incidentally after appendectomy, and the need for further right colectomy is an important question that is still debated. Both the North American and European Neuroendocrine Tumor Societies recommend right hemicolectomy due to high risk of metastases and improvement in prognosis. However, in several published analyses, there is evidence to suggest limited or no benefit of right colectomy, primarily in patients with low-grade disease and limited disease burden [50, 51]. Therefore, it is reasonable to consider appendectomy alone in those patients with tumor evidence. Several studies evaluating the extent of surgical resection in GCCs have suggested that there is no benefit in performing right hemicolectomy in those patients with small (<1 cm), localized, low-grade tumors without high-risk features such as positive resection margins [52].

To summarize, right colectomy is recommended for tumors >2 cm, pT3 or T4, with higher grade histology with signet rings, or with positive surgical margins on appendectomy. Lastly, despite lack of level 1 evidence, it is also recommended that adjuvant chemotherapy with a regimen based on 5-fluorouracil (FU) is offered to patients with stage II and stage III GCCs. Historically, the most commonly used regimens are FOLFOX (5-FU, leucovorin, oxaliplatin) or FOLFIRI (5-FU, folic acid, irinotecan) [53].

9.9.3 Neuroendocrine Tumors

Also, in this case, the debate is open on the choice between appendectomy and right colectomy.

In general, the following statements apply to the specific situations:

- T1 (ENETS) or T1a (UICC/AJCC) NETS (i.e., <1 cm): Appendicectomy is usually curative, if it obtains R0 resection margin. The only exception could be the extremely rare situation when the tumor is located at the base of the appendix or when a mesoappendiceal invasion of more than 3 mm is discovered with the histopathological examination. In these cases, a completion of the resection with right colectomy is recommended [54, 55].
- T2 (ENETS) or T1b (UICC/AJCC) NET (i.e., >1 cm but <2 cm): Right colectomy should be considered and discussed with the patient if one or more of the following risk factors coexist because of the increased risk for LN involvement or distant metastasis (WHO grading G2, vascular or lymph vascular invasion, mesoappendiceal infiltration >3 mm).
- T3 (ENETS) or T2 (UICC/AJCC) or higher stage NET (i.e., >2 cm): Right colectomy is recommended [26, 33].

Appendiceal NETs <1 cm with R0 resection margin require no follow-up. For all other patients, long-term follow-up is advised [56].

9.9.4 Mucinous Tumors

Appendiceal mucinous neoplasms are a heterogeneous group of tumors with a rising incidence. Treatment is based on stage and histology.

Patients with Tis (LAMN) are usually treated with complete resection of the appendix without the risk for recurrent disease. Given the uncertainty regarding the risk of peritoneal dissemination of patients with T3 LAMN, a close and long-lasting follow-up over 10 years, even if not standardized, should be recommended. Obvious intraperitoneal contamination, histologically confirmed extraperitoneal mucin, appendiceal perforation, and peritoneal free cancer cells are considered significant risk factors for the development of PMP or peritoneal recurrence.

For patients with LAMN T4a with acellular mucin on the visceral peritoneal surface, a close follow-up is recommended similarly to patients with LAMN T3 [26]. Low-grade tumors in advanced disease require debulking and HIPEC to reduce the rate of peritoneal recurrence. However, the roles of additional surgery and HIPEC therapy are still uncertain.

Patients with HAMNs should have an appendectomy with negative margins and should have long-term follow-up. High-grade appendiceal mucinous carcinomas should be considered for systemic preoperative chemotherapy, and in case of benefit, surgical resection and HIPEC treatment should be considered [27].

Funding This research received no specific grant from any funding agency in the public, commercial, or not-for-profit sectors.

Conflicts of Interest The authors declare no conflict of interest.

Informed Consent Not required.

References

1. Berger A. Ein Fall von Krebs des Wurmfortsatzes. Ber Klin Wochenschr. 1882;19:610.
2. Masson P. Carcinoids (Argentaffin-cell tumors) and nerve hyperplasia of the appendicular mucosa. Am J Pathol. 1928;4(3):181–212.
3. Hanna M, Hwang G, Moghadamyeghaneh Z, et al. Incidental appendiceal cancer at appendectomy: an analysis of incidence, trends and risk factors. Dis Colon Rectum. 2015;58:E339.
4. Connor SJ, Hanna GB, Frizelle FA. Appendiceal tumors: retrospective clinicopathologic analysis of appendiceal tumors from 7970 appendectomies. Dis Colon Rectum. 1998;41(1):75–80. https://doi.org/10.1007/BF02236899.
5. Turaga KK, Pappas SG, Gamblin T. Importance of histologic subtype in the staging of appendiceal tumors. Ann Surg Oncol. 2012;19(5):1379–85. https://doi.org/10.1245/s10434-012-2238-1.
6. Marmor S, Portschy PR, Tuttle TM, Virnig BA. The rise in appendiceal cancer incidence: 2000–2009. J Gastrointest Surg. 2015;19(4):743–50. https://doi.org/10.1007/s11605-014-2726-7.

7. O'Donnell ME, Badger SA, Beattie GC, Carson J, Garstin WI. Malignant neoplasms of the appendix. Int J Color Dis. 2007;22(10):1239–48. https://doi.org/10.1007/s00384-007-0304-0.
8. Stinner B, Rothmund M. Neuroendocrine tumors (carcinoids) of the appendix. Best Pract Res Clin Gastroenterol. 2005;19:729–38.
9. Smeenk RM, van Velthuysen ML, Verwaal VJ, Zoetmulder FA. Appendiceal neoplasms and pseudomyxoma peritonei: a population based study. Eur J Surg Oncol. 2008;34(2):196–201. https://doi.org/10.1016/j.ejso.2007.04.002.
10. Cerame MA. A 25-year review of adenocarcinoma of the appendix. A frequently perforating carcinoma. Dis Colon Rectum. 1988;31(2):145–50. https://doi.org/10.1007/BF02562650.
11. Sandor A, Modlin IM. A retrospective analysis of 1570 appendiceal carcinoids. Am J Gastroenterol. 1998;93(3):422–8. https://doi.org/10.1111/j.1572-0241.1998.00422.x.
12. Cortina R, McCormick J, Kolm P, Perry RR. Management and prognosis of adenocarcinoma of the appendix. Dis Colon Rectum. 1995;38(8):848–52. https://doi.org/10.1007/BF02049842.
13. Murphy EM, Farquharson SM, Moran BJ. Management of an unexpected appendiceal neoplasm. Br J Surg. 2006;93(7):783–92. https://doi.org/10.1002/bjs.5385.
14. Smith JW, Kemeny N, Caldwell C, Banner P, Sigurdson E, Huvos A, Pseudomyxoma peritonei of appendiceal origin. The Memorial Sloan-Kettering Cancer Center experience. Cancer. 1992;70(2):396–401.
15. Didolkar MS, Fanous N. Adenocarcinoma of the appendix: a clinicopathologic study. Dis Colon Rectum. 1977;20(2):130–4. https://doi.org/10.1007/BF02587328.
16. Ussia A, Vaccari S, Gallo G, Grossi U, Ussia R, Sartarelli L, Minghetti M, Lauro A, Barbieri P, Di Saverio S, Cervellera M, Tonini V. Laparoscopic appendectomy as an index procedure for surgical trainees: clinical outcomes and learning curve. Updates Surg. 2021;73(1):187–95. https://doi.org/10.1007/s13304-020-00950-z.
17. Guaitoli E, Gallo G, Cardone E, Conti L, Famularo S, Formisano G, Galli F, Giuliani G, Martino A, Pasculli A, Patini R, Soriero D, Pappalardo V, Casoni Pattacini G, Sparavigna M, Meniconi R, Mazzari A, Barra F, Orsenigo E, Pertile D. Consensus Statement of the Italian Polispecialistic Society of Young Surgeons (SPIGC): diagnosis and treatment of acute appendicitis. J Investig Surg. 2021;34(10):1089–103. https://doi.org/10.1080/08941939.2020.1740360.
18. Di Saverio S, Podda M, De Simone B, Ceresoli M, Augustin G, Gori A, Boermeester M, Sartelli M, Coccolini F, Tarasconi A, De' Angelis N, Weber DG, Tolonen M, Birindelli A, Biffl W, Moore EE, Kelly M, Soreide K, Kashuk J, Ten Broek R, Gomes CA, Sugrue M, Davies RJ, Damaskos D, Leppäniemi A, Kirkpatrick A, Peitzman AB, Fraga GP, Maier RV, Coimbra R, Chiarugi M, Sganga G, Pisanu A, De' Angelis GL, Tan E, Van Goor H, Pata F, Di Carlo I, Chiara O, Litvin A, Campanile FC, Sakakushev B, Tomadze G, Demetrashvili Z, Latifi R, Abu-Zidan F, Romeo O, Segovia-Lohse H, Baiocchi G, Costa D, Rizoli S, Balogh ZJ, Bendinelli C, Scalea T, Ivatury R, Velmahos G, Andersson R, Kluger Y, Ansaloni L, Catena F. Diagnosis and treatment of acute appendicitis: 2020 update of the WSES Jerusalem guidelines. World J Emerg Surg. 2020;15(1):27. https://doi.org/10.1186/s13017-020-00306-3.
19. O'Donnell ME, Carson J, Garstin WI. Surgical treatment of malignant carcinoid tumors of the appendix. Int J Clin Pract. 2007;61:431–7.
20. Stark C, Jousi M, Enholm B. Preoperative assessment and treatment of appendiceal mucocele complicated by acute torsion: a case report. BMC Res Notes. 2014;7:1. https://doi.org/10.1186/1756-0500-7-1.
21. Moertel CG, Weiland LH, Nagorney DM, Dockerty MB. Carcinoid tumor of the appendix: treatment and prognosis. N Engl J Med. 1987;317(27):1699–701. https://doi.org/10.1056/NEJM198712313172704.
22. Feldman JM, Jones RS. Carcinoid syndrome from gastrointestinal carcinoids without liver metastasis. Ann Surg. 1982;196(1):33–7. https://doi.org/10.1097/00000658-198207000-00008.
23. Baskin LS, Stoller ML. Unusual appendiceal pathology presenting as urologic disease. Urology. 1991;38(5):432–6. https://doi.org/10.1016/0090-4295(91)80232-v.
24. Young RH, Gilks CB, Scully RE. Mucinous tumors of the appendix associated with mucinous tumors of the ovary and pseudomyxoma peritonei. A clinicopathological analysis of 22

cases supporting an origin in the appendix. Am J Surg Pathol. 1991;15(5):415–29. https://doi.org/10.1097/00000478-199105000-00001.
25. Gamble HA 2nd. Adenocarcinoma of the appendix: an unusual case and review. Dis Colon Rectum. 1976;19(7):621–5. https://doi.org/10.1007/BF02590980.
26. Van de Moortele M, De Hertogh G, Sagaert X, Van Cutsem E. Appendiceal cancer: a review of the literature. Acta Gastroenterol Belg. 2020;83(3):441–8.
27. Glasgow SC, Gaertner W, Stewart D, Davids J, Alavi K, Paquette IM, Steele SR, Feingold DL. The American Society of Colon and Rectal Surgeons, clinical practice guidelines for the management of appendiceal neoplasms. Dis Colon Rectum. 2019;62(12):1425–38. https://doi.org/10.1097/DCR.0000000000001530.
28. Nagtegaal ID, Odze RD, Klimstra D, Paradis V, Rugge M, Schirmacher P, Washington KM, Carneiro F, Cree IA, WHO Classification of Tumors Editorial Board. The 2019 WHO classification of tumors of the digestive system. Histopathology. 2020;76(2):182–8. https://doi.org/10.1111/his.13975.
29. Leonards LM, Pahwa A, Patel MK, Petersen J, Nguyen MJ, Jude CM. Neoplasms of the appendix: pictorial review with clinical and pathologic correlation. Radiographics. 2017;37(4):1059–83. https://doi.org/10.1148/rg.2017160150.
30. Amin MB, Greene FL, Edge SB, Compton CC, Gershenwald JE, Brookland RK, Meyer L, Gress DM, Byrd DR, Winchester DP. The eighth edition AJCC cancer staging manual: continuing to build a bridge from a population-based to a more "personalized" approach to cancer staging. CA Cancer J Clin. 2017;67(2):93–9. https://doi.org/10.3322/caac.21388.
31. Carr NJ, Cecil TD, Mohamed F, Sobin LH, Sugarbaker PH, González-Moreno S, Taflampas P, Chapman S, Moran BJ. Peritoneal surface oncology group international. A consensus for classification and pathologic reporting of pseudomyxoma peritonei and associated appendiceal neoplasia: the results of the peritoneal surface oncology group international (PSOGI) modified Delphi process. Am J Surg Pathol. 2016;40(1):14–26. https://doi.org/10.1097/PAS.0000000000000535.
32. https://documents.cap.org/protocols/cp-appendix-net-17protocol-4001.pdf.
33. Pape UF, Niederle B, Costa F, Gross D, Kelestimur F, Kianmanesh R, Knigge U, Öberg K, Pavel M, Perren A, Toumpanakis C, O'Connor J, Krenning E, Reed N, O'Toole D, Vienna Consensus Conference Participants. ENETS consensus guidelines for neuroendocrine neoplasms of the appendix (excluding goblet cell carcinomas). Neuroendocrinology. 2016;103(2):144–52. https://doi.org/10.1159/000443165.
34. Deshmukh S, Verde F, Johnson PT, Fishman EK, Macura KJ. Anatomical variants and pathologies of the vermix. Emerg Radiol. 2014;21(5):543–52. https://doi.org/10.1007/s10140-014-1206-4.
35. Pickhardt PJ, Levy AD, Rohrmann CA Jr, Kende AI. Primary neoplasms of the appendix manifesting as acute appendicitis: CT findings with pathologic comparison. Radiology. 2002;224(3):775–81. https://doi.org/10.1148/radiol.2243011545.
36. Pickhardt PJ, Levy AD, Rohrmann CA Jr, Kende AI. Primary neoplasms of the appendix: radiologic spectrum of disease with pathologic correlation. Radiographics. 2003;23(3):645–62. https://doi.org/10.1148/rg.233025134.
37. Low RN, Barone RM, Gurney JM, Muller WD. Mucinous appendiceal neoplasms: preoperative MR staging and classification compared with surgical and histopathologic findings. AJR Am J Roentgenol. 2008;190(3):656–65. https://doi.org/10.2214/AJR.07.2018.
38. Misdraji J. Mucinous epithelial neoplasms of the appendix and pseudomyxoma peritonei. Mod Pathol. 2015;28(Suppl 1):S67–79. https://doi.org/10.1038/modpathol.2014.129.
39. Misdraji J, Young RH. Primary epithelial neoplasms and other epithelial lesions of the appendix (excluding carcinoid tumors). Semin Diagn Pathol. 2004;21(2):120–33. https://doi.org/10.1053/j.semdp.2004.11.005.
40. Low RN, Barone RM, Lucero J. Comparison of MRI and CT for predicting the peritoneal cancer index (PCI) preoperatively in patients being considered for cytoreductive surgical procedures. Ann Surg Oncol. 2015;22(5):1708–15. https://doi.org/10.1245/s10434-014-4041-7.

41. Tchana-Sato V, Detry O, Polus M, Thiry A, Detroz B, Maweja S, Hamoir E, Defechereux T, Coimbra C, De Roover A, Meurisse M, Honoré P. Carcinoid tumor of the appendix: a consecutive series from 1237 appendectomies. World J Gastroenterol. 2006;12(41):6699–701. https://doi.org/10.3748/wjg.v12.i41.6699.
42. Bayhan Z, Yildiz YA, Akdeniz Y, Gonullu E, Altintoprak F, Mantoglu B, Capoglu R, Kahyaoglu AZ. Appendix neuroendocrine tumor: retrospective analysis of 4026 appendectomy patients in a single center. Emerg Med Int. 2020;2020:4030527. https://doi.org/10.1155/2020/4030527.
43. Squires MH 3rd, Volkan Adsay N, Schuster DM, Russell MC, Cardona K, Delman KA, Winer JH, Altinel D, Sarmiento JM, El-Rayes B, Hawk N, Staley CA 3rd, Maithel SK, Kooby DA. Octreoscan versus FDG-PET for neuroendocrine tumor staging: a biological approach. Ann Surg Oncol. 2015;22(7):2295–301. https://doi.org/10.1245/s10434-015-4471-x.
44. van Eeden S, Offerhaus GJ, Hart AA, Boerrigter L, Nederlof PM, Porter E, van Velthuysen ML. Goblet cell carcinoid of the appendix: a specific type of carcinoma. Histopathology. 2007;51(6):763–73. https://doi.org/10.1111/j.1365-2559.2007.02883.x.
45. Lee KS, Tang LH, Shia J, Paty PB, Weiser MR, Guillem JG, Temple LK, Nash GM, Reidy D, Saltz L, Gollub MJ. Goblet cell carcinoid neoplasm of the appendix: clinical and CT features. Eur J Radiol. 2013;82(1):85–9. https://doi.org/10.1016/j.ejrad.2012.05.038.
46. Guo J, Wu G, Chen X, Li X. Primary appendiceal lymphoma presenting as suspected perforated acute appendicitis: clinical, sonography and CT findings with pathologic correlation. Int J Clin Exp Pathol. 2014;7(10):7068–71.
47. Pickhardt PJ, Levy AD, Rohrmann CA Jr, Abbondanzo SL, Kende AI. Non-Hodgkin's lymphoma of the appendix: clinical and CT findings with pathologic correlation. AJR Am J Roentgenol. 2002;178(5):1123–7. https://doi.org/10.2214/ajr.178.5.1781123.
48. McCusker ME, Coté TR, Clegg LX, Sobin LH. Primary malignant neoplasms of the appendix: a population-based study from the surveillance, epidemiology and end-results program, 1973–1998. Cancer. 2002;94(12):3307–12. https://doi.org/10.1002/cncr.10589.
49. https://www.nccn.org/patients/guidelines/content/PDF/colon-patient.pdf.
50. Bucher P, Gervaz P, Ris F, Oulhaci W, Egger JF, Morel P. Surgical treatment of appendiceal adenocarcinoid (goblet cell carcinoid). World J Surg. 2005;29(11):1436–9. https://doi.org/10.1007/s00268-005-7958-y.
51. Varisco B, McAlvin B, Dias J, Franga D. Adenocarcinoid of the appendix: is right hemicolectomy necessary? A meta-analysis of retrospective chart reviews. Am Surg. 2004;70(7):593–9.
52. Shaib W, Krishna K, Kim S, Goodman M, Rock J, Chen Z, Brutcher E, Staley CI, Maithel SK, Abdel-Missih S, El-Rayes BF, Bekaii-Saab T. Appendiceal neuroendocrine, goblet and signet-ring cell tumors: a spectrum of diseases with different patterns of presentation and outcome. Cancer Res Treat. 2016;48(2):596–604.
53. Gilmore G, Jensen K, Saligram S, Sachdev TP, Arekapudi SR. Goblet cell carcinoid of the appendix—diagnostic challenges and treatment updates: a case report and review of the literature. J Med Case Rep. 2018;12(1):275. https://doi.org/10.1186/s13256-018-1789-6.
54. Shapiro R, Eldar S, Sadot E, Papa MZ, Zippel DB. Appendiceal carcinoid at a large tertiary center: pathologic findings and long-term follow-up evaluation. Am J Surg. 2011;201(6):805–8. https://doi.org/10.1016/j.amjsurg.2010.04.016.
55. Boxberger N, Redlich A, Böger C, Leuschner I, von Schweinitz D, Dralle H, Vorwerk P. Neuroendocrine tumors of the appendix in children and adolescents. Pediatr Blood Cancer. 2013;60(1):65–70. https://doi.org/10.1002/pbc.24267.
56. Murray SE, Lloyd RV, Sippel RS, Chen H, Oltmann SC. Postoperative surveillance of small appendiceal carcinoid tumors. Am J Surg. 2014;207(3):342–5. https://doi.org/10.1016/j.amjsurg.2013.08.038.

Left Colon

10

Nikolaos Pararas, Andreas Pikoulis,
Dimitris Papakonstantinou, and Emmanouil Pikoulis

10.1 Introduction

Colorectal cancer accounts for about 1.5 million new cases per year and is the third most commonly diagnosed malignancy. Worldwide, it represents the second most common type of cancer in women (614,000 cases, 9.2% of the total) and the third most common cancer in men (746,000 cases, 10.0% of the total), while it is the fourth leading cause of death from cancer in the world, with almost 700,000 deaths in 2012 [1, 2].

The incidence of colorectal cancer fluctuates by geographic region: the incidence in Europe is higher than that in North America, followed by Oceania, Latin America, and Africa. In North America, a decreasing rate is reported, as well as in Europe and in Oceania and particularly in New Zealand, the USA, and France; on the other side, an increasing incidence is observed in Latin America, Asia, and Eastern Europe [3]. Nevertheless, the trend of colorectal cancer seems to fluctuate according to the Human Development Index (HDI), with a variable due to changes in diet, activity patterns, smoke attitude, and screening programs. An increasing incidence of colorectal cancer is observed in the population younger than 50 years: this could potentially encourage an update in the screening programs [4, 5].

Nevertheless, up to 33% of patients with colorectal cancer will present with symptoms requiring acute or emergent surgical intervention despite the increased screening efforts [6, 7]. Large bowel obstruction, perforation, and hemorrhage are common emergency presentations. Rates of morbidity, mortality, and stoma formation are higher for patients who require an emergency intervention than those who are managed electively [8, 9]. Worse outcomes are related to the emergency itself and to baseline differences in the two patient groups, with the emergency patients

N. Pararas (✉) · A. Pikoulis · D. Papakonstantinou · E. Pikoulis
3d Department of Surgery, Attikon General Hospital, National and Kapodistrian University of Athens (NKUA), Faculty of Medicine, Athens, Greece
e-mail: dimpapa7@hot.mail; mpikoul@med.uoa.gr

A. Tarasconi et al. (eds.), *Oncologic Surgical Emergencies*, Hot Topics in Acute Care Surgery and Trauma, https://doi.org/10.1007/978-3-031-36860-8_10

having dehydration, electrolyte abnormalities, poor nutrition, neglected comorbidities, and more physiologic derangements.

Tumor biology may also play a significant role in their presentation and outcome. Cancers resected in an emergency setting are more likely to present lymphovascular invasion of a more advanced T stage, and a higher histologic grade and contemporary liver metastases are a common finding [6–10]. If it is required to operate at the patient's acute presentation, the diagnosis and accurate staging information may not be available or complete. When the initial findings suggest generalized metastatic disease, the necessity for an emergency intervention may have long-term implications.

The difficulties of patients presenting with suboptimal physiology and limited information require individualization of their surgical management. The principles of an oncologic resection for colorectal cancer surgery include wide proximal and distal margins and high ligation of the vascular pedicle for extended lymphadenectomy (≥12 nodes). These oncologic principles should be maintained even in emergency operations for colorectal cancer.

The objectives of the treatment of colon cancer-related emergencies according to the American Society of Colon and Rectal Surgeons clinical guidelines committee are as follows: (1) avoid the negative effect of any immediate complications; (2) accomplish the best possible tumor control; and (3) make sure timely recovery to permit the initiation of appropriate adjuvant chemotherapy or systemic treatment [11].

In this chapter, the authors discuss specific emergency situations related to left colon cancer and their management options.

10.2 Left Colon Obstruction

Obstruction is a very common symptom of colorectal cancer, with the incidence ranging from 15 to 29% [11]. It is also the most common indication for emergency surgery for colorectal carcinoma, making up to 77% of emergencies in a recent series [3]. Likewise, the most common cause of large bowel obstruction in adults is colon malignancy [1, 12, 13]. By itself, surgery for large bowel obstruction in a patient that presents acutely should be performed oncologically, even if an official diagnosis of malignancy has not yet been reached. The patients presenting with obstruction and with no evidence of metastatic disease should be operated upon with curative intent [1]. The clinical presentation of complete bowel obstruction from colorectal carcinoma is usually delayed by a gradual onset of symptoms. The patients may describe an increasing difficulty with their bowel movements or self-medication with laxatives. They can develop significant abdominal distension before complete obstipation occurs, and it results in the need for emergent medical attention. Such an insidious and subtle onset of symptoms can result in relatively stable patients. Typically, late signs consist of severe dehydration and electrolyte abnormalities. In certain cases, symptoms can be sudden in onset, with severe persistent colicky abdominal pain [14]. Absence of passage of flatus and/or feces and abdominal distension are the most common symptoms and physical signs [15].

Physical examination of the abdomen shows abdominal distension, tenderness, and absent or hyperactive bowel sounds. Initial complaint of bloody stools and passage of blood per rectum, despite the absence of bowel movement, can be associated with colon cancer. A rectal cancer may be palpable as an intrinsic lesion [16, 17].

Laboratory tests are directed at evaluating the electrolyte imbalances, elevated urea nitrogen, and metabolic alkalosis that may occur due to vomiting and dehydration.

Computerized tomography (CT) has become the golden standard imaging modality for patients presenting with symptoms of obstruction of the colon. It is quickly available in emergency departments and can localize, with a sensitivity of 96% and specificity of 93%, an obstructing lesion [18, 19]. Especially with the use of a triple-contrast protocol with oral, rectal, and intravenous (IV) contrast, CT can make an accurate diagnosis in up to 89% of the cases. CT also offers precise staging information of both locoregional and distant disease spread [15–19].

Although less commonly used in current practice, the hydrosoluble contrast enema is also a valuable imaging technique. In colonic obstructions, sensitivity and specificity are 80% and 100%, respectively [15–17]. CT may not be able to identify a small intraluminal lesion that is readily apparent on contrast enema in a stool-filled colon.

When possible, colonoscopy offers the ability to identify and localize an obstructing lesion as well as to confirm a diagnosis with tissue sampling. Colonoscopy also offers the possibility for relief of obstruction with the placement of endoluminal stents. Endoscopy is often not appropriate nor available in the emergency setting, and patients presenting in critical condition might require surgical intervention before an endoscopic procedure and evaluation is arranged. When faced outside the emergency setting, a lesion that cannot be overlapped with a standard colonoscope (diameter 11.8–13.0 mm) is more likely to necessitate an emergency operation, with a hazard ratio of 6.9 (1.6–29.7) [4]. This finding demands a quick referral to a surgeon.

Obstructing colon cancers can be identified as occurring either proximal or distal to the splenic flexure, with the site of the disease having a significant impact on treatment options. The left colon is more susceptible to obstruction, most commonly in the sigmoid colon [20]. The reasons for this are a relatively narrow colonic luminal diameter, a tendency toward morphologically more annular lesions, and thicker stool consistency [21].

10.3 Management of Obstruction of the Left Colon

The most common sites for obstruction by colon cancer are the descending and sigmoid colon because of the narrow bowel diameter and thicker stool consistency. Compared to the proximal lesions, there are significantly more options for the surgeon addressing such patients. Even though it is generally accepted that a specific approach must be individualized to each patient, according to the surgeon's expertise and the available resources, significant controversy remains on the best possible emergency management of these obstructing left colon cancers. The treatment alternatives are reported in a 2010 guideline statement, which was updated in 2017, from the World Society for Emergency Surgery (WSES) and Peritoneum and Surgery Society [22, 23].

10.4 Loop Colostomies

An established component of the surgical treatment options for obstructing distal colon cancer is the loop colostomy, with the intent of providing definitive oncologic resection in a staged approach. The obstruction is therefore controlled in the first stage with a proximal loop colostomy formation. In a second stage, the cancer is then resected, and the stoma is reversed. Otherwise, the colostomy reversal can be performed as a third stage. The transverse or descending colon could be utilized depending on the patient and tumor-specific factors. Most of the time, a loop ileostomy is not suggested because the presence of a functional ileocecal valve may prevent sufficient relief of the obstruction.

The loop colostomy approach is a safe option best suited to patients who are too fragile to undergo resection. The application of this staged approach has the advantage that it minimizes the operative time and the surgical trauma during the acute presentation of such patients, when tissue integrity is not optimal and physiologic derangements exist. In some cases, the initial colostomy may even be performed with only local analgesia [24]. It also decreases the risk of contamination from an unprepared bowel and allows complete staging and multidisciplinary review of the patients before definitive treatment [25, 26]. Still, loop colostomies are frequently associated with high complication rates, including hernia, stomal prolapse, and dehydration, and additionally this approach does not allow an oncologic resection. Loop colostomy might also be suitable when the cancer invades adjacent organs and is locally advanced, limiting the feasibility of a correct oncologic resection in the emergency setting.

10.5 Hartmann Procedure

The classic Hartmann procedure requires the resection of the primary lesion with the creation of an end colostomy and closing of the distal colon/rectum. Large reviews have established the feasibility of an emergency resection following the standard oncological principles of high ligation of the vascular pedicle, and retrieval of at least 12 regional lymph nodes, and en bloc resection of other adjacent tissues for negative margins [27, 28]. Like a loop colostomy, this approach alleviates the risk of an anastomotic leak. Hartmann resection is currently considered as the most common operation performed for distal colon carcinomas presenting in an emergency setting [29–31].

The literature has not shown any worse short- or long-term outcomes in patients undergoing formal Hartmann resection compared with the staged approach, despite the longer operative time for a formal resection. A randomized study by Kronborg [32] showed no difference in mortality, recurrence rate, and cancer-specific survival between colostomy and Hartmann's procedure in the emergency-setting patients. The only significant difference found in this study was the longer hospital stay in the patient group that received the staged approach due to the multiple subsequent operations needed. Notably, this study has been criticized for its long accrual period, the heterogeneous underlying pathology, and the incomplete follow-up. A Cochrane systematic review in 2004, that did not include the Kronborg study due to methodological flaws, made the same conclusions [33]. The WSES guidelines concluded that colostomy formation (staged approach) should be reserved for "damage control" cases, unresectable tumors, and cases where multimodal treatment is anticipated before formal resection [28].

A contradictory conclusion was made by another randomized controlled trial (RCT) that found no difference in outcomes, transfusion rates, or duration of hospitalization between Hartmann's procedure and a staged approach [34]. The investigators of this study claim rather that colostomy for staged approach is ideal for healthier, younger patients who will undergo a definitive surgery in as little as 2–3 weeks when less inflammation and bowel distension will allow a technically easier and more oncological resection [34]. However, most investigators agree that the Hartmann's resection is the procedure of choice for older patients with a high American Society of Anesthesiologists (ASA) score, advanced obstructions, and proximal bowel distension and whose underlying medical comorbidities might preclude definitive surgery in a staged manner [28, 32–34].

The main disadvantage of the Hartmann procedure is the residual stoma. The rate of Hartmann's reversal is only 20% among patients with colon cancer, for reasons including complications from treatment, advanced disease, and poor performance status [35, 36]. Operations to restore intestinal continuity are also associated with significant morbidity and mortality rates [15]. Colostomies are not without their own complications, and rates increase the longer they are in place, unfavorably affecting the quality of life of these patients [37, 38].

10.6 Single-Stage Primary Resection and Anastomosis

For several years, a single-stage oncologic resection with primary anastomosis was considered high risk in the emergency setting. Concerns included increased extent of surgery and operating room time, difficulty in manipulating and mobilizing a distended colon, potential for contamination of the peritoneal cavity, and further physiologic derangement to a critically ill patient. Patients may be severely malnourished due to poor oral intake before their presentation with an obstruction. Going forward with an operation before nutritional optimization might increase the risk for postoperative complications, especially if the proximal bowel is ischemic, dilated, or otherwise not appropriate for anastomosis. Of paramount importance are the complications from an anastomotic leak, which can be catastrophic and delay adjuvant systemic chemotherapy. Recent extensive studies have established the feasibility of primary resection and anastomosis (PRA) in appropriately selected patients. Resection with primary anastomosis can reduce the length of stay and the number of operations needed, with similar morbidity and mortality rates. Retrospective data and non-randomized reviews show the rate of anastomotic leak in the emergency settings to be 2.2–12%, which is almost the same as the rates in elective colon resection of 1.9–8% [28]. Thus, in the position statement from the Association of Coloproctologists of Great Britain and Ireland, PRA is recommended even in acutely symptomatic distal colon cancers [37, 39].

The appropriate patient selection is critical for the success in this high-risk environment. Specific factors related to poor outcomes in obstructing colon cancer operations include surgery within 24 h of presentation, advanced cancer stage, age greater than 70, ASA grades III–IV, and preoperative renal failure. For any of these factors, either a primary anastomosis with a protecting loop ileostomy or a Hartmann resection with end colostomy should be carried out.

10.7 Total Abdominal Colectomy

For selected patients, another option is total abdominal colectomy with ileorectal anastomosis (TAC/IRA). It removes the distended and potentially ischemic proximal colon by resecting back to the healthy terminal ileum for a primary anastomosis. This approach is particularly suitable for cases with suspected synchronous tumors or hereditary colorectal cancer syndromes. Another very significant indication for TAC/IRA is a cecal perforation or impending perforation, which is common in advanced distal obstructions.

Overall, leaving the transverse colon intact and performing a double resection to remove the cecum and the distal tumor separately are not recommended [40].

10.8 Self-Expanding Stents

Self-expandable metal stents (SEMSs) represent a nonoperative modality to deal with distal colon malignant obstructions. These stents were initially developed in the 1990s in patients considered as poor candidates for resection surgery or for palliation of obstructions from unresectable tumors [41, 42]. They are also used as a temporary "bridge to surgery" therapy, with the goal of allowing elective resection, possibly laparoscopic.

SEMSs require the endoscopic placement of a guidewire across the obstructing lesion, often with the assistance of fluoroscopy, followed by an uncovered, self-expanding metal stent. Balloon dilation is not usually necessary. Once the stent has been positioned, success is confirmed by the passing of air and fluid past the obstruction. If required, the endoscope can be advanced through the stent to visualize the proximal colon. Even though stenting is technically feasible for all areas of the colon, it is better studied and more successful for lesions of the left colon. Stenting is an attractive option for emergency surgery. Supporters claim that stenting can allow the treating team to stabilize the patient, optimize medical comorbidities and nutritional status, correct dehydration and other electrolyte imbalances, complete the oncologic staging, and engage a multidisciplinary team. Early studies that supported the use of SEMS in this situation discussed that as a bridge to surgery, stents might lower stoma rates and reduce morbidity and mortality if compared to surgery alone [42–47]. Not all published data, though, have supported these claims, as in a recent observational study that compared SEMS to surgery as a bridge to surgery.

Despite relatively low rates of complications (micro-perforation rate 13%) and high technical success rates with stent placement (91%), there was no difference in rates of primary anastomosis or stoma creation and no difference in perioperative mortality [47].

In a large meta-analysis and systematic review, the clinical success rate by relieving the obstruction with SEMS placement was only 52.5% overall, compared with the 99% achieved with surgery. The morbidity and mortality were again similar between groups; however, the rates of primary anastomoses were unexpectedly low in the bridge-to-surgery group, only 64.9% compared with 55% in the surgery-first group, with no statistical difference. Anastomotic leak rates were marginally better in the stented patients but also not statistically significant [48].

Stent placement is not without a risk. In fact, of the six RCTs comparing up-front surgery to SEMS in left colon obstructing cancers, half stopped enrollment early due to high rates of stent-related complications, most notable perforation during deployment [49]. Other complications include migration, failure to relieve the obstruction, and subsequent stent occlusion. Tumor perforation during stent deployment likely mandates emergency surgeries. The peritoneal spillage adds further physiologic stress to the patients and might limit the surgical options in the setting of feculent peritonitis. Some authors argue that even following uncomplicated positioning, the local trauma from a stent may boost tumor cell dissemination and worsen oncological outcomes [50]. A retrospective comparative study using SEMS for a bridge-to-surgery therapy found a higher cancer-specific mortality in the SEMS group (48% vs. 21% for surgery only) and a significantly lower overall 5-year survival in the SEMS group when compared to surgery alone (25% vs. 62%, respectively). There were also nonsignificant benefits for the surgery-only group in recurrence rates, disease-free survival, and mean time to a recurrence. Stent insertion, in fact, in the study's multivariate analysis, was the only modifiable factor affecting the poor outcomes in that arm. In general, success rates are higher and complication rates lower in the SEMS case series when experienced endoscopists are involved. Yet, further studies are needed before SEMS is considered the standard of care for malignant left colon obstructions. Stents may prevent a morbid operation in the existence of the metastatic disease or short life expectancy and allow faster initiation of systemic chemotherapy. To limit complication rates, SEMS should only be performed by endoscopists with an adequate expertise.

10.9 Perforation

Perforation is the second most common cause for urgent or emergent surgery associated with colorectal cancer, with an incidence range of 2.6–12% [51, 52]. The perforations most commonly occur at the site of the primary tumor due to necrosis and friable tissue. They may progress to either free or contained perforations, depending on the position.

Perforation can also happen proximal to an obstructing cancer. Distension and increasing pressure from a complete obstruction distally follow the law of Laplace, which can eventually result in ischemia of the proximal bowel and perforations at distant proximal sites. The most common site of this type of perforation is the cecum [6]. This clinical presentation has been described as an independent prognostic factor for morbidity and mortality [7]. An obstructing carcinoma increases the risk of a perforation, with rates ranging from 12 to 19% [53]. Perforation is described to be the most lethal complication of colorectal cancer. In some studies, the mortality associated with a secondary peritonitis from perforation is as high as 30–50% [1, 54].

10.10 Free Perforation

Free perforation with spillage into the peritoneum is suggested by the classic findings of generalized peritonitis, including involuntary guarding and rebound tenderness. CT imaging may show free fluid, air at the perforation site, free air, portal venous air, or pneumatosis intestinalis. Colorectal perforation seeding in the peritoneal cavity is a surgical emergency with a poor outcome. The golden standard in the diagnosis of a perforation from colorectal carcinoma is the CT with a specificity of 95–97%, sensitivity of 95–98%, and accuracy of 95% [1]. These patients can rapidly progress into disseminated intravascular coagulation, septic shock, multisystem organ failure, and death. Even though emergency surgical intervention is usually required, outcomes have been generally poor, with mortality ranging from 6 to 33% in older studies [55–57]. Even in the most recent series highlighting advanced critical care management, by Yamamoto and colleagues [55], the mortality is 12%. Risk factors included low preoperative blood pressure and older age. Patients and families should be thoroughly instructed about the poor prognosis before any kind of operation in the emergency setting of a perforated colorectal cancer.

The surgical approach is typically an open exploration and thorough washout with the identification of the perforation site. Even without the established diagnosis of malignancy, resection of the perforated site should follow the principles of oncologic resection with extended lymphadenectomy for a precise pathology staging.

Despite the poor perioperative mortality, patients that present with perforation from a colorectal carcinoma, without findings of extensive metastatic lesions, should still be treated with a curative intent. Tumor perforation does not directly impact the M stage but upstages the lesion's T stage to T4. An oncologic resection typically concludes with the creation of an end stoma. Primary anastomosis may be considered in the carefully selected patient, given that the anastomosis is protected with a diverting loop ileostomy [29].

Lesions proximal to the splenic flexure, when they cause perforation, are twice more probable to result in peritonitis rather than to localized abscess [58]. As well, poorly contained leaks should also be expected when the perforations mentioned above happen at a distal obstructing carcinoma, which ends in ischemia and perforation of the proximal bowel, most of the time, the cecum. The operation of choice in these situations is subtotal colectomy. An ileorectal or ileocolic anastomosis may be considered in low-risk patients.

10.11 Abscess

Contained perforations may possibly present with localized tenderness. Imaging could reveal a phlegmon or an abscess, which is more common than free perforation in the descending and sigmoid colon lesions [59]. Many cases of perforated colorectal carcinomas presenting as abscesses are not diagnosed preoperatively and can mimic diverticulitis or appendicitis on CT imaging.

The role for percutaneous drainage of a contained perforation from a carcinoma differs from that of a benign disease. In the presence of extensive metastatic disease, treatment with antibiotics and percutaneous drainage avoids the morbidity of an operation. In some cases, however, drawn-out infectious complications can delay systemic chemotherapy.

In the absence of widely disseminated disease, percutaneous drainage of a contained perforation may result in seeding tumor cells along the drainage tract, making the disease metastatic [59]. When malignancy is suspected, drains should be placed in a manner where the drain tract and the skin can be resected en bloc with the cancer in a later stage. Definitive surgical management involves the en bloc resection of the mass and any invaded adjacent organs and/or percutaneous drains whenever it is technically possible [1].

10.12 Bleeding

In patients with colorectal cancer, gastrointestinal bleeding is reported in up to 50% of the cases [1, 60]. Most of these bleedings, however, are self-limited, are of low volume, and do not require an emergency surgical intervention. Bleeding is frequently an early symptom of a colorectal tumor, which is associated with a lower risk of advanced stage at presentation. Patients often remember precisely, to the day, when the bleeding began, unlike the insidious onset of an obstructing cancer [61]. Bleeding is sometimes complicated by the fact that most acute tumor bleeding is likely to happen in the setting of chronic anemia due to cancer and blood loss from the tumor. Massive, acute gastrointestinal bleeding from a colorectal tumor is rare. The initial management is targeted at resuscitation, establishing large-bore IV access, stabilizing the patient with crystalloid, and correcting any underlying coagulopathy or other metabolic abnormalities. Localization of the source of bleeding should be attempted before any surgical treatment whenever possible in the clinically stable patient. 1 Endoscopy can identify the source in 74–89% of cases, although this technique may be limited in an unprepared colon [62, 63]. A less sensitive modality is the tagged red blood cell scan, which localizes the source of bleeding in 26–72% of the cases. Nevertheless, it cannot detect bleeding at rates as low as 0.1 mL/min, making it a potential screening test before angioembolization. Embolization has documented success rates of 42–86%; however, it has the risk of worsening, if present, intestinal ischemia [1, 64]. This option might be more attractive in the case of a metastatic disease to avoid laparotomy and associated delays in starting systemic chemotherapy.

Surgery is still the most effective and definitive approach when dealing with a bleeding colorectal cancer. Some general indications for surgical intervention include (a) slow bleeding requiring more than three units of blood products per day, (b) hemodynamic instability despite transfusion of more than six units of blood products, (c) inability to stop the bleeding with endovascular or endoscopic techniques, or (d) recurrent and persistent episodes of hemorrhagic shock [65]. Resection should follow the oncologic principles with a curative intent when the site of hemorrhage has been localized. The decision to perform a PRA with or without proximal diversion or form a stoma should be carefully considered in light of any coagulopathy, anemia, and unstable hemodynamics that often come with the bleeding patient.

10.13 Minimally Invasive Surgery

Several case series and case-control studies have described an emergency laparoscopic colectomy for symptomatic colorectal cancer. Laparoscopy typically requires longer operative times but is associated with lower blood loss, shorter hospital stay, and similar morbidity and mortality when compared with open surgery. The rates of conversion to open surgery range from 0 to 17% in emergency colectomies [63, 66].

Appropriate patient selection is central to the safety and feasibility of minimally invasive techniques in the emergency setting. A prerequisite is the surgeon's experience with elective laparoscopic colectomy techniques.

The first case report of an emergency robotic colectomy was recently published for a hemorrhagic right-sided colon cancer, with good postoperative and oncologic outcome [63].

10.14 Outcomes

The feasibility and effectiveness of oncologic resections in the emergency setting have been well demonstrated. Teixeira et al. [7] documented that R0 resections are possible in up to 92% of emergency colectomies. Patients for whom R0 resections were not achieved had bulky T4 lesions or could not tolerate more radical en bloc resections. Adequate lymphadenectomy (>12 nodes) was documented in 71% of the cases. The oncologic and long-term outcomes for colorectal cancers presenting with emergency complications are worse than their elective counterparts. A recent retrospective review from Ireland included 34% of colon resections performed emergently and collected during the long-term follow-up to assess oncologic outcomes. Emergency resections were performed with perforation as the diagnosis for 8% of the cases, in which the lesions were more often T4 (38% vs. 13%) and lymph node positive (58% vs. 38%). Positive margin rate was much higher compared to the elective cases and found in 10% of emergency cases compared with only 1% of elective cases. The median survival for emergency cases was 59 months compared with 82 months for elective cases during the same time for a 5-year follow-up [10]. Other investigators showed similar results [67], although precisely the cause for these worse outcomes is still under debate [68].

High complication rates have been associated with urgent or emergent colectomy.

One retrospective review of 209 consecutive colectomies in a single institution found higher rates of wound infections and wound dehiscence and a higher rate of intra-abdominal abscesses in emergency colectomies [67]. The perioperative mortality rates for emergency colorectal cancer resections range from 5 to 34% [68–71]. The imminent threats to life will dictate how resources are assigned to the resuscitation and preoperative workup. The liberal use of stomas is encouraged and demonstrated in most series.

10.15 Conclusion

Specific complications occur frequently in patients with left colon cancer and threaten immediate survival and long-term oncological outcomes. Multidisciplinary management (surgeons, radiologists, endoscopists, oncologists) is required, and oncological principles should be respected during emergency treatment.

References

1. Arnold M, Sierra MS, Laversanne M, Soerjomataram I, Jemal A, Bray F. Global patterns and trends in colorectal cancer incidence and mortality. Gut. 2017;66(4):683–91.
2. Torre LA, Siegel RL, Ward EM, Jemal A. Global cancer incidence and mortality rates and trends—an update. Cancer Epidemiol Biomark Prev. 2016;25(1):16–27.
3. Benson AB 3rd, Venook AP, Cederquist L, et al. Colon cancer, version 1.2017, NCCN clinical practice guidelines in oncology. J Natl Compr Cancer Netw. 2017;15(3):370–98.
4. Bailey CE, Hu CY, You YN, Bednarski BK, Rodriguez-Bigas MA, Skibber JM, Cantor SB, Chang GJ. Increasing disparities in the age-related incidences of colon and rectal cancers in the United States, 1975–2010. JAMA Surg. 2015;150(1):17–22.
5. Barnett A, Cedar A, Siddiqui F, et al. Colorectal cancer emergencies. J Gastrointest Cancer. 2013;44(2):132–42.
6. Gunnarsson H, Holm T, Ekholm A, et al. Emergency presentation of colon cancer is most frequent during summer. Color Dis. 2011;13(6):663–8.
7. Teixeira F, Akaishi EH, Ushinohama AZ, et al. Can we respect the principles of oncologic resection in an emergency surgery to treat colon cancer? World J Emerg Surg. 2015;10:5.

8. Chalieopanyarwong V, Boonpipattanapong T, Prechawittayakul P, et al. Endoscopic obstruction is associated with higher risk of acute events requiring emergency operation in colorectal cancer patients. World J Emerg Surg. 2013;8:34.
9. Bayar B, Yilmaz KB, Akinci M, et al. An evaluation of treatment results of emergency versus elective surgery in colorectal cancer patients. Ulus Cerrahi Derg. 2016;32:11–7.
10. Bass G, Fleming C, Conneely J, et al. Emergency first presentation of colorectal cancer predicts significantly poorer outcomes: a review of 356 consecutive Irish patients. Dis Colon Rectum. 2009;52(4):678–84.
11. Alvarez JA, Baldonedo RF, Bear IG, et al. Presentation, treatment, and multivariate analysis of risk factors for obstructive and perforative colorectal carcinoma. Am J Surg. 2005;190:376–82.
12. Phillips RK, Hittinger R, Fry JS, et al. Malignant large bowel obstruction. Br J Surg. 1985;72:296–302.
13. Garcia-Valdecasas JC, Llovera JM, deLacy AM, et al. Obstructing colorectal carcinomas: prospective study. Dis Colon Rectum. 1991;34(9):759–62.
14. Chang GJ, Kaiser AM, Mills S, et al. Practice parameters for the management of colon cancer. Dis Colon Rectum. 2012;55:831–43.
15. Ohman U. Prognosis in patients with obstructing colorectal carcinoma. Am J Surg. 1982;143:742–7.
16. De Dombal FT, Matharu SS, Staniland JR, et al. Presentation of cancer to the hospital as "acute abdominal pain". Br J Surg. 1980;67:413–6.
17. Peterson M. Large intestine. In: Marx JA, Hockberger RS, Walls RM, editors. Rosen's emergency medicine: concepts and clinical practice. 6th ed. Philadelphia: Elsevier; 2006. p. 1332–4.
18. Gordon PH. Malignant neoplasms of the colon. In: Gordon PH, Nivatvongs S, editors. Principles and practice of surgery for the colon, rectum and anus. 3rd ed. New York: Informa Healthcare; 2007. p. 534–5.
19. Markogiannakis H, Messaris E, Dardamanis D, Pararas N, Tzertzemelis D, Giannopoulos P, Larentzakis A, Lagoudianakis E, Manouras A, Bramis I. Acute mechanical bowel obstruction: clinical presentation, etiology, management and outcome. World J Gastroenterol. 2007;13(3):432–7.
20. Cappell MS, Batke M. Mechanical obstruction of the small bowel and colon. Med Clin N Am. 2008;92(3):575–97.
21. Lopez-Kostner F, Hool GR, Lavery IC. Management and causes of acute large-bowel obstruction. Surg Clin N Am. 1997;77(6):1265–90.
22. Frago R, Ramirez E, Millan M, et al. Current management of acute malignant large bowel obstruction: a systematic review. Am J Surg. 2014;207:127–38.
23. Frager D, Rovno HD, Baer JW, et al. Prospective evaluation of colonic obstruction with computed tomography. Abdom Imaging. 1998;23(2):141–6.
24. Gainant A. Emergency management of acute colonic cancer obstruction. J Visc Surg. 2012;149:e3–10.
25. Kleespies A, Fuessl KE, Seeliger H, et al. Determinants of morbidity and survival after elective non-curative resection of stage IV colon and rectal cancer. Int J Colorectal Dis. 2009;24:1097–109.
26. Wolmark N, Wieand HS, Rockette HE, et al. The prognostic significance of tumour location and bowel obstruction in Dukes' B and C colorectal cancer. Ann Surg. 1983;198:743–50.
27. Ansaloni L, Andersson RE, Bazzoli F, et al. Guidelines in the management of obstructing cancer of the left colon: consensus conference of the World Society of Emergency Surgery (WSES) and Peritoneum and Surgery (PnS) Society. World J Emerg Surg. 2010;5:29.
28. Pisano M, Zorcolo L, Merli C, et al. 2017 WSES guidelines on colon and rectal cancer emergencies: obstruction and perforation. World J Emerg Surg. 2018;13:36.
29. Kelley WE Jr, Brown PW, Lawrence W Jr, Terz JJ. Penetrating, obstructing, and perforating carcinomas of the colon and rectum. Arch Surg. 1981;116(4):381–4.
30. McArdle CS, Hole DJ. Emergency presentation of colorectal cancer is associated with poor 5-year survival. Br J Surg. 2004;91(5):605–9.

31. Meyer F, Marusch F, Koch A, et al. Emergency operation in carcinomas of the left colon: value of Hartmann's procedure. Tech Coloproctol. 2004;8(suppl):s226.
32. Kronborg O. Acute obstruction from tumour in the left colon without spread. A randomized trial of emergency colostomy versus resection. Int J Color Dis. 1995;10:1–5.
33. De Salvo GL, Gava C, Lise M, et al. Curative surgery for obstruction from primary left colorectal carcinoma: primary or staged resection? Cochrane Database Syst. 2004;2:CD002101.
34. Krstic S, Resanovic V, Alempijevic T, et al. Hartmann's procedure vs loop colostomy in the treatment of obstructive rectosigmoid cancer. World J Emerg Surg. 2014;9:52.
35. Zorcolo L, Covotta L, Carlomagno N, et al. Safety of primary anastomosis in emergency colorectal surgery. Color Dis. 2003;5:262–9.
36. Desai DC, Brennan EJ, Reilly JF, et al. The utility of the Hartmann procedure. Am J Surg. 1998;175:152–4.
37. Kavanagh DO, Nolan B, Judge C, et al. A comparative study of short- and medium-term outcomes comparing emergent surgery and stenting as a bridge to surgery in patients with acute malignant colonic obstruction. Dis Colon Rectum. 2013;56:433–40.
38. Sprangers MA, Taal BG, Aaronson NK, et al. Quality of life in colorectal cancer. Stoma vs. nonstoma patients. Dis Colon Rectum. 1995;38:361–9.
39. Tekkis PP, Kinsman R, Thompson MR, et al. The Association of Coloproctology of Great Britain and Ireland study of large bowel obstruction caused by colorectal cancer. Ann Surg. 2004;204:76–81.
40. The SCOTIA Study Group. Single-stage treatment for malignant left-sided colonic obstruction: a prospective randomized clinical trial comparing subtotal colectomy with segmental resection following intraoperative irrigation. Br J Surg. 1995;82:1622–7.
41. Kwak MS, Kim WS, Lee JM, et al. Does stenting as a bridge to surgery in left-sided colorectal cancer obstruction really worsen oncological outcomes? Dis Colon Rectum. 2016;59:725–32.
42. Dohmoto M, Hünerbein M, Schlag PM. Palliative endoscopic therapy of rectal carcinoma. Eur J Cancer. 1996;32a:25–9.
43. Khot UP, Lang AW, Murali K, et al. Systematic review of the efficacy and safety of colorectal stents. Br J Surg. 2002;89:1096–102.
44. Cennamo V, Luigiano C, Coccolini F, et al. Meta-analysis of randomized trials comparing endoscopic stenting and surgical decompression for colorectal cancer obstruction. Int J Color Dis. 2013;28:855–63.
45. Sebastian S, Johnston S, Geoghegan T, et al. Pooled analysis of the efficacy and safety of self-expanding metal stenting in malignant colorectal obstruction. Am J Gastroenterol. 2004;99:2051–7.
46. Matsuda A, Miyashita M, Matsumoto S, et al. Comparison of long-term outcomes of colonic stent as "bridge to surgery" and emergency surgery for malignant large-bowel obstruction: a meta-analysis. Ann Surg Oncol. 2015;22:497–504.
47. Zhang Y, Shi J, Shi B, et al. Self-expanding metallic stent as a bridge to surgery versus emergency surgery for obstructive colorectal cancer: a meta-analysis. Surg Endosc. 2012;26:110–9.
48. Cuffy M, Abir F, Audisio RA, Longo WE. Colorectal cancer presenting as surgical emergencies. Surg Oncol. 2004;13(2–3):149–57.
49. Maruthachalam K, Lash GE, Shenton BK, et al. Tumour cell dissemination following endoscopic stent insertion. Br J Surg. 2007;94:1151–4.
50. Sabbagh C, Browet F, Diouf M, et al. Is stenting as "a bridge to surgery" an oncologically safe strategy for the management of acute, left-sided, malignant, colonic obstruction? A comparative study with a propensity score analysis. Ann Surg. 2013;258:107–15.
51. Tsai HL, Hsieh JS, Yu FJ, et al. Perforated colonic cancer presenting as intraabdominal abscess. Int J Colorectal Dis. 2007;22(1):15–9.
52. Saegesser F, Sandblom P. Ischemic lesions of the distended colon. A complication of obstructive colorectal cancer. Am J Surg. 1975;129:309–15.
53. Umpleby HC, Williamson RCN. Survival in acute obstructing colorectal carcinoma. Dis Colon Rectum. 1984;27:299–304.

54. Langell JT, Mulvihill SJ. Gastrointestinal perforation and the acute abdomen. Med Clin N Am. 2008;92(3):599–625.
55. Yamamoto T, Kita R, Masui H, et al. Prediction of mortality in patients with colorectal perforation based on routinely available parameters: a retrospective study. World J Emerg Surg. 2015;10:24.
56. Horiuchi A, Watanabe Y, Doi T, et al. Evaluation of prognostic factors and scoring system in colonic perforation. World J Gastroenterol. 2007;13:3228–31.
57. Komatsu S, Shimomatsuya T, Nakajima M, et al. Prognostic factors and scoring system for survival in colonic perforation. Hepato-Gastroenterology. 2005;52:761–4.
58. Yeo ES, Ng KH, Eu KW. Perforated colorectal cancer: an important differential diagnosis in all presumed diverticular abscesses. Ann Acad Med Singap. 2011;40(8):375–8.
59. Adelstein BA, Macaskill P, Chan SF, et al. Most bowel cancer symptoms do not indicate colorectal cancer and polyps: a systematic review. BMC Gastroenterol. 2011;11:65.
60. Zuccaro G Jr. Management of the adult patient with acute lower gastrointestinal bleeding. Am J Gastroenterol. 1998;93(8):1202–8.
61. Davila RE, Rajan E, Adler DG, et al. ASGE guideline: the role of endoscopy in the patient with lower-GI bleeding. Gastrointest Endosc. 2005;62(5):656–60.
62. Tavakkolizadeh A, Ashley S. Acute gastrointestinal hemorrhage. In: Townsend CM, Beauchamp RD, Evers BM, et al., editors. Sabiston textbook of surgery: the biological basis of modern surgical practice. 19th ed. Philadelphia: Elsevier; 2012. p. 1139–59.
63. Felli E, Brunetti F, Disabato M, et al. Robotic right colectomy for hemorrhagic right colon cancer: a case report and review of the literature of minimally invasive urgent colectomy. World J Emerg Surg. 2014;9:32.
64. Ji WB, Hahn KY, Kwak JM, Kang DW, Baek SJ, Kim J, Kim SH. Mechanical bowel preparation does not affect clinical severity of anastomotic leakage in rectal cancer surgery. World J Surg. 2017;41(5):1366–74. https://doi.org/10.1007/s00268-016-3839-9.
65. Oliphant R, Mansouri D, Nicholson GA, et al. Emergency presentation of node-negative colorectal cancer treated with curative surgery is associated with poorer short and longer-term survival. Int J Color Dis. 2014;29:591–8.
66. Weixler B, Warschkow R, Ramser M, et al. Urgent surgery after emergency presentation for colorectal cancer has no impact on overall and disease-free survival: a propensity score analysis. BMC Cancer. 2016;16:208.
67. Kim J, Mittal R, Konyalian V, et al. Outcome analysis of patients undergoing colorectal resection for emergent and elective indications. Am Surg. 2007;73:991–3.
68. Boyle DJ, Thorn C, Saini A, et al. Predictive factors for successful colonic stenting in acute large-bowel obstruction: a 15-year cohort analysis. Dis Colon Rectum. 2015;58:358–62.
69. Breitenstein S, Rickenbacher A, Berdajs D, et al. Systematic evaluation of surgical strategies for acute malignant left-sided colonic obstruction. Br J Surg. 2007;94(12):1451–60.
70. Tan CJ, Dasari BV, Gardiner K. Systematic review and meta-analysis of randomized clinical trials of self-expanding metallic stents as a bridge to surgery versus emergency surgery for malignant left-sided large bowel obstruction. Br J Surg. 2012;99:469–76.
71. Trompetas V. Emergency management of malignant acute left-sided colonic obstruction. Ann R Coll Surg Engl. 2008;90:181–6.

Rectum 11

Ga-ram Han, Justin T. Brady, Mohamad B. Sonbol,
and Vanessa P. Ho

11.1 Introduction

Colorectal cancer patients present as emergencies in approximately 30% of cases, despite screening with colonoscopy, computed tomography (CT) colonography, fecal occult blood tests, fecal immunochemical tests, and fecal deoxyribonucleic acid (DNA) test [1, 2]. Unfortunately much of the literature on colorectal emergencies is not specific to rectal cancer. However, there are three common types of surgical emergencies encountered in rectal cancers: obstruction, perforation, and bleeding. When feasible, management of these emergencies should address life-threatening acute disease while still optimizing oncologic outcomes [3]. In the elective setting, rectal cancer workup includes a full colonoscopy; staging computed tomography of the chest, abdomen, and pelvis; magnetic resonance imaging (MRI) of the pelvis with rectal cancer protocol; and serum carcinoembryonic antigen (CEA) level [4]. Unfortunately, this is not feasible in an emergency presentation. In addition, patients requiring emergency interventions tend to present with more advanced disease and subsequently have increased morbidity and mortality [5]. In cases of advanced rectal cancer warranting palliative treatment, a multidisciplinary approach should be taken with shared decision-making, taking into consideration the patient's priorities and anticipated life expectancy.

G.-r. Han · J. T. Brady
Department of Surgery, Mayo Clinic Arizona, Phoenix, AZ, USA

M. B. Sonbol
Department of Hematology and Oncology, Mayo Clinic Arizona, Phoenix, AZ, USA
e-mail: Sonbol.Mohamad@mayo.edu

V. P. Ho (✉)
Department of Surgery, The MetroHealth System, Cleveland, OH, USA
e-mail: vho@metrohealth.org

A. Tarasconi et al. (eds.), *Oncologic Surgical Emergencies*, Hot Topics in Acute Care Surgery and Trauma, https://doi.org/10.1007/978-3-031-36860-8_11

11.2 Obstruction

11.2.1 Clinical Presentation

The initial presentation of 8–29% of patients with colorectal cancer is with obstructive symptoms [6]. Patients with obstructing rectal cancers may present with crampy abdominal pain, distension, or obstipation. History may also reveal constipation, hematochezia, unintentional weight loss, mucoid stools, or change in the caliber of the stool. Emesis tends to be a late finding and may not occur in the presence of a competent ileocecal valve. In patients with low rectal cancer, patients may have a history of tenesmus or sensation of incomplete evacuation with bowel movements [7].

11.2.2 Workup

A focused history should include the date of last colonoscopy and a family plus personal history of colon polyps or cancer. In the absence of complications, the abdominal exam is usually non-tender. Focal tenderness may be suggestive of ischemia or localized perforation. Generalized tenderness with guarding and rebound is suspicious for a bowel perforation. Patients with a competent ileocecal valve and a complete large bowel obstruction are at particular risk for cecal perforation due to closed loop physiology. Tachycardia can reflect intravascular dehydration or impending bowel compromise. Digital rectal examination should evaluate for a hard mass, although malignancy in the proximal rectum may not be palpable. The size, distance from the anal verge, top of the anal sphincters, and presence of fixation to the surrounding structures should be noted. Lastly, patients should be examined for signs of lymph node or distant metastases by evaluation for jaundice, scleral icterus, and inguinal or supraclavicular lymphadenopathy [7].

Workup should include complete blood count and comprehensive metabolic panel. Results may reveal evidence of fluid sequestration in the intestines causing hypovolemia and electrolyte derangements. Leukocytosis is a worrisome finding and could suggest near or complete obstruction or associated complications such as perforation.

An upright and supine abdominal radiograph is a reasonable choice for the first imaging study as it is quick, easy, and cost-effective to identify surgical emergencies including free air or pneumatosis coli. It has been shown to have a sensitivity of 84% and specificity of 72% for diagnosing large bowel obstructions [8]. Abdominal X-rays may also be used to estimate the cecal diameter; a diameter greater than 9–12 cm is worrisome for impending perforation.

In a patient with an acute large bowel obstruction suspected to be related to rectal cancer, CT of the abdomen and pelvis with intravenous contrast is the diagnostic test of choice. It has a sensitivity of 91–96% and a specificity of 91–93% in the diagnosis of colonic obstruction [9, 10]. It can diagnose large bowel obstruction and provide valuable information about the tumor including location, extent of tumor involvement, and presence of lymphadenopathy or distal metastases. It may also define the size of the colonic diameter, reveal whether the ileocecal valve is competent based upon the presence of small bowel dilation, and identify the presence of complications including perforation, ischemia, and/or necrosis.

Contrast enemas may provide further information with a sensitivity of 80–96% and specificity of 98–100% for diagnosing colonic obstructions, although these may be deferred in the acute setting in favor of cross-sectional CT imaging [8, 11]. For enemas, the preferred contrast material in these cases is an air contrast or water-soluble contrast study, as barium increases the risk of peritonitis and mortality if a bowel perforation is present [7, 12]. Localization of the level of obstruction is more accurate than with standard plain films, and an "apple-core" lesion may be identified. Water-soluble contrast enemas may also detect small intraluminal lesions that can be challenging to identify on CT scans of a stool-filled colon although these are unlikely to cause obstruction [11]. Despite these benefits, contrast enemas are infrequently obtained as they may increase abdominal pain and risk of perforation.

TNM staging is not required in the emergent setting but may be completed after management of the acute disease; most patients presenting with obstructive rectal cancers have already progressed to stage III or IV disease [3]. If possible, obtaining a CT scan of the chest for staging may be helpful to anticipate the needs for adjuvant chemotherapy if lung metastases are present.

11.2.3 Treatment

Obstructive rectal cancers pose a challenging scenario; treatment goals are to relieve the obstruction while optimizing the overall oncologic outcomes. Obstructing tumors tend to be locally advanced, and it can be difficult to achieve the desired oncologic margin with emergent resection [13]. The presence of an obstructing tumor has been suggested by some to be an indication for neoadjuvant therapy [14]. We advocate avoiding oncologic resection in the emergent setting for an obstructing rectal cancer to permit the administration of neoadjuvant therapy prior to resection (Fig. 11.1). However, this remains an area of debate.

Management should begin with resuscitation and correction of any electrolyte derangements. Treatment of the obstruction must be performed expeditiously to avoid progression to ischemia or perforation. In patients with a competent ileocecal valve, the obstructing mass causes a "closed loop" configuration, and therefore, these patients are at the highest risk of perforation [15]. Patients with emesis or evidence of an incompetent ileocecal valve may benefit from decompression with a nasogastric tube while awaiting more definitive management. Signs of generalized peritonitis, perforation, or closed loop physiology with ischemia or necrosis mandate emergent surgical intervention. The tumor distance from the anal verge should be characterized to determine options for further management. Proximal tumors are 10–15 cm from the anal verge, while distal tumors are 0–5 cm from the anal verge.

In patients with proximal rectal cancer, there are two options available: endoscopic stent placement and proximal diverting stoma creation. Several case series

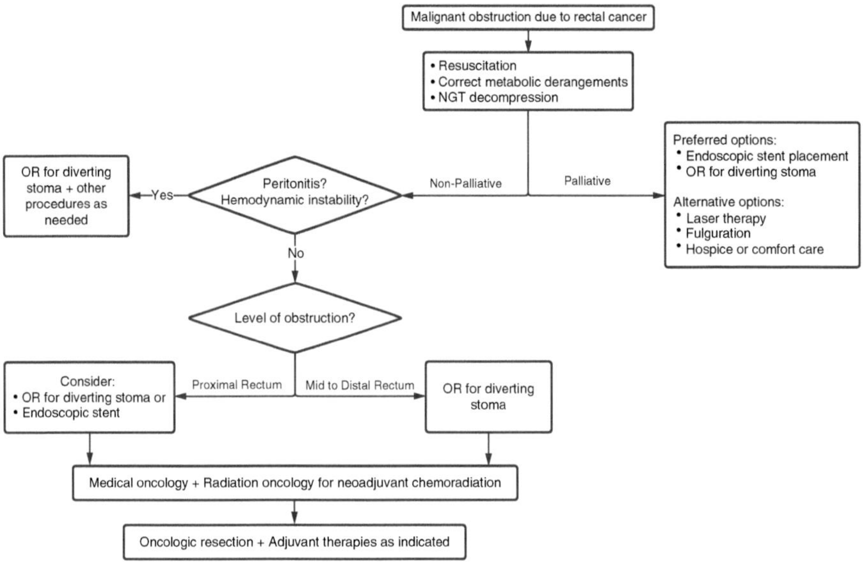

Fig. 11.1 Management of malignant obstruction due to rectal cancer

have suggested that there may be a higher local rectal cancer recurrence rate in patients who undergo stent placement although this has not yet been definitively demonstrated in the literature. Possible reasons for the increased local recurrence rates could be due to the risk of perforation with endoscopic stent placement and shedding of tumor cells during stent deployment or secondary to local inflammation from the presence of the stent [16, 17]. If the patient is expected to have a limited life expectancy, then stenting may be the better palliative option. There is the risk that endoscopic insufflation for stent placement could make colonic distention worse and present an increased risk for perforation for patients with a competent ileocecal valve, so patients must be chosen carefully. If, however, the small bowel distension suggests an incompetent ileocecal valve and/or the cecum is not dilated as a result of obstruction, stent placement as a bridge to surgery is a reasonable option.

In patients with distal rectal cancer, decompression with a proximal diverting stoma is strongly recommended [3]. Endoscopic stent placement is not anatomically feasible in the lower rectum as the distal extent of the stent must be placed above the anorectal ring. Failure to do so could cause chronic perianal pain, fecal urgency, tenesmus, fecal incontinence, poor quality of life, and increased risk of stent migration [18].

11.2.4 Creation of a Diverting Ostomy

Emergent fecal diversion may be achieved through creation of a proximal diverting loop ostomy. The loop configuration allows for fecal passage through the afferent limb as well as venting of the bowel between the stoma site and the obstruction [19]. In addition, a loop ostomy permits endoscopic evaluation of the entire colon for synchronous lesions prior to the definitive oncologic resection. It is pertinent to note that emergent surgery due to obstructing colorectal cancer is associated with a mortality rate of 15–34% and a morbidity of 32–64% [20].

If feasible, preoperative stoma site marking should be performed. In the setting of obstruction, it may be difficult to assess for sites of skin folds, but it is important to make sure that the patient can see the stoma in cases of a large pannus. Preoperative preparation should include broad-spectrum antibiotics, a urinary catheter, and lithotomy positioning to allow access to the rectum. Depending on the patient's degree of abdominal distension and body habitus, a laparoscopic approach may be considered. Minimally invasive surgery has been shown to have a shorter recovery time and reduced rates of infectious complications, both of which may facilitate timely initiation of neoadjuvant therapy. However, bowel distension causing loss of abdominal domain may preclude a laparoscopic approach. In addition, open surgery may result in increased adhesion formation, rendering the subsequent resection longer or more challenging.

Diversion via a sigmoid loop colostomy is recommended. In the subsequent oncologic resection, the sigmoid colostomy may serve as the proximal end of the anastomosis. Other stoma options include a transverse loop colostomy or a diverting loop ileostomy. A transverse loop colostomy has an increased risk of prolapse, making it difficult for the patient to manage, and subsequent colostomy takedown can be technically more challenging. A diverting loop ileostomy could theoretically cause a closed loop obstruction between a competent ileocecal valve and the obstructing tumor and would not alleviate the risk of cecal perforation. Patients who have had prior mobilization of the right colon or who have distended small bowel on preoperative imaging may have an incompetent ileocecal valve, and therefore this theoretical risk may not be relevant. However, increased risk of fluid loss via an ileostomy is still a consideration. To date, there is no data to indicate which type of diversion—colostomy or ileostomy—is superior. We recommend against creation of a right-sided colostomy as it is more challenging to reverse than an ileostomy and provides no functional benefit over loop ileostomy.

11.2.5 Endoscopic Stent Placement

An alternative option for the stable patient with proximal to mid-rectal tumors who have no signs of ischemia or perforation is endoscopic placement of self-expanding metal stents. This procedure is performed under moderate sedation in the endoscopy suite with the assistance of fluoroscopy. The stent should have at least a 2 cm overlap with normal colon on either side of the lesion and have a diameter of at least

24 mm [21]. Endoluminal stenting can provide decompression of the bowel, eliminate the need for a surgical procedure under general anesthesia, and serve as a bridge to a semi-elective oncologic resection [22]. It has a success rate of 83–99% and a short recovery time which allows rapid initiation of neoadjuvant therapy [23, 24].

Stent placement must be carefully utilized, as it has a major complication rate of 23–32% including ulceration, bleeding, tenesmus, occlusion, stent migration, and perforation [24, 25]. Stent placement is not recommended in patients who are on an antiangiogenic agent such as bevacizumab because of the heightened risk of perforation [26]. Dilation of the narrowing prior to stent placement is also discouraged due to an increased risk of perforation [23]. Stents that are placed too far distally may cause symptoms of anorectal pain that are prohibitive. It is therefore recommended that the lesion be at least 3 cm proximal to the top of the anal sphincters to undergo stenting [27].

After stent placement, the obstructive symptoms should subside within a few days. Abdominal radiograph may be used to evaluate stent position and to confirm appropriate bowel decompression.

11.2.6 Palliative Care

Endoscopic placement of self-expanding metal stents is the recommended treatment for patients that present emergently with an acute large bowel obstruction but have widely metastatic disease, terminal life expectancy, or comorbidities that preclude resection. In this subset of patients, stenting can be successfully placed in up to 97% with a short hospital length of stay and with relatively low rates of morbidity and mortality [27]. Repeat treatment may be needed such as endoscopic interventions, re-stenting, or subsequent fecal diversion [27, 28]. Palliative stenting does not change long-term survival but does improve quality of life with equally effective decompression compared to surgical management in this population [29].

Other palliative options are laser therapy or fulguration. If these less invasive procedures are unable to decompress the large bowel, a palliative diverting stoma may be considered [15]. In the stable patient with a partial bowel obstruction due to rectal cancer and without proximal bowel dilatation, chemoradiotherapy may be a reasonable option for symptomatic management and to prevent progression to complete obstruction.

In patients unable to undergo stent placement, laser therapy is a viable palliative option with a 65–91% rate of achieving long-term relief of obstructive symptoms [30–34]. Treatment usually requires multiple sessions to be effective; thus, for patients with an acute obstruction, in general, this is not an option. Advantages of laser therapy include simple application, cost-efficiency, and minimal morbidity or mortality [35]. Furthermore, laser therapy can treat obstruction and bleeding, whereas a diverting stoma does not address bleeding symptoms [36]. The risk of complications increases with multiple therapy sessions and includes bleeding, perforation, fistula formation, and pain [33]. Laser therapy can be used after self-expanding metal stent placement for tumor ingrowth causing reocclusion.

Endocavitary fulguration involves debulking of the rectal tumor under regional or general anesthesia and is another option for palliation of obstructing rectal cancers that is now rarely used.

11.3 Perforation

11.3.1 Clinical Presentation and Workup

Perforation in colorectal cancer is overall rare, occurring in 2.6–12% of patients, but has significant negative implications for patient outcomes [37]. The mortality rate for tumor-related perforation presenting emergently is as high as 65% [3]. Surgeons should have a keen suspicion that perforation often represents locally advanced disease and potentially metastatic disease. The presentation can be quite variable based on if the perforation is intraperitoneal, extraperitoneal, a free perforation, or contained. Additional factors to consider are if the patient is currently receiving chemotherapy as this may affect clinical presentation and therapeutic options. Regardless of the situation, the immediate priority is to control sepsis, followed by optimization of oncologic outcomes. Rectal cancer is best treated in a multimodal fashion; thus, definitive resection is usually reserved for a later date and temporizing surgery may be preferred.

11.3.2 Intraperitoneal Perforation

Patients with a high rectal cancer with intraperitoneal perforation will present with the typical signs of a perforated viscus including tachycardia, fever, generalized peritonitis, altered mental status, and tachypnea. Patients with contained perforation may present with focal peritonitis. In patients with perforated cecum due to a downstream obstruction, the symptoms may resemble late appendicitis with generalized peritonitis [7].

We recommend CT scan of the abdomen and pelvis with IV contrast for diagnostic imaging. CT scan has a sensitivity and specificity greater than 95% for detection of perforation [38]. In general, oral contrast has a limited role when there is concern for perforation from rectal cancer and will provide an undue delay in obtaining the scan. Rectal contrast may be helpful in defining patient anatomy and the extent of perforation but does have the theoretical risk of worsening intraperitoneal contamination. The additional benefit of CT scan is that it allows for staging of the abdomen for evidence of liver metastasis or carcinomatosis. If CT scan is unavailable or the patient is hemodynamically unstable, an acute abdominal X-ray series (including an upright chest radiograph to assess for free air) can be combined with contrast enema radiograph to evaluate for obvious extravasation. If there is concern for perforation, it is important to notify the performing radiologist so that water-soluble contrast is used instead of barium due to the risk of barium peritonitis.

11.3.3 Extraperitoneal Perforation

Patients with an extraperitoneal perforation will often present with symptoms of rectal pain and may also have tachycardia and fever. On physical exam, they may have minimal discomfort on abdominal exam due to a low perforation. On digital rectal exam, a defect may be felt for a low-lying tumor or elicit pain due to local inflammation if a defect is not palpated.

For imaging evaluation, we again recommend CT scan of the abdomen and pelvis with IV contrast. The use of rectal contrast in this setting may further define the perforation anatomy but often is not tolerated due to pain. If CT is not available, plain-film X-rays to rule out intra-abdominal perforation are helpful. Contrast enema in the setting in which CT is not available is the best imaging test to delineate the rectal anatomy. Although rectal MRI is the local staging imaging of choice, in addition to CT, it should be deferred until after control of sepsis.

11.3.4 Treatment

Management of tumor-related perforation begins with resuscitation, correction of metabolic derangements, and administration of IV antibiotics. Further treatment depends on the level of perforation as well as the stability of the patient (Fig. 11.2).

11.3.5 Intraperitoneal Perforation

Perforation of high rectal cancers that are intraperitoneal can be treated similarly to perforation due to colon cancers. Emergent surgery is generally required, with the

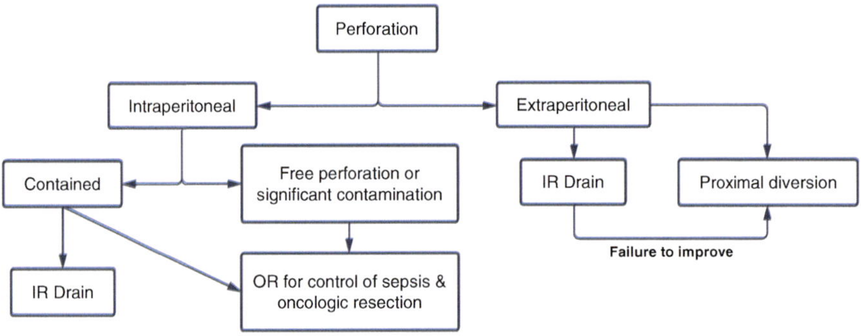

Fig. 11.2 Management of bowel perforation due to rectal cancer

primary goal of controlling contamination [3]. A well-placed clamp or suture across the site of perforation is the first step of the operation. The next steps depend on patient stability and site of perforation. Patients may perforate at the site of the tumor due to locally advanced disease. They may also perforate upstream from the tumor due to obstruction as mentioned previously [7]. If the perforation occurs immediately proximal to the malignancy, an extended resection to include both areas of pathology may be considered [3]. If the proximal perforation is far removed from the tumor site (i.e., the cecum), we recommend resection of the perforated segment with creation of a proximal end stoma and mucous fistula. We advise against trying to anastomose the colon and create a more proximal stoma as the intervening segment of bowel is often attenuated from the obstruction and not amenable to anastomosis. Options for reconstruction and closure also depend upon the patient's clinical status at the time of surgery.

We will focus on perforation at the site of tumor for the discussion below. In the unstable patient, simple bowel resection at the site of perforation with the bowel left in discontinuity and temporary abdominal closure may be all that is possible. After aggressive resuscitation in the intensive care setting, the patient can be brought back to the operating room for a more definitive surgery.

For contained perforations, one can consider drainage by interventional radiology (IR), but this is a temporizing measure as tumor does not tend to seal itself as compared to IR drainage of diverticular abscesses. This may allow for complete staging of the patient and/or transfer to a higher volume rectal cancer center for more definitive treatment.

For the stable patient, a definitive operation is preferred. Surgeons should aim for an oncologic resection with 5 cm proximal and distal margins for upper rectal cancers and 1–2 cm for more distal rectal cancers. In general, a high ligation of the inferior mesenteric artery near the takeoff from the aorta allows for appropriate yield of at least 12 lymph nodes [4]. The distal dissection will involve entering into the avascular mesorectal plain for an oncologic total mesorectal excision (TME). It is easiest to enter this plane posteriorly and carry the dissection around anteriorly. It is important to identify and protect the ureters during this dissection. Most patients in this situation are best served with an end colostomy. Factors to be considered when deciding whether to perform an anastomosis include patient stability, medical comorbidities, tissue quality, technical challenges in performing a tension-free anastomosis, and duration and extent of fecal contamination [15]. Carefully selected patients may undergo primary anastomosis, but in that scenario, strong consideration should be made for a diverting loop ileostomy. If the surgeon is unfamiliar with this anatomy, it may be better to transfer the patient to a tertiary center with an available colorectal surgeon rather than perform an oncologically inadequate surgery or risk injuring neighboring structures.

11.3.6 Extraperitoneal Perforation

For extraperitoneal perforations, the septic source is somewhat confined within the mesorectum. These patients are most likely to benefit from a multidisciplinary approach for their lower rectal cancer including neoadjuvant chemoradiotherapy. Thus, surgical interventions should aim to minimize further contamination. Some patients may be managed with percutaneous drainage, but there is concern for seeding the drainage tract with tumor cells which could make the patient unresectable. Therefore, any drain should be placed such that the drain and tract can be later excised. Because of this concern, many patients undergo proximal diversion as a method to control sepsis.

Similar to the management of tumor-related obstruction, the preferred stoma is a diverting loop sigmoid colostomy. In the setting of nonreconstructible rectal cancer, the distal limb can be transected, and the proximal sigmoid stoma limb left in situ as the definitive stoma. If a sigmoid colostomy cannot be fashioned, a loop ileostomy is preferred as these patients will often require ileostomy following oncologic rectal cancer resection after neoadjuvant therapy.

After the patient has been treated with neoadjuvant chemoradiation, the oncologic resection should include the usual margins as well as all tissues that have been exposed to the malignant cells by the contained perforation and drainage tracts. This may require a more extensive procedure such as a pelvic exenteration or extramesorectal dissection [15].

11.4 Bleeding

11.4.1 Clinical Presentation

Rectal cancer is a relatively rare cause of emergent, severe lower gastrointestinal bleeding, accounting for under 10% of all bleeding episodes in patients greater than 50 years of age [39]. It is more likely to present as a low-volume, transient, or intermittent bleed that prompts evaluation with an outpatient colonoscopy, leading to the diagnosis of rectal malignancy [11, 39]. However, it is not uncommon for patients with rectal bleeding or rectal cancer to have a delayed presentation. Patients may attribute rectal bleeding to hemorrhoids and defer proper evaluation [15]. A study by Forbes et al. looking at the risk factors for delay in symptomatic presentation in patients with malignancies found that 37% of patients with rectal cancer sought medical care over 3 months after the onset of symptoms, ranking this disease as the second most common type of malignancy to have a delayed presentation [40].

When rectal cancer presents with lower gastrointestinal bleeding in the emergency department, patients report bright red blood per rectum and other symptoms of acute blood loss anemia including lightheadedness, unsteadiness, fatigue, palpitations, nausea, thirst, diaphoresis, clammy skin, visual changes, irritability, lethargy, confusion, or syncope. They may complain of other symptoms of rectal cancer such as change in bowel habits, malaise, weight loss, abdominal pain, or pelvic pain [7].

11.4.2 Workup

A focused history should be obtained to characterize the rectal bleeding including the volume of blood loss and any recent rectal trauma. History-taking should include previous GI bleeding, prior colonoscopy results, prior diagnoses of colorectal malignancy or anorectal pathology, previous abdominopelvic surgeries or procedures, and any family history of colorectal cancer and/or inflammatory bowel disorder. It should also include screening for factors that may cause prolonged bleeding such as anticoagulant or antiplatelet use, liver failure, chronic renal disease, or bleeding disorders.

Severe hematochezia is defined as continued bleeding in the first 24 h of admission, a fall in hemoglobin by at least 2 g/dL, and requirement of at least 2 units of packed red blood cell (PRBC) transfusions. Severe bleeding may cause hemodynamic changes that reflect the degree of blood loss. Patients with <15% blood loss in Class I hemorrhage exhibit mild tachycardia. With 15–30% blood loss (Class II), patients become tachypneic and the pulse pressure narrows. Class III hemorrhage with 30–40% blood loss leads to hypotension and pale, cool skin. Class IV hemorrhage with >40% blood loss causes hypotension with end-organ effects such as altered mental status, loss of consciousness, and, eventually, cardiac arrest.

In patients with rectal tumor-associated bleeding, patients often have painless hematochezia with a benign abdominal examination. External perianal examination should be performed to evaluate for significant hemorrhoids, anal fissure, or rectal prolapse. On digital rectal examination, a rectal mass may be palpated. If it is not obviously apparent that the hematochezia is due to a lower gastrointestinal source, a nasogastric tube should be placed for examination of the color of the gastric fluid. If the gastric aspirate is bloody, evaluation for an upper GI source should commence.

Workup should include complete blood count, comprehensive metabolic panel, coagulopathy panel, and type and screen. Depending on the duration and severity of the tumor-associated hemorrhage, patients may have a normal hemoglobin or may exhibit normocytic anemia. The acute bleeding episode may be superimposed on anemia of chronic disease due to malignancy or on chronic anemia secondary to low-volume tumor-associated bleeding, previously attributed to benign anorectal pathology such as hemorrhoids [11].

Anoscopy and rigid proctosigmoidoscopy are cheap, rapid diagnostic tools that can be performed at the bedside. Common anorectal causes for bleeding can be ruled out, such as hemorrhoids, rectal prolapse, diverticular bleeding, or proctitis, and bleeding rectal tumors can be visualized [41]. The distance of the rectal tumor from the anal verge should be noted for eventual surgical planning [41]. In patients with brisk, arterial bleeding, anoscopy and proctosigmoidoscopy can also guide application of packing to temporize the bleed. In stable patients, colonoscopy is the recommended diagnostic modality to localize the bleeding site and has the advantage of also being therapeutic. Although a bowel prep is helpful, it is not necessary in all patients. The bleeding rectal tumor can be identified, and synchronous colorectal lesions should be ruled out. Endoscopic treatment modalities are discussed in the next section.

Imaging modalities include CT angiography, tagged red blood cell scans, and traditional angiography, though for patients presenting in the emergency setting with rectal bleeding, the source may be more evident. CT angiography is the preferred initial imaging and can localize the area of hemorrhage with a sensitivity of approximately 92% with active bleeding [39]. In patients with intermittent bleeding, the sensitivity decreases to 45–47% [15]. It is quick, widely available, does not require a bowel prep, and can detect bleeds with a rate as low as 0.3 mL/min [15]. Only IV contrast should be given as oral, or rectal contrast may obscure localization. The arterial phase images are best for identifying active extravasation or vascular malformations, while the portal venous images are valuable in detecting bowel wall thickening or hypovascular lesions [39]. Disadvantages include the exposure to ionizing radiation, potential for kidney injury due to IV contrast, and low sensitivity of localization with intermittent bleeds. It also allows for planning for IR-guided interventions.

Tagged reg blood cell scans have a sensitivity of 93% and specificity of 95% and can be used with bleeding rates as low as 0.04 mL/min [42]. However, these scans take time to perform the red blood cell radiolabel. In addition, for patients presenting with emergent bleeding, the site should be easily found via rigid proctosigmoidoscopy.

Although traditional angiography is an option for bleeding localization, it is infrequently used for initial diagnosis due to its invasive nature and the efficacy of the other two forms of imaging. This method can localize the hemorrhage with a bleeding rate as low as 0.5–1.5 mL/min [15]. If interventional radiology treatments (e.g., angioembolization) are required, traditional angiography is performed at the beginning of the case to establish the target treatment site.

11.4.3 Treatment

Management of the patient presenting emergently with a bleeding rectal mass should begin with standard resuscitation, including two large-bore IVs with crystalloids or blood transfusions as needed. Underlying coagulopathy or metabolic derangements should be corrected. Direct pressure should be applied, if possible, to the area of hemorrhage. Control of the bleeding site may be achieved with local interventions, endoscopic therapies, interventional radiology therapies, radiation therapy, or surgical intervention (Fig. 11.3).

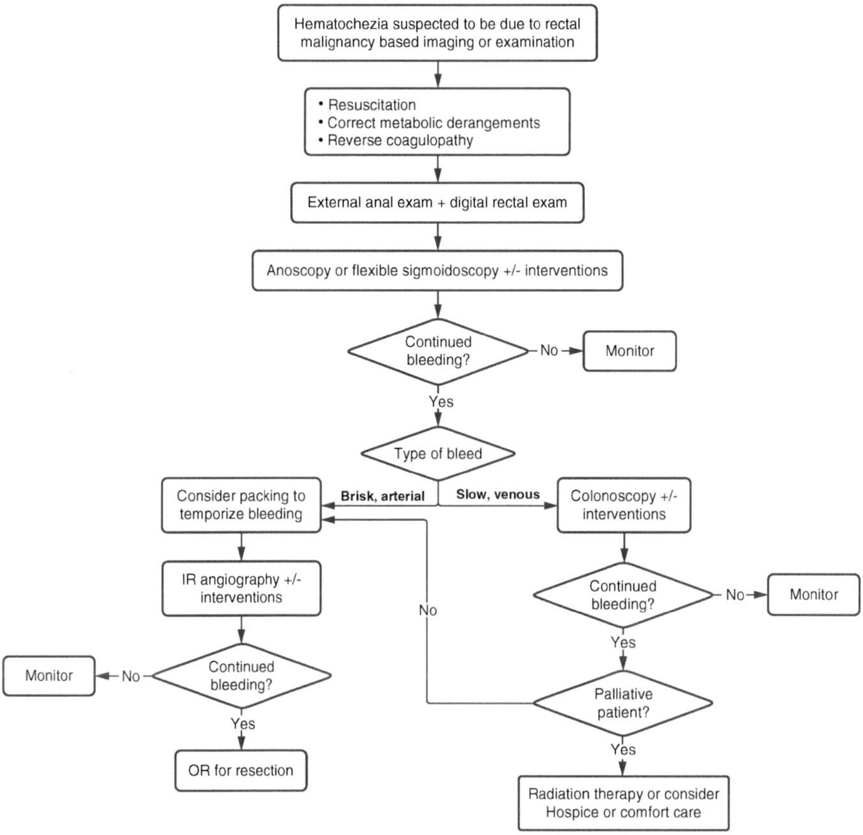

Fig. 11.3 Management of lower gastrointestinal bleeding due to rectal cancer

11.4.4 Local Interventions

If the patient can tolerate bedside examination with anoscopy or rigid proctoscopy, local interventions may be attempted to achieve hemostasis. Packing may be placed in the rectum to tamponade the bleeding and temporize the bleeding until more definitive treatment can be pursued. The packing material may be using Kerlix or topical thrombogenic materials such as Surgicel® (Ethicon, Cincinnati, OH, USA) or Gelfoam® (Pfizer, New York, NY, USA). Treatment of the bleeding site with formalin swabs may be considered. However, the application of formalin can cause a burning sensation if touching the perianal skin and be difficult to tolerate. In addition, care should be taken to avoid accidentally touching healthy tissue with the formalin swab.

11.4.5 Endoscopic Therapies

Colonoscopy is diagnostic and therapeutic and may localize the bleeding site in 74–100% of patients [15]. If patients are stable, this is the diagnostic and therapeutic modality of choice. A bowel prep is helpful but may not be necessary. Sometimes, a tap water enema may suffice. Overall, endoscopic therapies are effective in attaining hemostasis but are encumbered by significant rebleeding rates [43]. Nevertheless, these treatment modalities may help the patient avoid undergoing an emergent operation or may temporize the bleeding long enough to allow treatment with chemotherapy, radiation therapy, or an oncologic resection [43].

Depending on the tumor morphology and size, clips, bands, or Endoloops® (Ethicon, Cincinnati, OH, USA) may be used [44]. The rebleeding rate with clips is as high as 33%, and with bands, it is approximately 6% [15]. Tumor-associated bleeding is often diffuse. The bleeding surface may be sprayed with topical agents such as thrombin products or Hemospray® (Cook Medical, Bloomington, IN, USA), a hemostatic powder approved for hemostasis in non-variceal GI bleeds [44]. However, if there is persistent bleeding, the topical agent can obscure the site of bleeding, making it more difficult to target further therapies. Alternatively, ethanol, epinephrine, or hypertonic saline with epinephrine may be injected around the bleeding site to promote thrombogenesis [44]. Rebleeding rate with epinephrine injection has been reported to be as high as 35% [15].

Contact and noncontact thermal techniques may be used endoscopically. Contact thermal therapies include the use of monopolar or bipolar electrocautery, heater probes, or coagulation forceps. Although these methods have high rates of initial success, studies have shown a 33–80% risk of rebleeding within 30 days [44].

Noncontact thermal therapies include laser ablation and argon plasma coagulation (APC). Endoscopic laser coagulation is most often performed using the neodymium yttrium argon garnet (Nd:YAG) laser. The laser energy causes coagulative necrosis and tissue vaporization, and multiple sessions may be necessary for resolution of bleeding. It has been shown to take 2–5 sessions in 80–90% of patients to attain initial hemostasis and has a complication rate of 2–15% and a rebleeding rate of 10–80% [43, 45]. Laser ablation can be challenging in angulated areas of the rectum or with circumferential or long-segment lesions. Endoscopic laser therapy may be combined with other treatment modalities such as radiotherapy to improve its efficacy in palliating rectal bleeding [36, 46].

In APC, electrocautery is used to ionize argon gas, which is released from the probe to cause coagulative necrosis and fulguration of the tissues. It is highly effective at achieving initial hemostasis but has a rebleeding rate of approximately 33% [44]. When used properly, the effects are limited to a depth of 2–3 mm, and therefore, it is safer than laser ablation with a lower risk of causing perforation. It is also faster, less expensive, and simpler to use than laser ablation and, therefore, has become the favored noncontact thermal therapeutic modality for the management of gastrointestinal bleeding [45].

11.4.6 Interventional Radiology Therapies

If endoscopic therapies have failed to control the bleeding site or are not possible due to obscured visualization from significant ongoing hemorrhage, angiography with arterial interventions may be performed by the interventional radiologist. Angiography is completed to localize the area of bleeding, and the feeding artery is super-selectively catheterized as distally as possible for treatment [47]. Once the catheter has been placed at or beyond the mesenteric border, the vessel is embolized using coils or particulate, liquid, or gel embolic agents [42, 48]. Angioembolization may be successful in achieving hemostasis with active arterial bleeding in 50–100% of patients with a rebleeding rate of 22–24% [15]. The risk of ischemic complications from embolization is now rare due to the development of smaller catheters, able to super-select distal vessels.

When the distal artery is unable to be super-selectively catheterized or when there is a wide area of bleeding, intra-arterial vasopressin infusion may be administered to induce local vasoconstriction and clot formation [43]. It can be successful in 59–90% of cases but has a high rebleeding rate of 36–43% and may cause systemic hemodynamic changes, arrhythmias, or bowel ischemia. The catheter is left in place for 24–48 h, which introduces the risk of catheter dislodgement, infection, and line-associated thrombus formation [42, 47].

Risks of angiographic interventions include recurrent bleeding, bowel ischemia/perforation, access-site bleeding or hematoma, and arterial complications like dissection, perforation, or pseudoaneurysm [47].

11.4.7 Radiation Therapy

Radiation therapy is effective in causing hemostasis in 87–100% of patients with bleeding rectal tumors [3]. It is indicated with failure of other nonoperative interventions at obtaining hemostasis and is the first-line therapy for palliative treatment [3, 49]. Radiation therapy stimulates release of von Willebrand factor, causing improved platelet adhesion to the extracellular matrix of endothelial cells, resulting in platelet plug formation. It can cause vessel fibrosis and tumor shrinkage, resulting in long-term hemostasis [49]. In palliative radiation therapy for bleeding rectal cancers, there is a 78–87% complete response rate to therapy and up to a 100% partial response rate [50, 51]. In one study, 91% of those who had hemostasis after radiation therapy suffered no subsequent rebleeding events [50]. Radiation may be combined with chemotherapy for neoadjuvant treatment or for palliation. The side effects of radiation therapy appear to be mild to moderate in severity. Potential complications include radiation enteritis or proctitis, adhesive bowel obstruction, pelvic scarring, chronic pain, rectal stenosis, skin fibrosis or necrosis, and fistula formation [52].

11.4.8 Surgical Resection

Resection is the most definitive therapy for a bleeding rectal mass. In general, clinical indications for surgery are as follows, although risks and benefits must be weighed depending on the specific clinical scenario [11]:

- Hemodynamic instability despite administration of greater than 6 units of packed red blood cells (PRBCs)
- Transfusion requirement of greater than 3 units of PRBC daily
- Bleeding refractory to endoscopic or angiographic interventions
- Persistent bleeding with obstruction, perforation, intussusception, and/or peritonitis

Unless the patient's disease burden has already deemed this to be a palliative case, the resection should be performed with curative intent, in keeping with general oncologic principles. Surgical options with localized tumor-related bleeding include a Hartmann's procedure, an abdominoperineal resection, a resection with primary anastomosis with or without a proximal diverting loop ileostomy, or pelvic exenteration. The choice of surgical procedure depends on the extent of invasion to local structures and the level of the tumor in relation to the anal sphincter. The decision on whether to perform an anastomosis is determined by the operative hemodynamic stability of the patient, their comorbidities, and any anticipated technical challenges in creating a tension-free anastomosis. One must also consider the risk of anastomotic leak with resultant delay in adjuvant therapy. When primary anastomosis is performed in the emergent setting of rectal cancer, a protecting loop ostomy should be considered as well.

11.4.9 Experimental Therapies

Other promising treatment modalities for tumor-associated bleeding in rectal cancer include IV desmopressin and radiofrequency ablation [44, 53]. A study looking at the safety and preliminary efficacy of desmopressin in patients with moderate-to-severe hemorrhage due to rectal adenocarcinoma showed complete hemostasis in 58% and at least partial hemostasis in 92% of patients treated with the maximal tolerated dose. Most adverse events were mild to moderate in severity and reversible [53]. Randomized phase III clinical trials are needed for further investigation into the effectiveness of this medication for this purpose.

11.5 Outcomes of Emergency Surgery

Overall, patients undergoing emergency surgery have worse oncologic outcomes compared to patients undergoing elective surgery. Due to the physiologic strain from perforation, patients may not be able to undergo en bloc resection, precluding the best oncologic outcome [54]. Most of the literature on perforation does not distinguish between colon and rectal cancer patients. Mortality rates at 30 days are as high as 40.5%, but a more recent series found a mortality rate of 11.8% [55, 56]. Phang et al. compared outcomes of patients with rectal cancer presenting emergently vs. electively [5]. They found that disease-specific survival at 4 years for stage II cancers was 14% worse and for stage III cancers 13% worse in the emergent presentation population. Local recurrence was 5% higher in stage II emergent patients and 50% higher in stage III emergent patients.

11.6 Oncologic Considerations

Systemic treatment with chemotherapy and molecularly targeted agents is commonly used in the management of patients with rectal adenocarcinoma. The cytotoxic agents that are usually used are oxaliplatin, irinotecan, and fluoropyrimidines (fluorouracil or capecitabine). On the other hand, targeted agents are mainly used in the metastatic setting and can be mainly classified into agents targeting epidermal growth factor receptor (EGFR) and others targeting vascular endothelial growth factor (VEGF) inhibitors such as bevacizumab [57].

11.6.1 Perforation

VEGF inhibitors carry a black box warning for the risk of gastrointestinal perforation, wound healing complications, and hemorrhage. The incidence of gastrointestinal perforation with bevacizumab is estimated to be at 0.3–3% across different studies with highest incidence in patients with prior pelvic radiation [58]. Overall, majority of these perforations occur within 50 days of the first dose. A perforation episode is a contraindication for any subsequent use of VEGF inhibitors.

11.6.2 Bleeding

Both chemotherapy and VEGF inhibitors carry a risk of bleeding. However, VEGF inhibitors have been found to be associated with a fivefold increased risk of bleeding compared to chemotherapy alone [58]. Overall, severe bleeding (grades 3–5) ranges from 0.4 to 7% in patients receiving bevacizumab. Any grade 3–5 hemorrhage is considered a contraindication for subsequent use of VEGF inhibitors [58].

11.6.3 Wound Healing Complications and Timing of Restarting Systemic Therapies

The decision regarding the timing of restarting chemotherapy after surgery is based on multidisciplinary discussion between the treatment teams. Overall, this depends on the patient recovery from the surgery rather than a direct effect of the chemotherapy on the healing process. This is in contrast to VEGF inhibitors where such agents are known to interrupt would healing [59]. Therefore, it is recommended not to administer bevacizumab for at least 28 days after surgery and until the wound is fully healed.

Chemotherapy is usually started about 4 weeks after major surgery and preferably no longer than 8 weeks in the adjuvant setting, with some studies suggesting worse survival for patients who were started after 8 weeks [60].

11.7 Conclusion

Rectal cancer patients who present with acute obstruction, perforation, or bleeding must be managed to address life-threatening surgical disease, with attention to future oncologic treatments or options as able. For patients with complex oncologic disease, collaboration with colorectal surgery and/or oncology may be warranted for long-term treatment planning. Therapy may also require a multidisciplinary team, involving not only surgical and medical oncologists, but also gastroenterology, radiation oncology, interventional radiology, and palliative medicine specialists when indicated. Unfortunately, patients with emergent presentations have decreased long-term survival compared to patients who present non-emergently. Lastly, it is of utmost importance to consider palliation and symptom management throughout the course of treatment, to ensure alignment between patient priorities and medical goals.

Conflicts of Interest The authors have no conflicts of interest to disclose.

Authors Contributions All the authors contributed substantially to the literature review, analysis, and interpretation of data, drafting, and revising of the chapter.

References

1. Diggs JC, Xu F, Diaz M, Cooper GS. Failure to screen: predictors and burden of emergency colorectal cancer resection. Am J Manag Care. 2007;13(3):157.
2. Pisano M, Zorcolo L, Merli C, et al. 2017 WSES guidelines on colon and rectal cancer emergencies: obstruction and perforation. World J Emerg Surg. 2018;13(1):1–27.
3. You YN, Hardiman KM, Bafford A, et al. The American Society of Colon and Rectal Surgeons clinical practice guidelines for the management of rectal cancer. Dis Colon Rectum. 2020;63(9):1191–222.
4. National Comprehensive Cancer Network. NCCN Clinical Practice Guidelines in Oncology. Rectal Cancer. Version 2.2021. National Comprehensive Cancer Network. Updated 9/20/2021. 2021. https://www.nccn.org/professionals/physician_gls/pdf/rectal_blocks.pdf. Accessed 10 Sept 2021.
5. Phang PT, MacFarlane JK, Taylor RH, et al. Effect of emergent presentation on outcome from rectal cancer management. Am J Surg. 2003;185(5):450–4.

6. Deans G, Krukowski Z, Irwin S. Malignant obstruction of the left colon. J Br Surg. 1994;81(9):1270–6.
7. Gordon PH, Nivatvongs S. Neoplasms of the colon, rectum, and anus. Boca Raton: CRC Press; 2007.
8. Chapman A, McNamara M, Porter G. The acute contrast enema in suspected large bowel obstruction: value and technique. Clin Radiol. 1992;46(4):273–8.
9. Frager D, Rovno H, Baer J, Bashist B, Friedman M. Prospective evaluation of colonic obstruction with computed tomography. Abdom Imaging. 1998;23(2):141–6.
10. Beattie GC, Peters RT, Guy S, Mendelson RM. Computed tomography in the assessment of suspected large bowel obstruction. ANZ J Surg. 2007;77(3):160–5.
11. Baer C, Menon R, Bastawrous S, Bastawrous A. Emergency presentations of colorectal cancer. Surg Clin. 2017;97(3):529–45.
12. Alavi K, Friel CM. Large bowel obstruction. In: The ASCRS textbook of colon and rectal surgery. Cham: Springer; 2016. p. 669–95.
13. Lohsiriwat V. Anorectal emergencies. World J Gastroenterol. 2016;22(26):5867.
14. Enker WE. The elusive goal of preoperative staging in rectal cancer. Ann Surg Oncol. 2004;11(3):245.
15. Steele SR, Hull TL, Read TE, Saclarides TJ, Senagore AJ, Whitlow CB. The ASCRS textbook of colon and rectal surgery. Cham: Springer; 2016.
16. Gorissen KJ, Tuynman J, Fryer E, Wang L, Uberoi R, Jones OM, Cunningham C, Lindsey I. Local recurrence after stenting for obstructing left-sided colonic cancer. Br J Surg. 2013;100(13):1805–9.
17. Cao Y, Gu J, Deng S, Li J, Wu K, Cai K. Long-term tumour outcomes of self-expanding metal stents as 'bridge to surgery' for the treatment of colorectal cancer with malignant obstruction: a systematic review and meta-analysis. Int J Color Dis. 2019;34(11):1827–38.
18. Shimura T, Joh T. Evidence-based clinical management of acute malignant colorectal obstruction. J Clin Gastroenterol. 2016;50(4):273–85.
19. Malakorn S, Stein SL, Lee JH, You YN. Urgent management of obstructing colorectal cancer: divert, stent, or resect? J Gastrointest Surg. 2019;23(2):425–32.
20. Smothers L, Hynan L, Fleming J, Turnage R, Simmang C, Anthony T. Emergency surgery for colon carcinoma. Dis Colon Rectum. 2003;46(1):24–30.
21. Van Hooft JE, Van Halsema EE, Vanbiervliet G, et al. Self-expandable metal stents for obstructing colonic and extracolonic cancer: European Society of Gastrointestinal Endoscopy (ESGE) clinical guideline. Endoscopy. 2014;46(11):990–1053.
22. Ceresoli M, Allievi N, Coccolini F, et al. Long-term oncologic outcomes of stent as a bridge to surgery versus emergency surgery in malignant left side colonic obstructions: a meta-analysis. J Gastrointest Oncol. 2017;8(5):867.
23. Khot U, Lang AW, Murali K, Parker M. Systematic review of the efficacy and safety of colorectal stents. J Br Surg. 2002;89(9):1096–102.
24. Small AJ, Coelho-Prabhu N, Baron TH. Endoscopic placement of self-expandable metal stents for malignant colonic obstruction: long-term outcomes and complication factors. Gastrointest Endosc. 2010;71(3):560–72.
25. Choi JH, Lee YJ, Kim ES, et al. Covered self-expandable metal stents are more associated with complications in the management of malignant colorectal obstruction. Surg Endosc. 2013;27(9):3220–7.
26. Van Halsema EE, Van Hooft JE, Small AJ, et al. Perforation in colorectal stenting: a meta-analysis and a search for risk factors. Gastrointest Endosc. 2014;79(6):970–82.
27. Hünerbein M, Krause M, Moesta KT, Rau B, Schlag PM. Palliation of malignant rectal obstruction with self-expanding metal stents. Surgery. 2005;137(1):42–7.
28. Tomiki Y, Watanabe T, Ishibiki Y, et al. Comparison of stent placement and colostomy as palliative treatment for inoperable malignant colorectal obstruction. Surg Endosc Other Interv Tech. 2004;18(11):1572–7.

29. Darr H, Abbas MA. Novel treatment strategies for advanced and aggressive colorectal cancer—multidisciplinary solutions: stenting as a bridge to surgery or a palliative treatment. Clin Colon Rectal Surg. 2020;33(5):279.
30. Mandava N, Petrelli N, Herrera L, Nava H. Laser palliation for colorectal carcinoma. Am J Surg. 1991;162(3):212–4.
31. Daneker GW, Carlson GW, Hohn DC, Lynch P, Roubein L, Levin B. Endoscopic laser recanalization is effective for prevention and treatment of obstruction in sigmoid and rectal cancer. Arch Surg. 1991;126(11):1348–52.
32. Brunetaud JM, Maunoury V, Cochelard D. Lasers in rectosigmoid tumors. Semin Surg Oncol. 1995;11(4):319–27.
33. Gevers A-M, Macken E, Hiele M, Rutgeerts P. Endoscopic laser therapy for palliation of patients with distal colorectal carcinoma: analysis of factors influencing long-term outcome. Gastrointest Endosc. 2000;51(5):580–5.
34. Loizou L, Grigg D, Boulos P, Bown S. Endoscopic Nd: YAG laser treatment of rectosigmoid cancer. Gut. 1990;31(7):812–6.
35. Rao V, Al-Mukhtar A, Rayan F, Stojkovic S, Moore P, Ahmad S. Endoscopic laser ablation of advanced rectal carcinoma—a DGH experience. Color Dis. 2005;7(1):58–60.
36. Mischinger H, Hauser H, Cerwenka H, et al. Endocavitary Ir-192 radiation and laser treatment for palliation of obstructive rectal cancer. Eur J Surg Oncol. 1997;23(5):428–31.
37. Baer C, Menon R, Bastawrous S, Bastawrous A. Emergency presentations of colorectal cancer. Surg Clin N Am. 2017;97(3):529–45.
38. Barnett A, Cedar A, Siddiqui F, Herzig D, Fowlkes E, Thomas CR Jr. Colorectal cancer emergencies. J Gastrointest Cancer. 2013;44(2):132–42.
39. Raman SP, Horton KM, Fishman EK. MDCT and CT angiography evaluation of rectal bleeding: the role of volume visualization. Am J Roentgenol. 2013;201(3):589–97.
40. Forbes LJ, Warburton F, Richards M, Ramirez A. Risk factors for delay in symptomatic presentation: a survey of cancer patients. Br J Cancer. 2014;111(3):581–8.
41. Ferguson MA. Office evaluation of rectal bleeding. Clin Colon Rectal Surg. 2005;18(04):249–54.
42. Cherian MP, Mehta P, Kalyanpur TM, Hedgire SS, Narsinghpura KS. Arterial interventions in gastrointestinal bleeding. Semin Intervent Radiol. 2009;26(3):184–96.
43. Heller SJ, Tokar JL, Nguyen MT, Haluszka O, Weinberg DS. Management of bleeding GI tumors. Gastrointest Endosc. 2010;72(4):817–24.
44. Ofosu A, Ramai D, Latson W, Adler DG. Endoscopic management of bleeding gastrointestinal tumors. Ann Gastroenterol. 2019;32(4):346.
45. Ronnekleiv-Kelly SM, Kennedy GD. Management of stage IV rectal cancer: palliative options. World J Gastroenterol. 2011;17(7):835.
46. Chapuis P, Yuile P, Dent O, Sinclair G, Low L, Aggarwal G. Combined endoscopic laser and radiotherapy palliation of advanced rectal cancer. ANZ J Surg. 2002;72(2):95–9.
47. Ramaswamy RS, Choi HW, Mouser HC, et al. Role of interventional radiology in the management of acute gastrointestinal bleeding. World J Radiol. 2014;6(4):82.
48. Wang CY, Hu J, Sheth RA, Oklu R. Emerging embolic agents in endovascular embolization: an overview. Prog Biomed Eng. 2020;2(1):012003.
49. Shuja M, Nazli S, Mansha MA, et al. Bleeding in locally invasive pelvic malignancies: is hypofractionated radiation therapy a safe and effective non-invasive option for securing hemostasis? A single institution perspective. Cureus. 2018;10(2):e2137.
50. Chia D, Lu J, Zheng H, et al. Efficacy of palliative radiation therapy for symptomatic rectal cancer. Radiother Oncol. 2016;121(2):258–61.
51. Jain S, Engineer R, Ostwal V, et al. Addition of short course radiotherapy in newly diagnosed locally advanced rectal cancers with distant metastasis. Asia Pac J Clin Oncol. 2021;17(2):e70–6.
52. Cameron MG, Kersten C, Vistad I, Fosså S, Guren MG. Palliative pelvic radiotherapy of symptomatic incurable rectal cancer—a systematic review. Acta Oncol. 2014;53(2):164–73.

53. Iseas S, Roca EL, O'Connor JM, et al. Administration of the vasopressin analog desmopressin for the management of bleeding in rectal cancer patients: results of a phase I/II trial. Investig New Drugs. 2020;38(5):1580.
54. Teixeira F, Akaishi EH, Ushinohama AZ, et al. Can we respect the principles of oncologic resection in an emergency surgery to treat colon cancer? World J Emerg Surg. 2015;10(1):5.
55. Yamamoto T, Kita R, Masui H, et al. Prediction of mortality in patients with colorectal perforation based on routinely available parameters: a retrospective study. World J Emerg Surg. 2015;10:24. https://doi.org/10.1186/s13017-015-0020-y.
56. Anwar MA, D'Souza F, Coulter R, Memon B, Khan IM, Memon MA. Outcome of acutely perforated colorectal cancers: experience of a single district general hospital. Surg Oncol. 2006;15(2):91–6.
57. Sonbol MB, Mountjoy LJ, Firwana B, et al. The role of maintenance strategies in metastatic colorectal cancer: a systematic review and network meta-analysis of randomized clinical trials. JAMA Oncol. 2020;6(3):e194489.
58. FDA. Avastin FDA Label. 2011. Accessed 20 Dec 2021.
59. Scappaticci FA, Fehrenbacher L, Cartwright T, et al. Surgical wound healing complications in metastatic colorectal cancer patients treated with bevacizumab. J Surg Oncol. 2005;91(3):173–80.
60. Biagi JJ, Raphael MJ, Mackillop WJ, Kong W, King WD, Booth CM. Association between time to initiation of adjuvant chemotherapy and survival in colorectal cancer: a systematic review and meta-analysis. JAMA. 2011;305(22):2335–42.

Liver Oncologic Surgical Emergencies

12

Morgan Schellenberg, Sulaiman Nanji, Michael J. Raphael, and Chad G. Ball

12.1 Introduction

Liver malignancies are the third most common cause of death from cancer, after lung and colorectal malignancies, representing 8% of overall deaths from cancer worldwide in 2020 [1]. Despite being the third most common cause of cancer death, liver malignancy is only the seventh most common cancer diagnosis, comprising 5% of all new cancer diagnoses [1]. The discrepancy between frequency of death and diagnosis implies a particularly dismal prognosis after liver malignancy, with 20% relative survival [2]. This makes liver malignancies the second or third most lethal malignancy in the United States, after pancreatic cancer (10% relative survival) and esophageal cancer (20% relative survival) [2].

Liver tumors can arise from any of the hepatic cell types, most commonly the hepatocytes or cholangiocytes, and can be primary or metastatic. The most common primary liver malignancies are hepatocellular carcinoma (HCC) followed by

M. Schellenberg (✉)
Division of Acute Care Surgery, Department of Surgery, LAC+USC Medical Center, University of Southern California, Los Angeles, CA, USA
e-mail: Morgan.Schellenberg@med.usc.edu

S. Nanji
Division of Hepatobiliary Surgery, Department of Surgery, Kingston Health Sciences Center, Queen's University, Kingston, ON, USA
e-mail: sulaiman.nanji@kingstonhsc.ca

M. J. Raphael
Division of Gastrointestinal Oncology, Department of Medical Oncology, Sunnybrook Health Sciences Center, University of Toronto, Toronto, ON, USA
e-mail: michaelj.raphael@sunnybrook.ca

C. G. Ball
Division of Acute Care Surgery and Hepatobiliary Surgery, Department of Surgery, Foothills Medical Center, University of Calgary, Calgary, AB, USA

A. Tarasconi et al. (eds.), *Oncologic Surgical Emergencies*, Hot Topics in Acute Care Surgery and Trauma, https://doi.org/10.1007/978-3-031-36860-8_12

cholangiocarcinoma. There are a number of benign primary liver tumors as well, including hemangiomas, focal nodular hyperplasia lesions, and hepatic adenomas. Metastatic liver tumors are far more common than primary liver tumors. Gastrointestinal tract tumors, particularly colorectal malignancies, as well as breast, pancreas, lung, and kidney primary malignancies are particularly prone to liver metastasis.

Liver malignancies may be diagnosed incidentally or following investigations based on symptomatology, including jaundice, pain, bleeding, weight loss, or constitutional symptoms. Risk factors for liver malignancy may also be helpful to elicit because associated diagnoses can increase the likelihood of underlying liver malignancy. These include extrahepatic malignancies with the potential to metastasize to the liver; cirrhosis; hepatitis B infection, which can cause HCC in the absence of cirrhosis; nonalcoholic steatohepatitis (NASH); and other comorbidities known to increase the risk of cirrhosis and/or liver malignancy, such as hepatitis C infection, tobacco or alcohol use, and obesity.

Fortunately, liver masses infrequently pose a surgical emergency. It is important nonetheless for general surgeons to have an approach to hepatic surgical oncologic emergencies in order to be prepared for them when they do occur. Oncologic surgical emergencies of the liver may arise as the result of the tumor itself, either from a primary tumor or tumor metastases or as a sequela of tumor treatment, which can occur following operative intervention, locoregional therapies, or chemotherapy. This chapter explores these emergent complications and their surgical management after first providing an overview of the relevant hepatic anatomy and physiology as well as an approach to emergent liver surgery.

12.2 Anatomy and Physiology

The liver is an abdominal solid organ located in the right upper quadrant. It is affixed anteriorly to the abdominal wall by way of the falciform ligament and ligamentum teres; superolaterally to the diaphragm via the paired triangular and coronary ligaments; and posteriorly to the retroperitoneum and retrohepatic inferior vena cava (IVC).

The liver is divided into eight segments and three sectors, corresponding to areas of liver parenchyma with shared blood supply, lymphatics, and biliary drainage. These segments are particularly relevant when oncologic liver resections are planned. Segment I is synonymous with the caudate lobe posteriorly. Segments II–IV represent the left lobe of the liver, which is distinguished from the right lobe of the liver, comprised of segments V–VIII, by Cantlie's line. Cantlie's line is defined by the trajectory of the middle hepatic vein and bisects the gallbladder fossa.

Blood is supplied to the liver by way of the proper hepatic artery and portal vein. The proper hepatic artery is the continuation of the common hepatic artery after it spawns the gastroduodenal artery. The common hepatic artery, in turn, is a branch of the celiac trunk, which is the first unpaired branch off of the aorta. The proper hepatic artery provides approximately 50% of the oxygen delivery to the liver but 30% of blood inflow. It courses in the hepatoduodenal ligament to the porta hepatis with the portal vein and common bile duct before dividing into the right and left hepatic arteries. It must be noted that only approximately 80% of patients have this conventional hepatic arterial anatomy [3]. In the remaining 20% of individuals, the right and/or left hepatic arteries are aberrant and termed replaced or accessory.

Instead of dividing from the proper hepatic artery, a replaced right hepatic artery typically arises from the superior mesenteric artery and is the most common aberrancy in hepatic arterial anatomy [3]. A replaced left hepatic artery commonly branches off the left gastric artery. Because of the relative frequency of aberrant hepatic arterial anatomy, consideration should always be given to the possibility of replaced and accessory vessels during preoperative surgical planning and intraoperative dissection and in the presence of ongoing hemorrhage following standard vessel ligation/occlusion.

Portal venous anatomy is more consistent. The portal vein tributaries are the splenic vein and superior mesenteric vein, which converge behind the pancreatic head to form the portal vein. The portal vein supplies 50% of oxygenation to the liver but 70% of its blood flow. Within the hepatic parenchyma, the portal vein divides into the right and left portal veins to supply the respective lobes of the liver.

Venous drainage of the liver occurs through a separate pedicle, via the three hepatic veins (right, middle, and left), which are largely intraparenchymal short-segment veins that drain directly into the closely apposed retrohepatic IVC. The separation of blood inflow and outflow in the liver makes vascular exclusion of this abdominal solid organ more complicated than bleeding control of solid organs with a single vascular pedicle containing both inflow and outflow vessels, such as the kidney. This distinction is an important consideration in hemorrhage control for surgical oncologic liver emergencies, as discussed further below.

The biliary drainage of the liver occurs via the intrahepatic biliary tree, comprised of bile canaliculi present throughout the liver, which coalesce into interlobar bile ducts. In the right and left lobes of the liver, these join as tributaries to form the right and left hepatic bile ducts. These ducts become extrahepatic just below the hilar plate, where they course for a short segment before fusing to form the common hepatic duct. The common hepatic duct, in turn, is met by the cystic duct to form the common bile duct. The common bile duct is joined within the pancreatic head by the pancreatic duct, and these combined structures then empty together into the second stage of the duodenum via the ampulla of Vater through the sphincter of Oddi.

The liver serves a number of important physiologic functions. These include a central role in protein, carbohydrate, fat, and vitamin metabolism; protein and enzyme synthesis; detoxification and toxin excretion; fat digestion; and coagulation. Because of these numerous essential functions, the anhepatic state is incompatible with life.

12.3 Surgical Principles of Emergent Liver Surgery

In the discussion of emergent hepatic surgery, the operative considerations are preoperative preparations, patient positioning, choice of incision, exposure, and necessary interventions. Preoperative preparations begin with a history and physical examination and include obtaining a set of vital signs and establishing intravenous access. Any further presurgical workup hinges upon the clinical stability of the patient. Exsanguinating patients, for example from a ruptured hepatic adenoma or HCC, will have the inciting lesion diagnosed intraoperatively, and surgical hemorrhage control should not be delayed.

Stable patients, however, should undergo relevant laboratory investigations, including a complete blood count and coagulation profile, as well as any relevant tumor markers such as alpha-fetoprotein (AFP) and CA 19-9. Cross-sectional imaging typically begins with a computed tomography (CT) scan of the abdomen and pelvis with intravenous contrast. Arterial and venous phases will allow for the diagnosis of the majority of liver emergencies, including liver abscess or active extravasation of contrast, indicating ongoing bleeding. In a bleeding patient with the liver as a suspected source of hemorrhage, an arterial phase is a necessity.

More nuanced diagnosis of select liver lesions may necessitate a four-phase CT scan of the liver. These four phases are non-contrast, arterial, portal venous, and a delayed venous phase. In some circumstances, such as those involving an obstructing cholangiocarcinoma, magnetic resonance cholangiopancreatography (MRCP) is a useful imaging modality to specifically image the intra- and extrahepatic biliary tree.

Before proceeding with a discussion of surgical control of hepatic hemorrhage, it must be stated that the standard treatment for patients with ongoing hemorrhage from hepatic tumors remains nonoperative, including percutaneous-based angioembolization by interventional radiology. Most hepatic tumors are preferentially supplied by the hepatic artery, so selective embolization of the supplying arterial branch is often sufficient to achieve hemorrhage control. Not only can this process be more selective than surgical ligation of a hepatic artery, which can be treacherous in the hands of a non-hepatic/transplant surgeon, but it also avoids many of the associated risks of open surgical procedures, which is particularly beneficial in patients with chronic liver disease such as cirrhosis.

In the unstable patient, however, patient positioning for hepatic oncologic surgical emergencies is the same as for emergent surgical intervention for abdominal trauma and for most hepatic cases. The patient is positioned supine on the operating room table with the arms abducted and appropriate pressure points padded. In cases of significant bleeding as the cause for the oncologic emergency, it is prudent to proceed as one would for a bleeding trauma patient. This includes prepping and draping prior to induction of general anesthesia to facilitate prompt surgical hemorrhage control in case the patient becomes increasingly hypotensive or suffers cardiac arrest after induction. The abdomen and chest should both be prepped in case a thoracic incision is necessary for hemorrhage control.

The surgical incision for hepatic oncologic surgical emergencies will generally be a midline laparotomy. In select circumstances, such as intervention for a hepatic abscess, a right subcostal incision may be appropriate. A right subcostal incision is also best when the pathology is located in the right lobe of the liver as it improves ease of right lobe mobilization, particularly in obese patients and those with a deep peritoneal cavity. In patients with previous midline laparotomy incision, a right subcostal incision may also avoid adhesions or iatrogenic bowel injury upon abdominal entry. Although a right subcostal incision gives more immediate access to the liver, it provides limited exposure of the abdomen. For hemorrhage control cases and in general for hepatic surgical emergencies, a midline laparotomy is a more prudent selection since it affords broad and extensile exposure. Extension of a midline laparotomy to the patient's right side ("T-ing" off the incision) will improve exposure to all intra- and perihepatic anatomy. As a result, it represents the ultimate right upper quadrant surgical exposure. After gaining access to the peritoneal cavity, the next maneuvers hinge upon the indication for operative intervention.

12.3.1 Hemorrhage Control

For hemorrhage control cases, an intraoperative blood salvage device (cell saver) should be utilized if the inciting lesion is suspected to be nonmalignant, particularly in centers with limited access to blood products. After entering the abdomen, begin by inserting a self-retaining retractor and evacuate the intraperitoneal blood with suction or sponges. Rapidly divide the ligamentum teres between ties and/or energy instrumentation, and take down the falciform ligament. Next, use vectored packing above and below the liver to obtain temporary hemostasis. This typically provides at least a brief moment to apply a fixed-wall retractor while the next steps are planned. Communication with anesthesiology, the scrub technician, and the circulating nurse is critical throughout this process.

If the packing has temporarily controlled the bleeding, gently remove the packs next and inspect the underlying bleeding oncologic lesion. A variety of techniques can be used to achieve hemostasis, including electrocautery, sutures placed to the liver capsule, topical hemostatic agents (such as a combined saline/radiofrequency energy device [4]), liver resection (nonanatomic or anatomic), balloon catheter tamponade of the lesion [5], and tractotomy. In the context of a bleeding tumor, liver resection may be the most reasonable option to remove the inciting lesion if this is feasible and the surgeon has oncologic experience. However, surgical oncologic principles should never be prioritized over control of exsanguination. A large or deep location of the tumor, or the presence of abnormal surrounding liver parenchyma such as in the case of a cholestatic or cirrhotic liver, may preclude safe liver resection in the emergent setting. In these cases, achieving hemostasis without tumor resection will be the best approach.

If the bleeding is not controlled by packing or the hemorrhage control techniques presented above, locate the foramen of Winslow and apply a Pringle maneuver to occlude the porta hepatis. This will reduce inflow to the liver via the proper hepatic artery and the portal vein, unless there is a replaced left hepatic artery or accessory hepatic arteries. If packing and a Pringle maneuver do not abate the hemorrhage, the hemorrhage is significant and a rapid but organized approach must be undertaken. Before proceeding to total hepatic vascular exclusion, improve exposure via the addition of a right subcostal incision and/or by taking the right diaphragm off of the ribs, taking care to leave a cuff of diaphragm apposed to the chest wall to facilitate later reconstruction. In some cases, a sternotomy or right thoracotomy may be necessary to improve exposure and allow for direct hemorrhage control and/or total hepatic vascular exclusion.

This will provide a few minutes of abated hemorrhage in which the liver is rapidly mobilized along its ligamentous attachments to expose the area of bleeding and directly control it. In total hepatic vascular exclusion, there are four points of vascular occlusion: the porta hepatis, the aorta, the suprarenal infrahepatic inferior vena cava (IVC), and the suprahepatic IVC. Occlusion of the porta hepatis is often already accomplished from an earlier Pringle maneuver (e.g., Rummel tourniquet, vessel loop, or vascular clamp to free up space and hands).

The aorta should be clamped prior to IVC occlusion as the dramatic preload reduction that occurs from caval occlusion is likely to precipitate cardiac arrest unless it is preceded by removing the outflow needs to the body below the diaphragm. The suprahepatic IVC can be occluded infradiaphragmatically or intrapericardially. The selection of occlusion site depends on surgeon experience and the specific pathology encountered. Proponents of intrapericardial occlusion site ease of dissection, while opponents accurately point out that this requires a chest incision (sternotomy or thoracotomy). Surgeons who prefer to access the suprahepatic IVC below the diaphragm avoid the need for chest entry but may encounter a more challenging dissection in the setting of hemorrhage, albeit one that is comfortable and familiar for hepatobiliary and transplant surgeons.

The fourth point of occlusion is the infrahepatic IVC above the insertion of the renal veins. This exposure requires a Cattell-Braasch maneuver, in which the right colon is first medialized off the retroperitoneum by dividing the white line of Toldt and taking down the hepatic flexure. A Kocher maneuver follows to mobilize the duodenum. The third and final step is mobilization of the small bowel mesentery off the retroperitoneum along the line traced from the cecum to the ligament of Treitz. This provides complete exposure of the infrahepatic IVC, at which point the suprarenal portion is identified and occluded with a sponge stick (mobilization risks additional IVC injury).

Once total hepatic vascular exclusion is in place, rapidly begin to mobilize the liver off the retrohepatic IVC by dividing the right triangular and coronary ligaments with electrocautery. With this maneuver, the right lobe of the liver can be completely mobilized to the retrohepatic IVC, providing direct access to the area of bleeding in order to achieve hemorrhage control. This must occur quickly given the physiologic impact on the patient during vascular occlusion.

12.3.2 Infection Control

If the operation pursued is for the management of hepatic necrosis or abscess, access to the liver and initial division of the ligamentum teres and falciform ligament proceed in the same fashion. The liver can be mobilized as necessary to access the area of infection by using electrocautery to divide the ligamentous attachments as needed. Nonanatomic liver resection may be necessary to remove necrotic liver parenchyma, although consideration of anatomic resection with a neoplastic inciting lesion is appropriate with the same caveats as discussed above. If resection is not required and simple drainage will suffice, laparotomy pads should be placed around the abscess prior to drainage to avoid contaminating the peritoneal cavity with pus and/or tumor cells. The surgeon should always remember that the presence of neoplastic lesion as the underlying cause of an infective process has a significant impact on optimal patient management. While underlying malignancy should not prevent a surgeon from obtaining prompt source control in the context of life-threatening septic shock, it is prudent to involve a hepatobiliary surgeon or surgical oncologist in the care of non-critically ill patients with a malignancy-associated abscess. This allows for careful and deliberate management planning to avoid seeding tumor cells while treating the infective process.

Lastly, if the operation pursued is for the management of a biliary oncologic emergency, the incision and approach will depend upon the specific emergency. Emergent surgical decompression of the biliary tree, for example in the case of cholangitis from choledocholithiasis, biliary stricture, or obstruction from a tumor, should only be undertaken if percutaneous or endoscopic attempts to do so have failed or are unavailable and transport to another facility is unsafe or unavailable. This is particularly evident in the associated mortality rates of surgical versus percutaneous/endoscopic therapy for life-threatening cholangitis (50% vs. 5%). When surgical biliary diversion is necessary, it may be accomplished via bypass or T-tube insertion proximal to the area of obstruction.

12.3.3 Oncologic Surgical Emergencies in Patients with Chronic Liver Disease

Patients with chronic liver disease deserve special commentary. Perioperative patient care optimization before emergent general surgery is especially critical in this patient population and is well described elsewhere [6]. Surgical access (open or laparoscopic) and placement of retractors should be planned to avoid engorged abdominal wall veins and to optimize surgical exposure in anticipation to the most critical operative steps. Despite the lack of formal definitive evidence, bipolar and ultrasonic energy devices, mechanical vascular staplers, and topical hemostatics are highly useful adjuncts in attempting to decrease both operating time and blood loss. This seems particularly true for the surgeon entering the abdominal wall with associated dilated veins. Use of a concurrent ligating and cutting energy instrument in a careful and cautious manner can help prevent massive blood loss. Postoperative coagulopathy can easily facilitate bleeding from initially minor sources, so extra attention to hemostasis is required throughout the operation.

Utilization of intra-abdominal drains to help control postoperative ascites and prevent surgical wound complications is a controversial topic. Improved control of postoperative ascites and potential associated surgical wound complications presents a compelling rationale for prophylactic drainage. This must be balanced against the risk of contamination of ascites and increased postoperative fluid shifts.

As a general rule, the most expeditious and least invasive operation should be utilized, including a laparoscopic approach where feasible and safe. The safety of laparoscopy in cirrhotic patients has been historically challenged due to the theoretical risks of hemorrhage from abdominal wall varices during port placement, detrimental effects of pneumoperitoneum on hepatic perfusion, and technical limitations to approaching intraoperative hemorrhage. These concerns, however, have been vastly mitigated over the years by experience and energy technologies.

The superiority of emergent laparoscopic over open cholecystectomy in cirrhotic patients has been demonstrated in terms of operative blood loss, surgical time, postoperative pain, morbidity, and hospital length of stay. Technical difficulties must be expected in retracting the liver and identifying anatomic landmarks due to hepatic distortion.

In cirrhotic patients, an increased risk of intraoperative hemorrhage should be expected. In laparoscopic surgery, utilization of additional ports and meticulous operative technique assist in preventing iatrogenic injuries. Venous hemorrhage can be temporized by brief increases in pneumoperitoneum pressure and compression with sponges. If application of electrocautery is contemplated for gallbladder bed bleeding, a high setting (i.e., 100 units on the spray setting) and precise contact to the site of bleeding are recommended. In cases where this technique does not arrest ongoing bleeding, placement of a clip immediately beside the site of hemorrhage into the liver in a perpendicular manner can be helpful as an ignition tool for cauterization.

12.4 Tumor-Related Emergencies

12.4.1 Primary Tumor

Regardless of the specific tumor pathology, the underlying management principles of primary liver tumor-related surgical emergencies are the same. Circumstances necessitating emergent intervention may include hemorrhage, thrombosis, necrosis/abscess, and cholestasis.

12.4.1.1 Hemorrhage

Bleeding from a hepatic tumor, such as hepatocellular carcinoma (HCC) or a large hepatic adenoma, only necessitates emergent surgical intervention in the hemodynamically unstable patient who does not respond to resuscitation with blood products. Hemodynamically normal patients and patients who respond at least transiently to blood transfusion should undergo an appropriate diagnostic workup before establishing an appropriate treatment plan. In the acute setting, this diagnostic workup would include a CT scan with IV contrast and basic laboratory investigations including a coagulation profile. Hemodynamically stable patients with a bleeding liver tumor who have evidence of contrast extravasation on CT scan, and down-trending hemoglobin, and those who only transiently respond to blood transfusion may benefit from broad or selective angioembolization. This represents definitive hemorrhage control in the acute setting and allows time for further diagnostic workup, including biopsy once the bleeding has resolved if necessary, and referral to a hepatobiliary surgeon or surgical oncologist for definitive treatment. Bleeding is typically considered an indication for resection, even if a malignant component to the mass has not been definitively identified.

12.4.1.2 Thrombosis

Thrombosis of branches of the hepatic arterial, hepatic venous, and/or portal venous systems may occur as a result of a liver tumor. In the context of malignancy, however, this rarely represents an emergency as the thrombosis is then a chronic process which allows collateral flow to develop.

12.4.1.3 Necrosis/Abscess

Liver abscesses in the setting of hepatic oncology can occur from spontaneous or treatment-induced tumor necrosis or from hematologic spread of intra-abdominal infection. Tumor necrosis is the intended goal of locoregional therapies for liver tumors such as HCC. The induced cell death, which leads to necrosis, from therapies including thermal ablation such as radiofrequency ablation (RFA), transarterial chemoembolization (TACE), transarterial radioembolization (TARE), and others aims to prolong patient survival by diminishing tumor size and reducing tumor burden. It can, however, cause necrosis of healthy liver parenchyma and result in hepatic abscess formation. This is covered in further detail below under *Treatment-Related Emergencies*. Regardless of the etiology of the necrosis/abscess, nonoperative management with supportive care and antibiotics as appropriate should be pursued whenever possible. If percutaneous or surgical intervention is necessary and time permits, discussion and care coordination with an oncologist and hepatobiliary surgeon should be pursued to ensure that oncologic principles are respected while achieving source control of infection.

12.4.1.4 Cholestasis

Cholestasis can occur both as a treatment-related consequence, for example among patients with neuroendocrine tumors on somatostatin analogs [7], and as a result of the liver tumor itself. In the first scenario, somatostatin analogs function by inducing tumor cell apoptosis and inhibiting tumor angiogenesis to stop or slow tumor growth. However, cholestasis and cholelithiasis are consequences of somatostatin therapy, particularly when it is administered for a long term. Symptomatic cholelithiasis, for example acute cholecystitis or cholangitis, among liver oncology patients on somatostatin analogs is treated as in non-oncology patients, provided that usual criteria for safe surgical intervention are met such as the absence of coagulopathy.

When cholestasis occurs as a mechanical result of the tumor itself, for example in a patient with an unresectable Klatskin tumor, this is typically treated with endoscopic retrograde cholangiopancreatography (ERCP) or percutaneous transhepatic cholangiography (PTC) with internal/external biliary drains. If cholestasis occurs among patients with resectable disease, then biliary diversion can be accomplished during the surgical resection. Cholestasis in this context presents as an emergency if the patient develops cholangitis, which would typically be managed with ERCP or PTC, and not surgical bypass or drainage, in the acute setting. It should be specifically noted that with hilar cholangiocarcinoma, ERCP is generally avoided in preference of PTC. Infecting the biliary tree from below (ERCP access) often leads to clinical deterioration from cholangitis in frail patients. As a result, drainage from the top (PTC) is safer and also allows subsequent MRI/MRCP (i.e., without a biliary tube obstructing images of the adjacent tumor) for evaluating resectability. PTC also generally permits better biliary drainage of the liver bilaterally through the right and left lobes when compared to ERCP, a feature which makes PTC particularly useful for Klatskin tumors.

12.4.2 Metastatic Tumor

Tumor metastases to the liver can cause the same surgical emergencies as primary liver tumors, including bleeding, thrombosis, necrosis, and cholangitis. An additional surgical emergency that can occur from metastases includes liver failure, which is typically chronic as opposed to acute liver failure. In an appropriate patient, such as one with a metastatic neuroendocrine tumor whose disease would be completely resected with hepatectomy [8], this emergency may be treated with liver transplantation. More commonly, this complication would occur among patients with cirrhosis and HCC. Suitability for liver transplantation in this context is decided based on published guidelines, including the Milan [9] and University of California San Francisco (UCSF) [10] criteria.

12.5 Treatment-Related Emergencies

12.5.1 Surgical Intervention-Related Emergencies

Complications may ensue following biliary reconstruction or liver resection for hepatic tumors, including resection of liver metastases [11]. These include hemorrhage, bile leak, biliary stricture, abscess, liver failure, and vascular thrombosis. Of these, hemorrhage, biliary stricture resulting in cholangitis, liver failure, and vascular thrombosis are those that may present in an emergent fashion.

12.5.1.1 Hemorrhage

Bleeding following surgical resection of a liver mass is managed in the standard fashion, with correction of abnormal coagulation parameters, angioembolization, or reoperation as appropriate based on the patient's hemodynamic status. The earlier in the postoperative course that hemorrhage occurs, the more frequently a rapid return to the operating room is the best option.

12.5.1.2 Cholangitis

Cholangitis, which may present with Charcot's triad (fever, right upper quadrant pain, and jaundice) or Reynold's pentad (Charcot's triad plus hypotension and altered mental status), can occur as a result of biliary stricture at a previous biliary anastomosis following resection of a Klatskin tumor with biliary reconstruction. These patients should be managed with antibiotics and resuscitation and temporized with PTC to decompress the biliary tree. This will resolve the underlying sepsis and allow for referral to a hepatobiliary surgeon after resolution of the infection. Once the cholangitis is resolved, the options are biliary stenting across the stricture or reoperation, depending on patient factors such as life expectancy in the context of the hepatic malignancy as well as anatomic considerations such as stricture location.

12.5.1.3 Acute Liver Failure

Acute liver failure after hepatic resection can generally be avoided or at least anticipated by considering the health of the remaining liver parenchyma, extent of surgical resection required, and mitigation of risk factors for postoperative liver decompensation events [12]. In general, patients without cirrhosis may have up to 70–80% of their liver parenchyma removed without inducing liver failure [13]. Although the safety of any degree of resection among patients with cirrhosis is much less predictable, in general only patients with Child–Turcotte–Pugh (CTP) score A cirrhosis are given consideration for liver resection as the residual hepatocytes are less able to compensate for the necessary liver function.

Patients with acute liver failure following liver resection may be emergently listed for transplant if they meet King's College Criteria for non-acetaminophen-induced acute liver failure [14] or satisfy Milan or UCSF criteria for liver transplant in cirrhosis and HCC. Hepatic dialysis machines may also be an option depending upon capabilities at each transplantation center.

12.5.1.4 Thrombosis

Lastly, thrombosis is managed with systemic anticoagulation if it is acute. In the case of chronic thrombosis with collateralization, such as cavernous transformation of the portal vein, anticoagulation is unnecessary. If systemic anticoagulation is contraindicated or fails to resolve an acute thrombosis, thrombectomy may be necessary. This procedure should be pursued by experienced hepatobiliary and/or transplant surgeons or interventional radiologists, depending on an institution's capabilities.

12.5.2 Locoregional Intervention-Related Emergencies

There are a host of ablative and intra-arterial locoregional treatment options for liver tumors, including percutaneous radiofrequency or microwave ablation, TACE, transarterial radioembolization (TARE), yttrium-90 radioembolization (Y-90), percutaneous microwave ablation, and stereotactic body radiation therapy (SBRT). These treatment options all endeavor to induce tumor cell death via locoregional delivery of chemotherapy, radiation, thermal energy, or a combination thereof while preserving surrounding normal hepatocytes.

In practical terms, complications may occur following these locoregional therapies and include hemorrhage, from either the lesion itself, arterial access sites, and/or surrounding vasculature; hollow viscus perforation; injury to other adjacent structures, such as the gallbladder or diaphragm; abscess/necrosis; biliary stricturing; and hepatic decompensation and liver failure [15], particularly when these therapies are used in the context of underlying liver disease.

In general, these treatment-related complications in the liver oncology patient are managed as they would be in a patient without a hepatic malignancy. However, the underlying malignancy must always be considered after recognition of the complication in decisions about the management plan. For example, any prior intervention involving the portal venous or arterial blood supply of the liver must be noted prior to embolization for bleeding, in order to ensure that adequate blood supply of the healthy liver parenchyma is preserved; residual healthy liver mass must be considered prior to resection; and any coagulopathy induced by the liver malignancy should be corrected prior to intervention to avoid further bleeding complications.

12.5.3 Chemotherapy-Related Emergencies

The options for systemic anticancer therapies (SACTs) available for patients living with liver cancer are expanding. Although many of these agents are associated with the potential for drug-induced liver injury (DILI) [16] or SACT-related biliary tree disease, chemotherapy-related hepatic surgical emergencies are fortunately rare.

12.5.3.1 Systemic Anticancer Therapy-Related Liver Emergencies

Broadly, hepatic surgical emergencies may result from direct, indirect, or idiosyncratic DILI related to SACT [17]. Direct DILI is a result of agents, which are intrinsically toxic to the liver. DILI in this setting is predictable, commonly occurring among patients exposed to the given agent; dose related; rapid in onset, within hours to days of medication delivery; and reproducible in animal models [18]. Indirect DILI is a result of the action of the drug, and not related to an intrinsic hepatotoxic property or idiosyncratic, such as immunotherapy-related cholangiopathy or hepatitis. Idiosyncratic DILI, on the other hand, results from agents that are not intrinsically toxic to the liver. DILI in this setting is unpredictable and rare among patients exposed to the given agent, and not typically dose related, with a variable latency period of days to weeks [18].

Regardless of the specific type of DILI occurring in a patient with an underlying hepatic malignancy, the treatment consists of supportive therapy directed at correction of manifestations of liver dysfunction and cessation of the agent whenever possible.

12.5.3.2 Systemic Anticancer Therapy-Related Biliary Emergencies

Cholecystitis is a rare but potentially serious complications of SACT [19]. Somatostatin analogs are associated with biliary tract stone disease, which can cause acute calculous cholecystitis. In a retrospective, multicenter study of 754 patients with neuroendocrine neoplasms treated with somatostatin analogs, 27% were found to have developed gallstones, among whom 28% developed biliary complications, including biliary colic, acute cholecystitis, cholangitis, and obstructive jaundice [20]. As a result of the potential for biliary tract complications, the North American Neuroendocrine Tumor Society guidelines recommend considering prophylactic cholecystectomy at the time of small bowel resection in patients who have a high likelihood for long-term somatostatin analog treatment, such as patients with liver metastases, peritoneal metastases, or significant nodal involvement [21].

More rarely, acute acalculous cholecystitis and chemical cholecystitis have been reported as a side effect of SACT [22–26]. Acalculous cholecystitis has been described in an increasing number of case reports related to receptor tyrosine kinase inhibitors, including sunitinib [24], axitinib [22], bosutinib [27], and lenvatinib [23, 28], and as an immune-related adverse event following treatment with immune checkpoint inhibitors [29]. Chemical cholecystitis is an important potential complication of intrahepatic chemotherapy. Early studies evaluating regional intrahepatic chemotherapy delivery reported high rates of cholecystitis related to extrahepatic perfusion to the gallbladder through the cystic artery [30]. As a result, routine prophylactic cholecystectomy is not recommended when hepatic arterial infusion pumps are inserted [26, 31].

Biliary sclerosis is a rare but serious potential complication seen with intrahepatic administration of floxuridine chemotherapy for patients with colorectal cancer liver metastases [32]. Floxuridine is a prodrug of fluorouracil, which is infused directly into the hepatic artery via an implanted continuous infusion pump. The short half-life and 95% first-pass hepatic extraction of floxuridine allow administration of very high dose of floxuridine that results in tumor exposure 400 times greater than could be achieved with systemic administration [33–35]. Intrahepatic floxuridine is associated with very high response rates for colorectal liver metastases, but approximately 5% of patients may develop biliary sclerosis, which may necessitate the insertion of stents or percutaneous biliary drains [36, 37]. Although oxaliplatin has a lower hepatic extraction rate, its intrahepatic use has not been reported to be associated with biliary sclerosis.

12.6 Conclusions

Surgical oncologic emergencies of the liver may occur as the result of the primary tumor, tumor metastases, or tumor treatment following chemotherapy, locoregional interventions, or surgery. In general, these emergencies are managed using core acute care surgery principles, including hemorrhage control and source control of infection. Consideration of the underlying malignancy and implications for optimal patient management should be maintained, and care coordination with a hepatobiliary surgeon or surgical oncologist, when possible, is prudent.

Conflict of Interest The authors have no conflicts of interest or disclosures of funding to declare.

References

1. Sung H, Ferlay J, Siegel RL, Laversanne M, Soerjomataram I, Jemal A, Bray F. Global cancer statistics 2020: GLOBOCAN estimates of incidence and mortality worldwide for 36 cancers in 185 countries. CA Cancer J Clin. 2021;71(3):209–49. https://doi.org/10.3322/caac.21660.
2. National Cancer Institute. Reports on cancer. National Institutes of Health (NIH): Surveillance, Epidemiology, and End Results Program. 2021. https://seer.cancer.gov/statfacts/html/common.html. Accessed 1 Dec 2021.
3. Noussios G, Dimitriou I, Chatzis I, Katsourakis A. The main anatomic variations of the hepatic artery and their importance in surgical practice: review of the literature. J Clin Med Res. 2017;9(4):248–52. https://doi.org/10.14740/jocmr2902w.
4. Ball CG, Campbell A, Grondin SC, Dixon E. The efficacy of a novel saline/bipolar radiofrequency energy instrument for arresting ongoing solid and non-solid organ hemorrhage in a swine model. Injury. 2016;47(12):2706–8. https://doi.org/10.1016/j.injury.2016.09.038.
5. Ball CG, Wyrzykowski AD, Nicholas JM, Rozycki GS, Feliciano DV. A decade's experience with balloon catheter tamponade for the emergency control of hemorrhage. J Trauma. 2011;70(2):330–3. https://doi.org/10.1097/TA.0b013e318203285c.
6. Bleszynski MS, Bressan AK, Joos E, Hameed SM, Ball CG. Acute care and emergency general surgery in patients with chronic liver disease: how can we optimize perioperative care? A review of the literature. World J Emerg Surg. 2018;32:13.
7. Ahrendt SA, McGuire GE, Pitt HA, Lillemoe KD. Why does somatostatin cause gallstones? Am J Surg. 1991;161(1):177–82. https://doi.org/10.1016/0002-9610(91)90381-m.
8. Gedaly R, Daily MF, Davenport D, McHugh PP, Koch A, Angulo P, Hundley JC. Liver transplantation for the treatment of liver metastases from neuroendocrine tumors: an analysis of the UNOS database. Arch Surg. 2011;146(8):953–8.
9. Mazzaferro V, Regalia E, Doci R, Andreola S, Pulvirenti A, Bozzetti F, Montalto F, Ammatuna M, Morabito A, Gennari L. Liver transplantation for the treatment of small hepatocellular carcinomas in patients with cirrhosis. N Engl J Med. 1996;334(11):693–9. https://doi.org/10.1056/NEJM199603143341104.
10. Yao FY, Kerlan RK Jr, Hirose R, Davern TJ 3rd, Bass NM, Feng S, Peters M, Terrault N, Freise CE, Ascher NL, Roberts JP. Excellent outcome following down-staging of hepatocellular carcinoma prior to liver transplantation: an intention-to-treat analysis. Hepatology. 2008;48(3):819–27. https://doi.org/10.1002/hep.22412.
11. Nanji S, Cleary S, Ryan P, Guindi M, Selvarajah S, Al-Ali H, Grieg P, McGilvary I, Taylor B, Wei A, Moulton CA, Gallinger S. Up-front hepatic resection for metastatic colorectal

cancer results in favorable long-term survival [Erratum in: Ann Surg Oncol. 2013 Dec;20 Suppl 3:S751. Al-Ali, Hassan [added]]. Ann Surg Oncol. 2013;20(1):295–304. https://doi.org/10.1245/s10434-012-2424-1.
12. Mir ZM, Djerboua M, Nanji S, Flemming JA, Groome PA. Predictors of postoperative liver decompensation events after resection in patients with cirrhosis and hepatocellular carcinoma: a population-based study. Ann Surg Oncol. 2022;29(1):288–99. https://doi.org/10.1245/s10434-021-10801-9.
13. Guglielmi A, Ruzzenente A, Conci S, Valdegamberi A, Iacono C. How much remnant is enough in liver resection? Dig Surg. 2012;29(1):6–17. https://doi.org/10.1159/000335713.
14. McPhail MJ, Wendon JA, Bernal W. Meta-analysis of performance of King's college hospital criteria in prediction of outcome in non-paracetamol-induced acute liver failure. J Hepatol. 2010;53(3):492–9. https://doi.org/10.1016/j.jhep.2010.03.023.
15. Groupe d'Etude et de Traitement du Carcinome Hépatocellulaire. A comparison of lipiodol chemoembolization and conservative treatment for unresectable hepatocellular carcinoma. N Engl J Med. 1995;332(19):1256–61. https://doi.org/10.1056/NEJM199505113321903.
16. Bahirwani R, Reddy KR. Drug-induced liver injury due to cancer chemotherapeutic agents. In: Seminars in liver disease. Thieme Medical Publishers; 2014. p. 162–71.
17. Hoofnagle JH, Björnsson ES. Drug-induced liver injury—types and phenotypes. N Engl J Med. 2019;381:264–73.
18. Andrade RJ, Aithal GP, Björnsson ES, et al. EASL clinical practice guidelines: drug-induced liver injury. J Hepatol. 2019;70:1222–61.
19. Jayakrishnan TT, Groeschl RT, George B, et al. Review of the impact of antineoplastic therapies on the risk for cholelithiasis and acute cholecystitis. Ann Surg Oncol. 2014;21:240–7.
20. Brighi N, Panzuto F, Modica R, et al. Biliary stone disease in patients with neuroendocrine tumors treated with somatostatin analogs: a multicenter study. Oncologist. 2020;25:259.
21. Howe JR, Cardona K, Fraker DL, et al. The surgical management of small bowel neuroendocrine tumors: consensus guidelines of the North American Neuroendocrine Tumor Society (NANETS). Pancreas. 2017;46:715.
22. Kameda T, Nakano K, Yamazaki M, et al. Axitinib-induced pneumatosis intestinalis and acute acalculous cholecystitis in a patient with renal cell carcinoma. Urology. 2017;101:e7–8.
23. Nervo A, Ragni A, Gallo M, et al. Symptomatic biliary disorders during lenvatinib treatment for thyroid cancer: an underestimated problem. Thyroid. 2020;30:229–36.
24. Gomes da Fonseca L, Barroso-Sousa R, Sabbaga J, et al. Acute acalculous cholecystitis in a patient with metastatic renal cell carcinoma treated with sunitinib. Clin Pract. 2014;4:24–6.
25. Carrasco CH, Freeny PC, Chuang V, et al. Chemical cholecystitis associated with hepatic artery infusion chemotherapy. Am J Roentgenol. 1983;141:703–6.
26. Ottery FD, Scupham RK, Weese JL. Chemical cholecystitis after intrahepatic chemotherapy. Dis Colon Rectum. 1986;29:187–90.
27. Altshuler E, Case R. Acalculous cholecystitis with gallbladder necrosis in a patient presenting without abdominal pain. BMJ Case Rep. 2020;13:e238386.
28. Ishigaki K, Hamada T, Nakai Y, et al. Lenvatinib-induced acute acalculous cholecystitis in a patient with hepatocellular carcinoma. Clin J Gastroenterol. 2020;13:568–71.
29. Abu-Sbeih H, Tran CN, Phillip SG, et al. Case series of cancer patients who developed cholecystitis related to immune checkpoint inhibitor treatment. J Immunother Cancer. 2019;7:1–8.
30. Kemeny MM, Goldberg DA, Browning S, et al. Experience with continuous regional chemotherapy and hepatic resection as treatment of hepatic metastases from colorectal primaries. A prospective randomized study. Cancer. 1985;55:1265–70.
31. Muaddi H, D'Angelica M, Wiseman JT, et al. Safety and feasibility of initiating a hepatic artery infusion pump chemotherapy program for unresectable colorectal liver metastases: a multicenter, retrospective cohort study. J Surg Oncol. 2021;123:252–60.
32. Ito K, Ito H, Kemeny NE, et al. Biliary sclerosis after hepatic arterial infusion pump chemotherapy for patients with colorectal cancer liver metastasis: incidence, clinical features, and risk factors. Ann Surg Oncol. 2012;19:1609–17.

33. Ensminger W, Gyves J. Clinical pharmacology of hepatic arterial chemotherapy. Semin Oncol. 1983;10:176–82.
34. Ensminger WD, Rosowsky A, Raso V, et al. A clinical-pharmacological evaluation of hepatic arterial infusions of 5-fluoro-2′-deoxyuridine and 5-fluorouracil. Cancer Res. 1978;38:3784–92.
35. Power DG, Kemeny NE. The role of floxuridine in metastatic liver disease. Mol Cancer Ther. 2009;8:1015–25.
36. Ko Y, Karanicolas P. Hepatic arterial infusion pump chemotherapy for colorectal liver metastases: an old technology in a new era. Curr Oncol. 2014;21:e116.
37. Cercek A, D'Angelica M, Power D, et al. Floxuridine hepatic arterial infusion associated biliary toxicity is increased by concurrent administration of systemic bevacizumab. Ann Surg Oncol. 2014;21:479–86.

Pancreas

13

Riccardo Memeo, Francesca D'Errico, Letizia Laera, Roberto Calbi, and Riccardo Inchingolo

13.1 Oncologic Surgical Emergencies: Pancreatic Neoplasms

Most of the pancreatic cancer patients do not undergo surgical treatment, due to the locally advanced status or due to the presence of distance metastasis [1, 2]. This condition needs to be considered due to the large number of patients who are potentially treatable with chemotherapy or radiotherapy and could develop during the treatment some surgical complications, which could require intervention [3–5]. This subset of complications, differently from the surgical complications of patients who underwent curative surgery [6–8], requires a multidisciplinary management that must be considered in the set of fragile patients who are usually treated with chemotherapy.

These pancreatic emergencies can occur in different stages of the oncologic management of the pancreatic cancer patients and could sometimes be life-threatening for the patient.

R. Memeo (✉)
Department of HPB Surgery, Miulli Hospital, Bari, Italy
e-mail: r.memeo@miulli.it

F. D'Errico
Department of Endoscopy, Miulli Hospital, Bari, Italy
e-mail: f.derrico@miulli.it

L. Laera
Department of Oncology, Miulli Hospital, Bari, Italy
e-mail: l.laera@miullii.it

R. Calbi
Department of Radiology, Miulli Hospital, Bari, Italy
e-mail: r.calbi@miulli.it

R. Inchingolo
Department of Interventional Radiology, Miulli Hospital, Bari, Italy
e-mail: r.inchingolo@miulli.it

A. Tarasconi et al. (eds.), *Oncologic Surgical Emergencies*, Hot Topics in Acute Care Surgery and Trauma, https://doi.org/10.1007/978-3-031-36860-8_13

In this situation, it is very important that the diagnosis of the complications is rapid to find the best solution for the surgical treatment of the patient.

13.2 Pancreatitis

Acute pancreatitis is a rare manifestation in patients who undergo chemotherapy and can be defined as drug-induced pancreatitis (DIP), described in literature in a range of 0.1–2% of cases [9]. The main cause of this complication can be different and could be directly related to the toxicity of the chemotherapy (cytotoxicity, immune-mediated response) or pancreatic degeneration (Wirsung stenosis, vascular thrombosis, metabolic effects). Balani et al. [10] identified some risk factors for this kind of complications, identifying children, women, elderly patients, those with CD4+ T cell count for <200 cells/mm^3 of advanced AIDS, and those with Crohn's disease as the potential population of patients who could develop DIP.

The typical manifestation of this complications is with epigastric pain, nausea, and vomiting, associated with reduction of weight and hunger. The manifestation of symptoms could vary, evolving up to necrotizing pancreatitis. The classification of the pancreatitis could follow the APACHE score classification [11], according to the radiologic asset and gravity of the patient. The onset of this complication could be very dangerous for the patient, according to the condition of a patient who developed this complication fragilized by the effect of systemic treatment.

The main treatment for this kind of patient should include intravenous fluid resuscitation and, if necessary, intensive care support. The use of antibiotic is recommended only in case of the presence of direct effects of infection. The use of nutritional support could be crucial and should be considered in cases with self-limiting symptoms, in order to achieve a rapid recovery of the oncologic patient.

13.3 Jaundice

Jaundice [12–14] is the typical manifestation of pancreatic cancer, considering the localization on the head and neck of pancreatic neoplasm, which can determine the compression of the distal part of the bile duct, with the onset of jaundice, determining malabsorption, malnutrition, and weight loss, in some cases associated with the onset of cholangitis. The persistence of nonthreatening jaundice could determine coagulation problems that could lead to other life-threatening complications.

In these cases, the preferred solution should be the placement of a metallic stent and, in case of failure, the positioning of a percutaneous external drainage or internal external drainage. Historically, this drainage was performed surgically, with a hepaticojejunostomy often associated with a gastroenteric anastomosis, called double bypass for locally advanced pancreatic cancer. In recent period, both techniques have been replaced by minimally invasive management with endoscopic or percutaneous treatment.

13.4 Occlusion

Gastric obstruction is often seen in patients with periampullary malignancies [15], often in progression after chemotherapy. The main symptoms are nausea, reduction in feeding, and vomiting, strongly impacting the quality of life of patients. This complication could be usually managed by surgery, with a surgical bypass with a gastroenteric anastomosis, which could be performed by open or minimally invasive approach, in order to allow the correct feeding of oncological patients, usually faced with malnutrition. An anastomose is performed among the stomach and the first jejunal loop, creating a new communication jumping the obstacle created by the pancreatic neoplasm.

In case of impossibility to perform surgical bypass, another solution is represented by endoscopic placement of duodenal metallic stent, to solve the problem of occlusion. The use of covered or uncovered self-expanding stent could be chosen case by case, in order to better identify the patient based on the location of occlusion and the type of duodenal involvement. The main problem of this stent is the possibility of displacement, and in most of the cases, this stent is placed in poor prognosis patient with short life expectance. This kind of stent should be placed only in symptomatic patients, avoiding placing them in asymptomatic patients in consideration of the high rate of complications that often occur in patients with duodenal stent. This endoscopic bypass is less invasive.

13.5 Perforation

The use of chemotherapy could be associated with gastrointestinal perforation [16], sometimes associated with the formation of fistula or abscess in abdominal portion. In some cases, considering the vascular alteration that could be induced by the oncological problem, some bleeding and arterial and venous thromboembolic events can occur. The complication related to gastrointestinal perforation could be related to severe peritonitis, which could evolve, according to the National Cancer Institute's common terminology criteria for adverse events, up to life-threatening complications. The management of this complication must have the objective to solve the problem of peritonitis, with the resolution of the septic problem. The management of the stoma could be complicated in such fragile patients, but priority should be given to the resolution of the septic event and allowing the patient to continue to be treated with chemotherapy.

References

1. Idachaba S, Dada O, Abimbola O, et al. A review of pancreatic cancer: epidemiology, genetics, screening, and management. Open Access Maced J Med Sci. 2019;7(4):663–71. https://doi.org/10.3889/oamjms.2019.104.

2. Turpin A, el Amrani M, Bachet JB, et al. Adjuvant pancreatic cancer management: towards new perspectives in 2021. Cancers. 2020;12(12):3866. https://doi.org/10.3390/cancers12123866.
3. Klose J, Ronellenfitsch U, Kleeff J. Management problems in patients with pancreatic cancer from a surgeon's perspective. Semin Oncol. 2021;48:76–83.
4. Shen Z, Tian L, Wang X. Treatment of pancreatic head cancer with obstructive jaundice by endoscopy ultrasonography-guided gastrojejunostomy: a case report and literature review. Medicine (United States). 2018;97(28):e11476. https://doi.org/10.1097/MD.0000000000011476.
5. Yang QJ, Zheng J, Dang FT, et al. Acute pancreatitis induced by combination chemotherapy used for the treatment of acute myeloid leukemia: a case report. Medicine. 2020;99:e21848.
6. Mauri G, Mattiuz C, Sconfienza LM, et al. Role of interventional radiology in the management of complications after pancreatic surgery: a pictorial review. Insights Imaging. 2015;6(2):231–9. https://doi.org/10.1007/s13244-014-0372-y.
7. Andrén-Sandberg Å. Complications of pancreatic surgery. N Am J Med Sci. 2011;3(12):531–5. https://doi.org/10.4297/najms.2011.3531.
8. Biondetti P, Fumarola EM, Ierardi AM, et al. Bleeding complications after pancreatic surgery: interventional radiology management. Gland Surg. 2019;8(2):150–63. https://doi.org/10.21037/gs.2019.01.06.
9. Vinklerová I, Procházka M, Procházka V, et al. Incidence, severity, and etiology of drug-induced acute pancreatitis. Dig Dis Sci. 2010;55(10):2977–81. https://doi.org/10.1007/s10620-010-1277-3.
10. Balani AR, Grendell JH. Drug-induced pancreatitis: incidence, management and prevention. Drug Saf. 2008;31(10):823–37. https://doi.org/10.2165/00002018-200831100-00002.
11. Knaus WA, Draper EA, Wagner DP, et al. APACHE II: a severity of disease classification system. Crit Care Med. 1985;13(10):818–29. https://doi.org/10.1097/00003246-198510000-00009.
12. Chi Z, Chen L, Huang J, et al. A novel combination of percutaneous stenting with iodine-125 seed implantation and chemotherapy for the treatment of pancreatic head cancer with obstructive jaundice. Brachytherapy. 2021;20(1):218–25. https://doi.org/10.1016/j.brachy.2020.09.009.
13. Kozarek R. Role of preoperative palliation of jaundice in pancreatic cancer. J Hepatobiliary Pancreat Sci. 2013;20(6):567–72. https://doi.org/10.1007/s00534-013-0612-4.
14. Shen Z, Zhang J, Chen H, et al. Does pre-operative biliary drainage influence long-term survival in patients with obstructive jaundice with resectable pancreatic head cancer? Front Oncol. 2020;10:575316. https://doi.org/10.3389/fonc.2020.575316.
15. Tradounsky G. Palliation of gastrointestinal obstruction. Can Fam Physician. 2012;58(6):648–52.
16. Hapani S, Chu D, Wu S. Risk of gastrointestinal perforation in patients with cancer treated with bevacizumab: a meta-analysis. Lancet Oncol. 2009;10:559–68.

Biliary Tract

14

Ariel W. Knight, Chia-Ching Wang, and Deborah M. Stein

14.1 Introduction

Biliary tract malignancies are relatively rare. In the United States, gallbladder cancer is the most common biliary tract malignancy, although fewer than 5000 cases are diagnosed annually [1]. Gallbladder cancer carries a poor overall prognosis as it is commonly diagnosed at an advanced, unresectable stage. Approximately 1–2% of patients undergoing clinical evaluation for cholelithiasis or acute cholecystitis will be diagnosed with gallbladder cancer [2, 3]. Five-year overall survival rates remains dismal at approximately 20%. However, when patients are diagnosed with localized disease and undergo appropriate oncologic resection, they have an improved 5-year overall survival rate of 65%.

Cholangiocarcinoma represents approximately 3% of all gastrointestinal malignancies, and most are advanced stage at the time of diagnosis [4]. The true incidence of cholangiocarcinoma in the United States is unclear, though, as oncologic databases have historically combined intrahepatic disease with other primary liver tumors and extrahepatic disease with gallbladder cancer. The global incidence of cholangiocarcinoma has increased over the past three decades, but the proportion of earlier stage disease has not [5]. Cholangiocarcinoma is more likely to be diagnosed in men and typically occurs between 50 and 70 years of age, except in patients with

A. W. Knight
Department of Surgery, Stanford University, Stanford, CA, USA
e-mail: awknight@stanford.edu

C.-C. Wang
Department of Hematology and Oncology, University of California, San Francisco, San Francisco, CA, USA
e-mail: Chia-ching.wang@ucsf.edu

D. M. Stein (✉)
Department of Surgery, University of Maryland School of Medicine, Baltimore, MD, USA
e-mail: dstein@som.umaryland.edu

A. Tarasconi et al. (eds.), *Oncologic Surgical Emergencies*, Hot Topics in Acute Care Surgery and Trauma, https://doi.org/10.1007/978-3-031-36860-8_14

primary sclerosing cholangitis (PSC) or choledochal cysts, when it may present up to two decades earlier [4, 6, 7].

Surgery is the only potentially curative treatment modality for both gallbladder cancer and cholangiocarcinoma. Unfortunately, only a minority of patients are appropriate operative candidates. In gallbladder cancer, appropriate surgical resection yields a 45–50% 5-year survival rate. Survival following cholangiocarcinoma resection depends upon the location of the primary tumor. Gallbladder cancer and cholangiocarcinoma frequently directly invade adjacent structures (most commonly the liver, but also the stomach, duodenum, pancreas, colon, omentum, and peritoneum), often precluding curative resection outside of high-volume institutions.

As biliary tract malignancies commonly present with vague, nonspecific symptoms that are also characteristic of benign biliary disease, they will be inevitably encountered by both general and acute care surgeons. Accordingly, a working knowledge of appropriate diagnostic workup, oncologic staging, prognosis, surgical therapy, neoadjuvant and adjuvant therapies, and subspecialty consultations is essential for timely and successful patient care.

14.2 Anatomy

The gallbladder rests on the cystic plate on the inferior margin of the right lobe of the liver and is comprised of the fundus, body, infundibulum, and neck. It drains into the biliary tree via the cystic duct, which joins the common bile duct. The gallbladder is supplied by the cystic artery, which is most commonly a branch of the right hepatic artery, and drains directly into the gallbladder fossa via the cystic veins.

Lymphatic drainage of the gallbladder is less predictable. In 95% of patients, lymphatic drainage of the gallbladder occurs via the cholecysto-retropancreatic route along the cystic duct, common bile duct, and portal vein, which then runs posterior to the pancreas to the para-aortic nodal basin [8]. Most remaining patients' lymphatic drainage occurs via the cholecysto-celiac pathway, which drains along the cystic duct before running medially along the hepatoduodenal ligament posterior to the head of the pancreas and culminating at the celiac axis [8].

Cholangiocarcinomas are classified as either intrahepatic (less than 10% of cases), perihilar (50% of cases), or distal/extrahepatic (40% of cases) [9–13]. Intrahepatic disease originates from either small intrahepatic ductules or larger intrahepatic bile ducts proximal to the bifurcation of the left and right hepatic ducts [14]. Lymphatic drainage of intrahepatic tumors typically demonstrates laterality. Left-sided intrahepatic cholangiocarcinoma tends to spread along the lesser curve of the stomach and to the inferior phrenic nodal basin. Regional lymph nodes include the inferior phrenic, hilar, and gastrohepatic basins. Conversely, right-sided tumors tend to spread to hilar and portocaval nodes. Both left- and right-sided intrahepatic cholangiocarcinomas can spread to celiac, periaortic, and pericaval lymph nodes. The involvement of pericaval nodes represents distant metastatic disease.

The extrahepatic bile ducts are divided into perihilar and distal segments. This transition occurs where the cystic duct drains into the common bile duct. Perihilar cholangiocarcinomas are further characterized by the Bismuth-Corlette classification [15]. In this system, type I tumors are found below the confluence of the right and left hepatic ducts, while type II tumors reach the confluence. Type IIIa and IIIb tumors refer to those that occlude the common hepatic duct and either the right or the left hepatic duct, respectively. Type IV tumors may either be multicentric or involve the confluence and both the right and left hepatic ducts. Cholangiocarcinoma tends to spread intrahepatically along the perineural and periductal lymphatics in addition to the hilar and pericholedochal lymph nodes in the hepatoduodenal ligament. Regional lymph nodes include the hilar, cystic duct, choledochal, portal, hepatic artery, and posterior pancreaticoduodenal basins. Involvement of the liver or any hepatoduodenal ligament lymph nodes represents distant metastatic disease.

Distal cholangiocarcinoma can also spread locoregionally to the pancreas, duodenum, stomach, colon, and omentum in addition to the common bile duct, common hepatic artery, portal vein, anterior and posterior pancreaticoduodenal, and superior mesenteric artery lymph node basins.

14.3 Risk Factors

Gallbladder cancer incidence increases with age and shows a predominance for Caucasian and female patients [16, 17]. Most cited risk factors are related to chronic gallbladder inflammation, including gallstones, porcelain gallbladder, gallbladder polyps, PSC, and certain chronic infections [18–21]. The overall incidence of gallbladder cancer associated with cholelithiasis is 0.5%, but the risk increases with larger stones and a longer duration of their presence [22–24]. Gallbladder polyps may be benign or malignant, although size greater than 1 cm is associated with an increased likelihood of underlying malignancy [25]. Approximately 6% of PSC patients have gallbladder masses, over half of which are malignant [26]. Chronic infections with *Salmonella typhi* and *Helicobacter pylori* have also been linked to the development of gallbladder cancer [26–28]. Additional risk factors for gallbladder cancer include congenital biliary cysts; exposure to cigarette smoke, radon, and aflatoxin; obesity; hyperglycemia; and anomalous pancreaticobiliary ductal anatomy [29–32].

Most patients diagnosed with cholangiocarcinoma do not have an identifiable risk factor despite numerous associations with chronic hepatobiliary disease, toxic exposures, lifestyle factors, and genetic predispositions [33]. Approximately 30% of cholangiocarcinoma cases are diagnosed in PSC patients, the risk of which further increases with concurrent tobacco and alcohol use [34–36]. Cholangiocarcinoma tends to develop at an earlier age with concomitant PSC, between 30 and 50 years of age. Any clinical deterioration, most commonly jaundice, weight loss, or new-onset abdominal pain in a PSC patient, should warrant prompt evaluation for cholangiocarcinoma.

Fibropolycystic liver disease, including Caroli disease, choledochal cysts, and congenital hepatic fibrosis, carries an approximately 15% risk of malignant degeneration [36–38]. Similar to PSC, cholangiocarcinoma tends to develop at a much earlier age in these patients. Chronic hepatitis C infection (more so than hepatitis B) also increases the risk of cholangiocarcinoma, as does cirrhosis of any etiology [39–41]. Intraductal and intraepithelial biliary neoplasms also carry a risk of malignant degeneration. Exposures to toxins including Thorotrast, cigarette smoke, alcohol, and iron are associated with cholangiocarcinoma development, as are chronic *Clonorchis* and *Opisthorchis* fluke infections [42–44]. Modifiable risk factors include hyperglycemia, obesity, metabolic syndrome, and long-term oral contraceptive use [45–47].

14.4 Clinical Presentation

Early-stage gallbladder cancers tend to either be asymptomatic or mimic symptomatic cholelithiasis. When symptomatic, gallbladder cancer tends to present with abdominal pain, nausea, vomiting, and anorexia. Symptoms that more closely mimic acute cholecystitis are more likely to represent earlier stage disease [24]. Many of these patients may, in fact, be diagnosed at the time of cholecystectomy for presumed benign disease. Conversely, more advanced disease may additionally present with weight loss and malaise. Patients may also present with obstructive jaundice due to direct invasion of the biliary tree or metastases to the hepatoduodenal ligament. These patients are ultimately less likely to have resectable disease. Gastric outlet obstruction may occur secondary to duodenal invasion, which is a contraindication to resection.

Extrahepatic cholangiocarcinoma typically becomes symptomatic with biliary obstruction, and thus may present with painless jaundice, pruritis, clay-colored stools, and dark urine output [48–50]. A smaller subset of patients may experience concomitant abdominal pain, weight loss, and/or fever in addition to malaise, fatigue, and night sweats. Cholangitis is an unusual presentation of extrahepatic disease.

Conversely, intrahepatic cholangiocarcinoma is less likely to present with jaundice. These patients are more likely to experience dull right upper quadrant abdominal pain and weight loss [48, 51]. Intrahepatic disease is much more likely to be discovered incidentally during hepatocellular carcinoma screening or further evaluation of abnormal liver function studies.

PSC patients who go on to develop cholangiocarcinoma classically present with rapid clinical deterioration accompanied by jaundice, weight loss, and abdominal pain. This subset of findings in a patient with known PSC warrants an urgent workup for cholangiocarcinoma.

14.5 Diagnostic Laboratory Studies

14.5.1 Basic Labs

Standard baseline laboratory tests should be obtained to further evaluate undifferentiated upper abdominal pain and/or jaundice, including a complete blood count, basic metabolic panel, coagulation studies, liver function tests (LFTs), amylase, and lipase. A cholestatic LFT pattern is expected in jaundiced patients and is more suggestive of an extrahepatic biliary obstruction. Chronic biliary obstruction will eventually lead to a transaminitis and elevated international normalized ratio (INR). Non-jaundiced patients with intrahepatic biliary malignancy may have a normal to slightly elevated bilirubin with an elevated alkaline phosphatase. Blood cultures and serum lactate should additionally be obtained if cholangitis is a concern.

Rarely, biliary tract tumors can present with hypercalcemia of malignancy, which is associated with severe hypercalcemia, hypophosphatemia, low parathyroid hormone levels, and low vitamin D levels [52].

14.5.2 Tumor Markers for Cholangiocarcinoma

14.5.2.1 Carbohydrate Antigen 19-9 (CA 19-9)

CA 19-9 is a widely established tumor marker for cholangiocarcinoma [53, 54]. Initially, elevated levels can be followed over time to evaluate for treatment effect and disease recurrence or progression. Higher levels prior to any treatment portend a poorer prognosis [55, 56]. Levels greater than 1000 U/mL are highly suggestive of advanced disease, including peritoneal carcinomatosis [57].

Additionally, serum levels are widely used to screen for and potentially diagnose cholangiocarcinoma in PSC patients [58, 59]. Levels above 129 U/mL in the setting of a dominant hilar stricture are highly concerning for cholangiocarcinoma [60]. A level greater than 100 U/mL is also included in the UNOS criteria for liver transplant eligibility for cholangiocarcinoma [61].

However, there are several limitations to the utility of CA 19-9 levels. Importantly, cholangitis and other benign causes of biliary obstruction leading to a direct hyperbilirubinemia above 3.0 mg/dL can falsely elevate serum CA 19-9 levels [54]. If a baseline level is obtained during such an episode, it is imperative to repeat the study once bilirubin levels have normalized. CA 19-9 expression also requires the presence of the Lewis blood group antigen, which is absent in 5–10% of patients, in whom trending CA 19-9 levels will not be clinically useful [62].

14.5.2.2 Carcinoembryonic Antigen (CEA)

CEA may be used in conjunction with CA 19-9 to evaluate for treatment effect and disease recurrence or progression [63]. However, by itself, it is neither sufficiently sensitive nor specific to diagnose cholangiocarcinoma but may be useful to trend if baseline CA 19-9 levels are not elevated [64]. Additionally, CEA levels may be elevated secondary to breast and other gastrointestinal malignancies in addition to benign causes, including peptic ulcer disease, gastritis, diverticulitis, chronic liver disease, and COPD.

14.5.2.3 Alpha Fetoprotein

Serum αFP levels are useful to differentiate an intrahepatic cholangiocarcinoma from a hepatocellular carcinoma. An αFP level should be obtained in all patients with a solid liver lesion.

14.6 Diagnostic Imaging

The utility of several diagnostic imaging studies for evaluation of underlying biliary malignancy is discussed below. The order in which these tests are pursued varies based upon the suspicion for an intrahepatic versus perihilar versus distal cholangiocarcinoma, which is outlined in Fig. 14.1.

14.7 Ultrasound

A formal abdominal ultrasound is the initial study of choice for evaluation of jaundice and/or right upper quadrant abdominal pain to evaluate for biliary dilation and potentially establish a level of obstruction, if present [65]. The addition of a duplex study can further evaluate the portal vasculature for thrombosis or disease involvement [66].

The overall staging accuracy of ultrasound for both gallbladder cancer and cholangiocarcinoma is limited [67]. Concerning findings that warrant additional evaluation for gallbladder cancer include a loss of interface between the gallbladder and liver, direct intrahepatic tumor infiltration, polyps greater than 1 cm, wall thickening

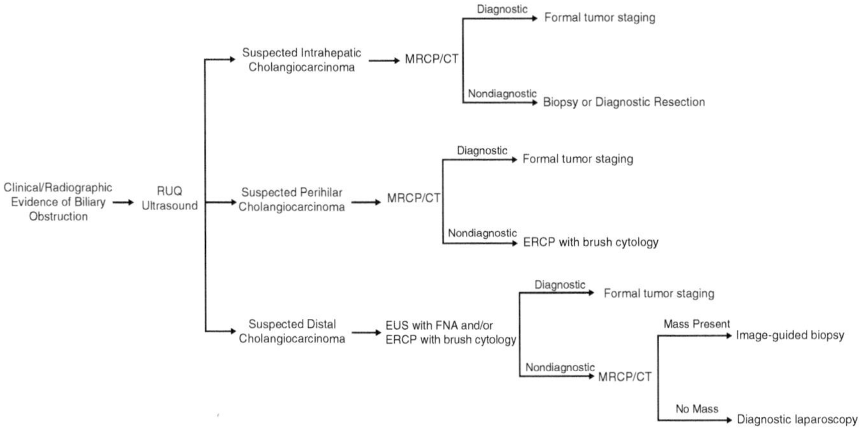

Fig. 14.1 Algorithm for diagnostic evaluation of suspected intrahepatic versus perihilar versus distal cholangiocarcinoma

not explained by cholecystitis, mural calcifications, or an intraluminal, fixed mass [68]. Cholangiocarcinoma may be suggested by intra- and/or extrahepatic biliary dilation that is not explained by another etiology [69]. More proximal lesions will demonstrate isolated intrahepatic ductal dilation, while more distal tumors may cause both intra- and extrahepatic ductal dilation [70]. Additionally, the location of a cholangiocarcinoma may be suggested by an abrupt change in ductal diameter.

Any ultrasound findings concerning for malignancy warrant further evaluation with cross-sectional imaging.

14.8 Computed Tomography

Detailed cross-sectional imaging is warranted if ultrasound is concerning for biliary malignancy. CT abdomen/pelvis should be performed with IV contrast and should include both arterial and delayed venous phases to assess for local, regional, and distant lymphadenopathy; vascular invasion; intrahepatic spread; peritoneal disease; and/or invasion of adjacent organs. CT chest should also be obtained in patients without intra-abdominal metastases who are good surgical candidates to evaluate for occult spread to the lungs and/or pleura.

On CT, gallbladder cancer classically appears as either an intraluminal mass or a focal or diffuse wall thickening [71, 72]. Additional features suggestive of more advanced disease include invasion of liver parenchyma, regional lymphadenopathy, or evidence of distant metastatic disease.

CT is useful in the evaluation of intrahepatic tumors, including cholangiocarcinoma, and can further clarify the level of a biliary obstruction, if present. Approximately 60% of intrahepatic cholangiocarcinomas will appear as a hypodense or infiltrating lesion without a defined capsule, commonly with associated biliary dilation [73, 74]. These lesions will peripherally enhance in both arterial and venous phases. Conversely, hepatocellular carcinoma will hyper-enhance in the arterial phase and wash out during the venous phase, although these differentiating features are not always present. CT more easily evaluates malignant involvement of the portal vasculature and adjacent structures compared to MRCP, although the evaluation of tumor extent and biliary dilation is similar between the two modalities.

Cross-sectional imaging may not directly visualize extrahepatic cholangiocarcinoma but may demonstrate indirect signs of disease. In general, the site of ductal dilation suggests the location of an obstructing lesion. More proximal lesions may only show intrahepatic ductal dilation, whereas more distal lesions may show a combination of intra- and extrahepatic ductal dilation. Any observed ductal dilation >6 mm in the absence of stones should raise strong suspicion for an underlying cholangiocarcinoma. Klatskin tumors may show bilateral intrahepatic ductal dilation with nonunion of the right and left hepatic ducts. Perihilar tumors arising from either the right or the left hepatic ducts tend to be larger and readily infiltrate the adjacent hepatic parenchyma.

14.9 Magnetic Resonance Imaging/Magnetic Resonance Cholangiopancreatography

MRI with MRCP readily evaluates both the intrahepatic and extrahepatic ducts as well as the pancreatic duct. MRI yields higher quality images of the liver parenchyma and allows for 3D reconstruction of the biliary tree and hepatobiliary vasculature. MRCP provides important information regarding potential resectability [75, 76]. It is superior to CT in defining the anatomic extent of an underlying tumor and/or other causes of jaundice. Additionally, it is particularly useful in distinguishing benign versus malignant gallbladder polyps [77]. It is also helpful in the evaluation of locoregional lymphadenopathy and invasion of the hepatoduodenal ligament and porta hepatis.

When MRCP is used to further evaluate a suspected cholangiocarcinoma in the setting of biliary obstruction, it is imperative that the study be performed prior to any biliary drainage procedure. Evaluation of underlying intraductal pathology becomes far more challenging once the ducts are decompressed.

14.10 Endoscopic Ultrasound

EUS may be useful in both detecting and differentiating benign versus malignant gallbladder polyps and in assessing tumor invasion through the gallbladder wall, into the adjacent liver parenchyma or peripancreatic tissue, and locoregional lymph nodes [78]. It is more predictive of an underlying diagnosis compared to transabdominal ultrasound and affords an opportunity for fine needle aspiration (FNA) of a visualized gallbladder mass or aspiration of bile for cytologic analysis [79, 80].

It may also be used to further evaluate the locoregional extent and regional lymph node basins in distal cholangiocarcinoma. It also allows for FNA of distal tumors and/or enlarged lymph nodes while avoiding manipulation of the biliary tree [81]. It is a more sensitive modality for detecting cholangiocarcinoma as compared to standard transabdominal ultrasound and CT, but has a limited role in the evaluation of more proximal lesions [82].

14.11 Cholangiography

Both endoscopic retrograde cholangiopancreatography (ERCP) and percutaneous transhepatic cholangiography (PTC) are of minimal additional diagnostic value in biliary malignancy evaluation, having largely been replaced by MRI/MRCP [83]. However, both modalities may facilitate biliary decompression to palliate obstructive jaundice. Brush cytology or bile samples may be obtained to attempt to yield a formal diagnosis. However, these tests have a relatively limited sensitivity, and a negative study does not rule out the presence of an underlying malignancy [84–86].

The role of preoperative biliary decompression in suspected cholangiocarcinoma remains a controversial practice [87, 88]. However, if biliary drainage is clinically indicated, an endoscopic approach is considered as first-line therapy [89, 90]. If this is unsuccessful or not technically feasible, percutaneous transhepatic drainage is a reasonable alternative [91]. In general, a total bilirubin level >10 mg/dL in the setting of intrahepatic or perihilar disease necessitates preoperative decompression, and surgery is typically subsequently deferred until levels are less than 2–3 mg/dL. It is paramount to obtain full preoperative imaging prior to decompression as collapsed bile ducts are less amenable to radiographic evaluation and metal stent placement creates artifact impedance. It is safe to pursue diagnostic staging laparoscopy (DSL) while bilirubin levels are normalizing so that alternative therapies may be planned if a tumor is deemed unresectable.

Some studies suggest that preoperative biliary decompression does not contribute to postoperative liver failure or mortality, while others associate preoperative drainage with higher postoperative morbidity, including the development of perihepatic abscess and biliary leak, without a mortality benefit. However, unrelieved biliary obstruction may rapidly lead to cholestasis, liver insufficiency, and biliary cirrhosis, and thus decompression should be considered on a case-by-case basis [92, 93]. Patients may also benefit from drainage of a future liver remnant less than 30% predicted volume regardless of other clinical features [94]. Notably, up to 6% of patients who undergo preoperative drainage will develop recurrent disease along prior catheter tracts, which must also be taken into consideration [95, 96].

14.12 Positron-Emission Tomography

The role of PET imaging in gallbladder cancer and cholangiocarcinoma staging continues to evolve as most biliary tract tumors are FDG-avid [97]. It is typically performed as an outpatient test for patients with good performance status who have been diagnosed with potentially resectable disease on full cross-sectional imaging to evaluate for occult metastatic disease. PET imaging leads to a change in surgical management in approximately 25% of patients and thus plays an important role in minimizing unnecessary procedures [98]. If imaging does not demonstrate distant metastases, patients should proceed next to DSL. However, PET imaging is not an adequate substitution for DSL. False-positive results may occur secondary to cholangitis and inflammatory lesions [98].

14.13 Additional Considerations in Primary Sclerosing Cholangitis

Radiographic diagnosis of cholangiocarcinoma can be notoriously difficult in patients with underlying PSC as benign and malignant strictures often have similar appearances and mass lesions are rare. As such, most patients do not develop new or worsening intrahepatic ductal dilation. Worrisome imaging findings include progression of a stricture on serial cholangiograms, marked biliary dilation proximal to a dominant stricture, or a greater than 1 cm ductal mass [99]. If MRCP is nondiagnostic and high suspicion for cholangiocarcinoma remains, ERCP should be pursued and brush cytology of a dominant stricture and/or abnormal-appearing tissue obtained. If further imaging or cytology is suggestive of cholangiocarcinoma, the patient should undergo a full staging workup. If the diagnosis remains in doubt, PET imaging should be obtained. If this remains nondiagnostic, the patient should be followed closely and a repeat MRCP obtained at 3 months.

14.14 Complete Staging Evaluation

14.14.1 Gallbladder Cancer

Gallbladder cancer is staged via a traditional TNM approach based upon the American Joint Committee on Cancer's eighth edition guidelines (Tables 14.1 and 14.2) [100, 101]. Overall staging distribution is approximately as follows: T1

Table 14.1 AJCC Eighth Edition Gallbladder Cancer TNM Staging. Adapted from Zhu AX, Pawlik TM, Kooby DA, Schefter TE, Vauthey JN. Gallbladder. In: AJCC Cancer Staging Manual, 8th ed, Amin MB (Ed). American College of Surgeons, Chicago 2017

Primary tumor (T)	
TX	Primary tumor cannot be assessed
T0	No evidence of primary tumor
Tis	Carcinoma in situ
T1	Tumor invades the lamina propria or muscular layer
T1a	Tumor invades the lamina propria
T1b	Tumor invades the muscular layer
T2	Tumor invades the perimuscular connective tissue on the peritoneal side without involvement of the serosa, or tumor invades the perimuscular connective tissue on the hepatic side without extension into the liver
T2a	Tumor invades the perimuscular connective tissue on the peritoneal side without involvement of the serosa
T2b	Tumor invades the perimuscular connective tissue on the hepatic side without extension into the liver
T3	Tumor perforates the serosa and/or directly invades the liver and/or one other adjacent organ or structure, including the stomach, duodenum, colon, pancreas, omentum, or extrahepatic bile ducts
T4	Tumor invades the main portal vein or hepatic artery or invades two or more extrahepatic organs or structures
Regional lymph nodes (N)	
NX	Regional lymph nodes cannot be assessed
N0	No regional lymph node metastasis
N1	Metastases to 1–3 regional lymph nodes
N2	Metastases to 4+ regional lymph nodes
Distant metastasis (M)	
M0	No distant metastasis
M1	Distant metastasis

Table 14.2 Eighth Edition AJCC Prognostic Stage Groups for Gallbladder Cancer. Adapted from Zhu AX, Pawlik TM, Kooby DA, Schefter TE, Vauthey JN. Gallbladder. In: AJCC Cancer Staging Manual, 8th ed, Amin MB (Ed). American College of Surgeons, Chicago 2017

Stage 0	TisN0M0
Stage I	T1N0M0
Stage IIA	T2aN0M0
Stage IIB	T2bN0M0
Stage IIIA	T3N0M0
Stage IIIB	T1-3N1M0
Stage IVA	T4N0-1M0
Stage IVB	Any T, N2M0
	Any T, any N, M1

disease 11%, T2 disease 58% (of these, 61% are T2a and 39% are T2b), T3 disease 30%, and T4 disease 2% [102]. Expectedly, higher T stage disease is more likely to correlate with nodal disease. For example, while only 17% of T2a tumors have nodal involvement, nearly 60% of T3 tumors demonstrate lymphatic spread. The most common distant sites of gallbladder cancer metastases are the peritoneal surface, liver, and occasionally lungs and pleura.

Full staging evaluation for gallbladder cancer includes CT abdomen/pelvis as described above in addition to CT chest to evaluate for metastatic disease. PET/CT may be used to evaluate for occult, advanced disease that may preclude surgical resection. Preoperative PET imaging alters staging and treatment recommendations in up to 23% of patients. However, it remains insensitive for peritoneal carcinomatosis and is generally not helpful in evaluating for potential re-resection following cholecystectomy. Ultimately, only 15–60% of patients will be resection candidates after appropriate staging due to the presence of distant metastatic disease [103].

14.14.2 Cholangiocarcinoma

Intrahepatic, perihilar, and distal cholangiocarcinomas have separate AJCC eighth edition TNM staging systems, as shown in Tables 14.3, 14.4, 14.5, 14.6, 14.7, and 14.8.

Full staging evaluation for cholangiocarcinoma includes cross-sectional imaging of the abdomen/pelvis via either CT abdomen/pelvis or MRCP as detailed above. Chest CT should also be obtained to evaluate for metastatic disease. PET imaging may also be used to evaluate for occult metastatic disease if there is otherwise no radiographic evidence of distant spread. If a PET scan is unrevealing and the patient is a good surgical candidate, DSL should be pursued [104]. If any cross-sectional imaging study is equivocal for vascular involvement, the addition of a duplex ultrasound may be useful to evaluate for unresectable disease.

Table 14.3 AJCC 8th Edition Intrahepatic Cholangiocarcinoma. Adapted from Aloia T, Pawlik TM, Taouli B, Rubbia-Brandt L, Vauthey JN. Intrahepatic Bile Ducts. In: AJCC Cancer Staging Manual, 8th ed, Amin MB (Ed). American College of Surgeons, Chicago 2017

Primary tumor (T)	
TX	Primary tumor cannot be assessed
T0	No evidence of primary tumor
Tis	Carcinoma in situ (intraductal tumor)
T1	Solitary tumor without vascular invasion
T1a	Solitary tumor ≤5 cm without vascular invasion
T1b	Solitary tumor >5 cm without vascular invasion
T2	Solitary tumor with intrahepatic vascular invasion or multiple tumors with or without vascular invasion
T3	Tumor perforates the visceral peritoneum
T4	Tumor directly invades local extrahepatic structures
Regional lymph nodes (N)	
NX	Regional lymph nodes cannot be assessed
N0	No regional lymph node metastasis
N1	Regional lymph node metastasis present
Distant metastasis (M)	
M0	No distant metastasis
M1	Distant metastasis

Table 14.4 AJCC Prognostic Stage Groups for Intrahepatic Cholangiocarcinoma. Adapted from Aloia T, Pawlik TM, Taouli B, Rubbia-Brandt L, Vauthey JN. Intrahepatic Bile Ducts. In: AJCC Cancer Staging Manual, 8th ed, Amin MB (Ed). American College of Surgeons, Chicago 2017

Stage 0	TisN0M0
Stage IA	T1aN0M0
Stage IB	T1bN0M0
Stage II	T2N0M0
Stage IIIA	T3N0M0
Stage IIIB	T4N0M0
	Any T, N1M0
Stage IV	Any T, any N, M1

A formal tissue diagnosis can be obtained via brush cytology, fine needle aspiration (FNA), or image-guided biopsy. Notably, potential surgical candidates with classic radiographic findings of cholangiocarcinoma and those with obviously unresectable disease do not require formal tissue diagnosis. Furthermore, FNA or image-guided percutaneous biopsy can seed the biopsy tract with malignant cells, which precludes otherwise eligible patients from undergoing liver transplantation. As such, perihilar cholangiocarcinoma cases should be carefully reviewed with a liver transplant program prior to tissue sampling.

Table 14.5 AJCC 8th Edition Staging for Perihilar Cholangiocarcinoma. Adapted from Nagorney DM, Pawlik TM, Chun YS, Ebata T, Vauthey JN. Perihilar Bile Ducts. In: AJCC Cancer Staging Manual, 8th ed, Amin MB (Ed). American College of Surgeons, Chicago 2017

Primary tumor (T)	
TX	Primary tumor cannot be assessed
T0	No evidence of primary tumor
Tis	Carcinoma in situ/high-grade dysplasia
T1	Tumor confined to the bile duct, with extension up to the muscle layer or fibrous tissue
T2	Tumor invades beyond the wall of the bile duct to surrounding adipose tissue, or tumor invades adjacent hepatic parenchyma
T2a	Tumor invades beyond the wall of the bile duct to surrounding adipose tissue
T2b	Tumor invades adjacent hepatic parenchyma
T3	Tumor invades unilateral branches of the portal vein or hepatic artery
T4	Tumor invades the main portal vein or its branches bilaterally, or the common hepatic artery, or unilateral second-order biliary radicals with contralateral portal vein or hepatic artery involvement
Regional lymph nodes (N)	
NX	Regional lymph nodes cannot be assessed
N0	No regional lymph node metastasis
N1	1–3 positive lymph nodes (typically involving the hilar, cystic duct, common bile duct, hepatic artery, posterior pancreaticoduodenal, and portal vein lymph nodes)
N2	4+ positive lymph nodes from the sites described for N1
Distant metastasis (M)	
M0	No distant metastasis
M1	Distant metastasis

Table 14.6 AJCC Prognostic Stage Groups for Perihilar Cholangiocarcinoma. Adapted from Nagorney DM, Pawlik TM, Chun YS, Ebata T, Vauthey JN. Perihilar Bile Ducts. In: AJCC Cancer Staging Manual, 8th ed, Amin MB (Ed). American College of Surgeons, Chicago 2017

Stage 0	TisN0M0
Stage I	T1N0M0
Stage II	T2aN0M0
	T2bN0M0
Stage IIIA	T3N0M0
Stage IIIB	T4N0M0
Stage IIIC	Any T, N1M0
Stage IVA	Any T, N2M0
Stage IVB	Any T, any N, M1

Tissue diagnosis of cholangiocarcinoma is important in a few select circumstances [105]. Indeterminate strictures may require biopsy to evaluate for underlying malignancy. Additionally, some patients are reluctant to accept a diagnosis or proceed with treatment without a formal diagnosis.

Table 14.7 AJCC 8th Edition Staging for Distal Cholangiocarcinoma. Adapted from Krasinkas A, Pawlik TM, Mino-Kenudson M, Vauthey JN. Distal Bile Duct. In: AJCC Cancer Staging Manual, 8th ed, Amin MB (Ed). American College of Surgeons, Chicago 2017

Primary tumor (T)	
TX	Primary tumor cannot be assessed
T0	No evidence of primary tumor
Tis	Carcinoma in situ/high-grade dysplasia
T1	Tumor invades the bile duct wall with a depth <5 mm
T2	Tumor invades the bile duct wall with a depth of 5–12 mm
T3	Tumor invades the bile duct wall with a depth >12 mm
T4	Tumor involves the celiac axis, superior mesenteric artery, and/or common hepatic artery
Regional lymph nodes (N)	
NX	Regional lymph nodes cannot be assessed
N0	No regional lymph node metastasis
N1	Metastasis in 1–3 regional lymph nodes
N2	Metastasis in 4+ regional lymph nodes
Distant metastasis (M)	
M0	No distant metastasis
M1	Distant metastasis

Table 14.8 AJCC Prognostic Stage Groups for Distal Cholangiocarcinoma. Adapted from Krasinkas A, Pawlik TM, Mino-Kenudson M, Vauthey JN. Distal Bile Duct. In: AJCC Cancer Staging Manual, 8th ed, Amin MB (Ed). American College of Surgeons, Chicago 2017

Stage 0	TisN0M0
Stage I	T1N0M0
Stage IIA	T1N1M0
	T2N0M0
Stage IIB	T2N1M0
	T3N0M0
	T3N1M0
Stage IIIA	T1N2M0
	T3N2M0
Stage IIIB	T4N0M0
	T4N1M0
	T4N2M0
Stage IV	Any T, any N, M1

14.15 Histology

Greater than 90% of biliary tract malignancies are adenocarcinomas. The remainder tend to be squamous cell carcinomas. Gallbladder squamous cell carcinoma tends to be higher grade and diagnosed at a later stage, and thus is associated with worse survival outcomes [106]. While rarer still, papillary gallbladder carcinoma carries the most favorable histologic prognosis. Cholangiocarcinoma is divided into three subtypes—sclerosing, nodular, and papillary—all of which demonstrate slow growth, albeit with high rates of local invasion and mucin production [106]. Of these, the papillary subtype is the rarest, but carries the highest resectability rate as it tends to cause symptomatic biliary obstruction earlier in its clinical course. Distant metastases are uncommon.

14.16 Prognostic Factors

The most important prognostic factors for gallbladder cancer include T stage, N stage, tumor grade, lymphovascular and perineural invasion, CA 19-9 serum level, and status of surgical margins [102, 107–110]. Higher T stages predict a higher likelihood of both nodal and metastatic disease [103]. Disease recurrence is also associated with a worse prognosis and unfortunately occurs in up to 67% of patients [111, 112]. Two-thirds of these recurrences occur within 12 months, and most of the remainder occur within 24 months.

Cholangiocarcinoma prognosis is predominantly influenced by surgical margin status, lymphovascular invasion, and lymph node metastases [113–116]. R0 margins carry an improved 5-year survival rate of 19–47% compared to positive margins at 0–12% [114]. Node-positive disease carries a dismal 5–10% 5-year survival rate, even with adequate oncologic resection, whereas N0 disease carries an approximately 38% 5-year survival rate [117]. There is also an inverse relationship between survival and number of positive lymph nodes. Elevated CA 19-9 levels prior to any treatment also portend a poorer prognosis [55, 56].

14.17 Neoadjuvant Therapy

There is no defined role of neoadjuvant therapy in the treatment of gallbladder cancer, nor is it a standard approach to cholangiocarcinoma treatment [118]. However, on a case-by-case basis, neoadjuvant therapy may be considered for large, locally advanced, unresectable intrahepatic cholangiocarcinomas in an attempt to downstage disease to a resectable state. Neoadjuvant therapy may also be given to cholangiocarcinoma patients enrolled in a clinical trial or those being considered for liver transplantation.

14.18 Approach to Surgical Resection

14.18.1 Role of Staging Laparoscopy

Ultimately, in both gallbladder cancer and cholangiocarcinoma, not all unresectable disease is readily apparent on cross-sectional imaging. DSL allows identification of occult metastatic disease that precludes curative resection, and thus may spare patiens the morbidity of a laparotomy [119, 120]. Approximately 23% of patients with gallbladder cancer who undergo staging laparoscopy will have disseminated disease diagnosed intraoperatively. As such, DSL is recommended for all patients with suspected or known gallbladder cancer greater than stage T1b [119].

In cholangiocarcinoma, DSL effectively rules out peritoneal carcinomatosis, but does not always adequately evaluate vascular invasion. Nevertheless, it still identifies most patients with unresectable disease and substantially reduces the incidence of nontherapeutic laparotomy [120, 121]. Ultimately, true resectability of cholangiocarcinoma is only determined after complete abdominal exploration [92].

14.18.2 Unresectable Disease

Absolute contraindications to surgical resection of gallbladder cancer include peritoneal, liver, or hepatoduodenal ligament metastases; presence of malignant ascites; and encasement or occlusion of major vessels [101].

The presence of distant metastatic disease, including involvement of distant liver parenchyma, retropancreatic and paraceliac lymph node basins, and disseminated intra- or extra-abdominal disease, is a contraindication to cholangiocarcinoma resection [122, 123]. Traditionally, involvement of adjacent extrahepatic organs, portal vein, or hepatic artery was considered a contraindication to resection. However, some high-volume centers will proceed with en bloc resection of such locally advanced tumors with vascular and enteric reconstruction in select cases [124–126]. Additional contraindications to resection depend upon individual tumor characteristics.

Patients with unresectable disease should be referred to a medical oncologist for consideration of palliative chemotherapy as well as a palliative care specialist for optimization of symptom management and further definition of goals of care. There is no role for palliative or debulking, non-curative radical biliary surgery.

14.18.3 Resectable Gallbladder Cancer

14.18.3.1 Early-Stage Disease (Stage 0, I, or II)

Gallbladder cancer confined to the wall is potentially amenable to curative resection. T1a disease is successfully managed in 73–100% of cases with a simple cholecystectomy [2, 127–129]. T1b and higher disease, however, necessitates a more radical resection as higher T stages carry a higher incidence of lymph node metastases [127]. Patients with T1b disease who undergo an extended cholecystectomy and en bloc resection of the gallbladder with a rim of parenchyma of liver segments IVb and V have a longer median survival (9.8 vs. 6.4 years) than those who do not [127, 130–132]. Fifteen percent of these patients will have lymph node involvement. Unfortunately, less than 50% of T1b patients undergo an extended cholecystectomy, which subsequently leads to incomplete staging and thus undertreatment.

T2 disease also necessitates extended cholecystectomy [133–135]. Notably, patients with T2a disease carry a better prognosis than T2b disease. Over 60% of these patients will have lymph node metastases. Expectedly, when T2 disease is treated with simple cholecystectomy alone, there are high rates of local recurrence [136, 137]. Unfortunately, residual disease is also common following re-resection as well.

14.18.3.2 Locally Advanced or Node-Positive Disease

Some evidence suggests that radical resection of T3 and T4 disease in appropriately selected patients may provide a mortality benefit, but at the cost of high postoperative morbidity. T3 disease is treated with an extended cholecystectomy with en bloc resection of any involved adjacent organ(s) [138]. T4 disease is generally unresectable due to involvement of the portal vasculature or multiple adjacent extrahepatic organs.

Resection of node-positive disease may similarly be pursued in select patients. Locoregional lymphadenectomy removes the cystic duct, common bile duct, hepatic artery, and portal vein nodes and carries a 28–60% 5-year survival rate [127, 139]. Lymphadenectomy yields less favorable long-term survival when disease extends beyond the hepatoduodenal ligament [140].

14.19 Gallbladder Cancer Diagnosed During Cholecystectomy

If a malignant-appearing lesion is encountered intraoperatively and a surgeon who is formally trained in hepatobiliary surgical oncology is not immediately available, the incisions should be closed and the patient appropriately referred to a surgical oncologist. The lesion should not be biopsied, nor should simple cholecystectomy be performed in order to prevent peritoneal seeding or spillage and potential disease upstaging.

14.20 Gallbladder Cancer Diagnosed After Cholecystectomy

Of all patients undergoing laparoscopic cholecystectomy for presumed benign biliary disease, 0.25–1.5% will be diagnosed with an incidental gallbladder cancer on the final pathologic analysis [3, 136, 141]. These patients must undergo a full staging evaluation with cross-sectional imaging as detailed previously and should ideally be referred to a tertiary hepatobiliary center [142]. If re-resection is feasible for T1b and higher disease, it should ideally occur within 2 months of the patient's initial cholecystectomy [103, 143–146].

14.20.1 T1a Disease

T1a disease is cured with simple cholecystectomy alone. No survival benefit is achieved with re-resection [133, 147]. However, these patients should undergo full staging cross-sectional imaging at the time of diagnosis and again at 6 and 12 months postoperatively.

14.20.2 T1b Disease

Following staging, T1b disease is best treated with re-resection in the form of an extended cholecystectomy due to the 50–60% incidence of local recurrence following simple cholecystectomy alone. Some studies cite an increase in median survival by 3 years with re-resection of T1b disease [148]. Of those who undergo completion extended cholecystectomy, 12–20% will have lymph node metastases and around 13% will have hepatic involvement [144, 149].

14.20.3 T2 Disease

T2 disease is also best treated with extended cholecystectomy and regional lymphadenectomy. 40–76% of these patients will have some form of residual disease identified at re-resection [103, 143, 150, 151]. Five-year survival rate increases substantially with aggressive re-resection from 24–40% after simple cholecystectomy alone to 80–100% in some case series [152–157]. Lymphadenectomy for T2 disease is also associated with improved survival. A minimum of six lymph nodes must be removed in order for a gallbladder cancer to truly be staged as N0 disease [153].

14.20.4 T3/T4 Disease

Patients who receive a diagnosis of T3 disease following initial cholecystectomy should undergo a repeat DSL, as should those with poorly differentiated histology or a positive surgical margin. Ultimately, rates of residual disease are high with up to 46% of patients having nodal disease and 36% having hepatic involvement [144]. Nevertheless, median overall survival is nearly doubled with re-resection compared to no additional resection (23 vs. 12 months) [146].

T4 disease should be readily apparent on initial gallbladder evaluation for benign biliary disease, and thus should not be initially diagnosed on pathologic analysis following simple cholecystectomy.

14.21 Resectability of Localized Cholangiocarcinoma

No classification or staging system exists to accurately assess the ability to resect cholangiocarcinoma. Traditional criteria for resectability include the absence of retropancreatic and paraceliac nodal metastases, distant liver metastases, main portal vein or proper hepatic artery invasion, extrahepatic adjacent organ invasion, and disseminated disease [122–125]. More advanced disease may be considered for resection on a case-by-case basis at high-volume centers. Distal disease has the highest resectability rate, as high as 91% in some series, compared to intrahepatic and perihilar tumors [48]. Nevertheless, an R0 resection can only be obtained in 50% of distal cholangiocarcinomas and in only 20–40% of proximal tumors [154]. These percentages drop even further if a 5 mm negative margin is considered as an adequate oncologic resection [155].

Overall perioperative mortality for cholangiocarcinoma resection is approximately 5–6% [156]. Rates are highest for hepatectomy with biliary-enteric anastomosis and lowest for biliary-enteric anastomosis alone. Expectedly, the extent of postoperative liver dysfunction increases perioperative morbidity and mortality. Lowest complication rates are seen in patients younger than 60 years of age without preoperative jaundice, who do not receive neoadjuvant chemotherapy, who have T1a/b and N0 disease, and who do not require bile duct resection [157].

14.21.1 Intrahepatic Cholangiocarcinoma

Intrahepatic disease most commonly requires hepatic resection to achieve negative margins, which is successful in less than 30% of cases [9, 158, 159]. There is no demonstrable therapeutic benefit of lymphadenectomy, and thus this remains a controversial practice in the surgical management of intrahepatic cholangiocarcinoma [160–162]. Lymphadenectomy carries the risk of common bile duct devascularization and ideally is only performed for centrally located tumors where extrahepatic bile duct resection is required to achieve negative surgical margins. The presence of gross porta hepatis lymphadenopathy portends a poor prognosis and should only be resected on a case-by-case basis [160]. Five-year survival rate with an R0 resection of N0 disease may be as high as 44–63%, but ultimately, most patients will recur despite an adequate oncologic resection [9, 160, 163–165].

14.21.2 Perihilar Cholangiocarcinoma

Isolated bile duct resection, while technically feasible for certain perihilar tumors, is associated with higher rates of early disease recurrence [166, 167]. Less than 50% of patients with perihilar cholangiocarcinoma amenable to surgical therapy will actually have a curative resection. Type I, II, and III lesions require en bloc resection of the involved extrahepatic bile ducts and gallbladder with 5–10 mm bile duct margins, regional lymphadenectomy, and Roux-en-Y hepaticojejunostomy reconstruction [122, 166, 167]. Additional en bloc hepatectomy or trisegmentectomy is often required to achieve an R0 resection [168–172]. Type II and III tumors also commonly involve the caudate bile duct branches and thus necessitate a caudate lobectomy [122, 171]. Select type III and IV tumors are amenable to en bloc resection as detailed above plus portal vein resection and reconstruction. Highly select type II, III, and IV perihilar cholangiocarcinomas that are unresectable due to vascular invasion or underlying PSC should be referred for liver transplant evaluation (discussed later). Postoperative survival is adversely affected by transmural tumor extension to the gallbladder, mixed adenosquamous histology, hypoalbuminemia, and a preoperative total bilirubin level >10 mg/dL [14, 92, 173].

14.21.3 Distal Cholangiocarcinoma

Resectable distal disease is classically treated with either pylorus-resecting or pylorus-sparing pancreaticoduodenectomy. Five-year survival rate may be as high as 54–62% with an R0 resection of N0 disease but drops to below 20% for node-positive disease [113, 174, 175].

14.22 Role of Liver Transplantation in Cholangiocarcinoma Treatment

Some centers may consider liver transplantation as the standard therapy for patients with PSC and early-stage cholangiocarcinoma or those with early-stage, unresectable hilar cholangiocarcinoma who have completed rigorous neoadjuvant chemotherapy. Those patients who are evaluated for and eventually undergo liver transplantation for cholangiocarcinoma are more likely to have PSC and are more likely to have received neoadjuvant chemotherapy and/or chemoradiotherapy [176–181]. There are also some studies to suggest that liver transplantation yields better 3- and 5-year survival rates compared to resection for patients with initially resectable disease as well [182]. As such, the National Comprehensive Cancer Network (NCCN) recommends that transplant referral be placed for patients with locally advanced, unresectable cholangiocarcinoma [183].

There are no widely established patient selection criteria for curative liver transplantation for cholangiocarcinoma. The Mayo Clinic criteria include a formal cholangiocarcinoma diagnosis on cytology, a CA 19-9 level >100 U/mL and/or mass lesion on cross-sectional imaging and/or a malignant-appearing stricture on cholangiogram, tumor above the cystic duct, radial tumor diameter ≤3 cm, and no intra- or extrahepatic metastases in a patient who is otherwise clinically fit to undergo liver transplantation [176, 181]. The United Network for Organ Sharing (UNOS) has an established Model for End-Stage Liver Disease (MELD) score exception for early-stage, unresectable hilar cholangiocarcinoma patients who complete a protocolized neoadjuvant chemoradiotherapy regimen and undergo operative staging at a transplant center [184]. The baseline MELD score is set at 22 points and may increase every 3 months so long as selection criteria are still met.

As previously mentioned, FNA or percutaneous, image-guided biopsy of a suspected cholangiocarcinoma can seed the biopsy tract with malignant cells. This practice precludes otherwise eligible patients from undergoing transplant evaluation [184]. As such, perihilar cholangiocarcinoma cases should be carefully reviewed with transplant surgery prior to any tissue sampling.

14.23 Gallbladder Cancer Resection Techniques

14.23.1 Simple Cholecystectomy for Tis, T1a Disease

Simple cholecystectomy is considered curative for in situ or T1a gallbladder cancer. Notably, simple cholecystectomy may be selectively pursued as a palliative procedure in later disease stages to prevent recurrent cholecystitis episodes.

14.23.2 Extended Cholecystectomy for T2, T3 Disease

Extended cholecystectomy refers to the en bloc resection of the gallbladder with a 2 cm rim of liver segments IVb and V, most commonly performed via an open approach (midline laparotomy or right subcostal incision) [185–190]. It is important to avoid intraoperative bile spillage to minimize the risk of tumor dissemination [191]. Additionally, the cystic duct margin should be sent for frozen section analysis [144]. If this margin is negative, a portal lymphadenectomy completes the resection. However, if this margin is positive, further bile duct resection with portal and hepatoduodenal lymphadenectomy followed by biliary reconstruction is indicated [189, 192].

Indications for bile duct resection include tumor extension into the common bile duct and positive cystic duct margins [103, 189]. Reconstruction is most commonly performed via a Roux-en-Y hepaticojejunostomy. There is no survival benefit associated with routine bile duct resection [142, 144, 193]. Expectedly, bile duct reconstruction carries the increased risks of both biliary leak and anastomotic stricture.

Additionally, more extensive hepatic resection may be indicated for higher stage disease [194]. Typically, nonanatomic resection of at least a 2 cm margin of liver parenchyma of segments IVb and V is sufficient. For further disease infiltration, a formal IVb/V segmentectomy or even a formal hepatic lobectomy or extended right hepatectomy may be indicated. Overall, anatomic resection reduces the risk of bleeding and biliary leak compared to nonanatomic wedge resection [195]. However, there is ultimately no survival benefit to major hepatectomy or en bloc resection of adjacent organs in locally advanced gallbladder cancer [138].

Expectedly, perioperative morbidity and mortality are higher for those patients undergoing major hepatectomy [196–198]. The most commonly encountered complications include bleeding, biliary leak, and perihepatic abscess.

14.23.3 Role of Lymphadenectomy

Portal lymphadenectomy for gallbladder cancer is indicated for T1b and higher disease [143, 150, 199]. An adequate regional lymphadenectomy removes a minimum of six nodes in the porta hepatis and along the hepatoduodenal ligament, including the cystic duct, common bile duct, hepatic artery, and portal vein lymph nodes

[101]. Overall, the number of involved lymph nodes is of greater prognostic significance than their location [200].

14.23.4 Laparoscopic Port Site Excision

Port site recurrences are historically described following laparoscopic cholecystectomy for gallbladder cancer [201, 202]. Ultimately, the use of laparoscopic techniques does not adversely impact survival from gallbladder cancer, nor does radical re-section require excision of previous port sites [203]. Rather, tumor seeding at previous port sites represents disseminated disease and correlates well with the development of peritoneal metastases, and thus excision is neither beneficial nor curative [204].

14.24 Cholangiocarcinoma Resection Techniques

Typical surgical exposure for both intra- and extrahepatic cholangiocarcinoma is achieved through either an upper midline laparotomy or a right subcostal incision. From here, a wide Kocher maneuver is performed to expose the duodenum. This dissection is continued cephalad to expose the right side of the porta hepatis. Preoperatively placed stents may be palpated to help localize the common bile duct and ampulla of Vater. If the gallbladder is in situ, it is then removed from the cystic plate, but left attached to the common bile duct by the cystic duct.

Ultimately, further resection depends upon the location of the tumor. For example, surgical treatment of middle bile duct tumors depends upon the extent of superior and inferior involvement. Initially, uninvolved superior and inferior bile ducts are identified in addition to the adjacent vasculature. The use of intraoperative ultrasound can be useful in the identification of portal vasculature and tumor assessment. Traditionally, the right hepatic artery is found posterior to the common hepatic duct. Frozen section analysis should be performed on the inferior and superior margins. A positive inferior margin typically requires proceeding to pancreaticoduodenectomy, while a positive superior margin may require hepatic resection with biliary-enteric reconstruction.

Any suspicious or involved porta hepatis lymph nodes should be removed as well, although there is no clear consensus on the benefit of portal lymphadenectomy [205].

14.24.1 Roux-en-Y Biliary-Enteric Anastomosis

Routine biliary-enteric reconstruction is achieved via creation of either a Roux-en-Y choledochojejunostomy or a hepaticojejunostomy. The biliary blood supply is more robust proximal to the takeoff of the cystic duct. This is classically performed as an end-to-side anastomosis.

More specialized biliary reconstruction may occasionally be required due to tumor involvement, but more commonly due to iatrogenic or traumatic injury. Occasionally, multi-duct reconstruction may be necessary for multiply obstructed bile ducts. Preoperatively, PTC decompression should be attempted for all involved ducts. Intraoperatively, each orifice is identified and anastomosed to the Roux limb.

14.24.2 Distal Cholangiocarcinoma

Distal extrahepatic cholangiocarcinoma is nearly always surgically treated via pancreaticoduodenectomy. Consideration should also be given to distal enteral access.

14.25 Localized, Unresectable Gallbladder Cancer

Progression of gallbladder cancer is mostly locoregional, although gallbladder cancer has a greater propensity for distant metastases as compared to cholangiocarcinoma [111]. Locoregionally advanced, unresectable disease is most commonly managed with external beam radiation therapy with concurrent 5-fluorouracil infusion [206, 207]. Ultimately, the benefit of either chemotherapy or radiation therapy is unclear in this group of patients [118].

14.26 Localized, Unresectable Cholangiocarcinoma

Nonmetastatic, unresectable cholangiocarcinoma is initially treated with systemic chemotherapy, preferably with gemcitabine-cisplatin combination therapy [208, 209]. If patients demonstrate stable disease without progression after 3–4 months of systemic chemotherapy, locoregional therapies may be considered, including chemoradiotherapy, SBRT, and hepatic intra-arterial therapies [210–215]. These patients are treated with the goal of palliation, although a small minority may experience a sufficiently robust response to therapy to permit eventual surgical resection.

For unresectable intrahepatic disease, the NCCN recommends gemcitabine-cisplatin combination therapy, enrollment in a clinical trial, fluoropyrimidine-based chemotherapy, and/or capecitabine chemoradiotherapy [183]. For unresectable extrahepatic disease, patients may be referred to a transplant center as appropriate or may receive gemcitabine-cisplatin combination systemic chemotherapy, clinical trial enrollment, capecitabine chemoradiotherapy, and/or best supportive care.

14.27 Adjuvant Therapy for Resected Gallbladder Cancer and Cholangiocarcinoma

The overall survival of patients with biliary tract cancers is limited by disease recurrence after surgical resection, and therefore adjuvant therapy is often considered. While observation is an option for biliary tract cancers that have been completely resected, the limited study data that is available support the use of adjuvant therapy. The use of oral capecitabine is considered to be standard adjuvant therapy for resected biliary tract malignancies [216, 217]. Recently studied adjuvant therapeutic regimens have been well tolerated, and thus additional phase III studies are ongoing [218]. The greatest survival benefit with adjuvant therapy is observed in patients with N+ disease as well as those who have undergone an R1/R2 resection [219]. Accordingly, adjuvant therapy is strongly recommended for patients with these high-risk features.

14.28 Advanced, Unresectable Disease

As previously mentioned, biliary malignancy carries an exceptionally poor prognosis due to its commonly advanced stage at the time of diagnosis. The goals of treatment at this stage are to relieve pain, jaundice, and other symptoms and potentially prolong life. Ultimately, any palliative intervention depends upon the patient's symptoms and overall goals of care.

14.28.1 Obstructive Jaundice

Jaundice secondary to biliary obstruction is the presenting symptom of gallbladder cancer in 30–60% of patients, most commonly due to direct tumor infiltration of the common hepatic duct [220]. Stenting is the preferred treatment modality, either percutaneous or endoscopic, given patients' limited life expectancy, for both gallbladder cancer and unresectable, extrahepatic cholangiocarcinoma [221]. Ultimately, adequate drainage of as little as 30% of the liver is often sufficient to palliate jaundice and pruritis. More distal biliary obstructions are best treated via endoscopic drainage and stenting, while more proximal obstructions are often better served with percutaneous transhepatic drainage [222]. Both modalities carry similar rates of stent occlusion and median survival. As percutaneous drains often cannot be internalized and can be inconvenient for the patient, an initial endoscopic attempt at biliary decompression is typically pursued and is successful in 70% or more cases.

Unilateral versus bilateral stenting for hilar obstruction is debatable [223, 224]. Most cases require unilateral drainage only but may be inadequate and increase the risk of cholangitis in a handful of patients. Bilateral stent placement is more invasive but maximizes biliary drainage. In the event that only one side of the biliary tree can be technically drained, preprocedural imaging should be obtained to identify the dominant biliary system.

While there is much debate around the use of metal versus plastic stents, there is no associated survival benefit to either type [223, 225, 226]. Plastic stents are less expensive and more easily removed or exchanged but are more likely to occlude due to buildup of biliary sludge or bacterial biofilm [225]. Maintenance of patency typically requires serial ERCP every 3–6 months. Conversely, metal stents have a much longer duration of patency and are commonly placed in patients with unresectable disease who are expected to live beyond a few months [223, 227–233]. However, they may not be removable. As such, the diagnosis of an underlying malignancy should be firmly established prior to deployment.

There is also a similar debate around the use of covered versus uncovered stents, although they ultimately have similar patency rates [230]. In general, tumors that place extrinsic compression on the biliary tree are decompressed with uncovered stents, and those that are intraductal are decompressed with covered stents to minimize tumor ingrowth. Of note, in the setting of a distal malignant obstruction with an in situ gallbladder, placement of an uncovered bare metal stent is common to avoid occlusion of the cystic duct [231].

Surgical biliary or intestinal bypass may occasionally be considered in a handful of patients. However, even appropriately selected patients with good performance status and a longer estimated survival will ultimately fail these interventions due to disease progression. Palliative surgical bypass should be limited to patients who are found to have unresectable distal cholangiocarcinoma at the time of laparotomy, only if stenting is not a feasible option. Most commonly, this consists of a biliary-enteric bypass to either segment IV or left lateral sector of the liver with Roux-en-Y hepaticojejunostomy reconstruction.

14.28.2 Palliative Chemotherapy

Systemic chemotherapy is the primary treatment modality for unresectable biliary malignancies. It provides, at best, a modest benefit in treating advanced gallbladder cancer with approximately a 10–60% response rate [232–234]. First-line chemotherapeutic regimens are selected based upon the patient's performance status and degree of hyperbilirubinemia and are typically either gemcitabine or platinum based [100, 208, 209, 235–239]. Second-line chemotherapeutic agents are not well established.

14.29 Conclusion

Despite advances in surgical and medical therapies, the prognosis for biliary tract malignancies remains quite poor overall as these tumors are typically diagnosed at an advanced, unresectable stage. As initial presenting symptoms of both gallbladder cancer and cholangiocarcinoma can be vague and nonspecific, and thus may mimic benign biliary disease, these pathologies will be inevitably encountered by acute care surgeons upon initial patient evaluation as well as intraoperatively and postoperatively. It is imperative that non-hepatobiliary-trained surgeons be familiar with clinical, laboratory, and radiographic findings of biliary malignancies in order to best optimize patient outcomes.

References

1. Sharma A, Sharma KL, Gupta A, Yadav V, Kumar A. Gallbladder cancer epidemiology, pathogenesis and molecular genetics: recent update. World J Gastroenterol. 2017;23(22):3978.
2. Yamaguchi K, Chijiwa K, Ichimiya H, et al. Gallbladder carcinoma in the era of laparoscopic cholecystectomy. Arch Surg. 1996;131(9):981.
3. A prospective analysis of 1518 laparoscopic cholecystectomies. The Southern Surgeons Club. N Engl J Med. 1991;324(16):1073.
4. Vauthey JN, Blumgart LH. Recent advances in the management of cholangiocarcinomas. Semin Liver Dis. 1994;14(2):109.
5. Ouyang G, Liu Q, Wu Y, et al. The global, regional, and national burden of gallbladder cancer and biliary tract cancer and its attributable risk factors in 195 countries and territories, 1990 to 2017: a systematic analysis for the Global Burden of Disease Study 2017. Cancer. 2021;127(13):2238.
6. Van Dyke AL, Shiels MS, Jones GS, et al. Biliary tract cancer incidence and trends in the United States by demographic group, 1999-2013. Cancer. 2019;125(9):1489.
7. Broome U, Olsson R, Loof L, et al. Natural history and prognostic factors in 305 Swedish patients with primary sclerosing cholangitis. Gut. 1996;38(4):610.
8. Uesaka K, Yasui K, Morimoto T, et al. Visualization of routes of lymphatic drainage of the gallbladder with a carbon particle suspension. J Am Coll Surg. 1996;183(4):345–50.
9. DeOliveira ML, Cunningham SC, Cameron JL, et al. Cholangiocarcinoma: thirty-one-year experience with 564 patients at a single institution. Ann Surg. 2007;245(5):755.
10. Siegel RL, Miller KD, Fuchs HE, Jemal A. Cancer Statistics, 2021. CA Cancer J Clin. 2021;71(1):7.
11. Patel T. Increasing incidence and mortality of primary intrahepatic cholangiocarcinoma in the United States. Hepatology. 2011;33(6):1353.
12. Shaib YH, Davila JA, McGlynn K, El-Serag HB. Rising incidence of intrahepatic cholangiocarcinoma in the United States: a true increase? J Hepatol. 2004;40(3):472.
13. Patel N, Benipal B. Incidence of Cholangiocarcinoma in the USA from 2001 to 2015: a US Cancer Statistics Analysis of 50 States. Cureus. 2019;11(1):e3962.
14. Nagorney DM, Pawlik TM, Chun YS, et al. Perihilar bile ducts. In: Amin MB, editor. AJCC cancer staging manual. 8th ed. Chicago: American College of Surgeons; 2017.
15. Bismuth H, Nakache R, Diamond T. Management strategies in resection for hilar cholangiocarcinoma. Ann Surg. 1992;215(1):31.
16. Rahman R, Simoes EJ, Schmaltz C, et al. Trend analysis and survival of primary gallbladder cancer in the United States: a 1973-2009 population-based study. Cancer Med. 2017;6(4):874.
17. Scott TE, Carroll M, Cogliano FD, Smith BF, Lamorte WW. A case-control assessment of risk factors for gallbladder carcinoma. Dig Dis Sci. 1999;44(8):1619.
18. Strom BL, Soloway RD, Rios-Dalenz JL, et al. Risk factors for gallbladder cancer: an international collaborative case-control study. Cancer. 1995;76(10):1747.
19. Hsing AW, Gao YT, Han TQ, et al. Gallstones and the risk of biliary tract cancer: a population-based study in China. Br J Cancer. 2007;97(11):1577.
20. Maranghini A, Moreau JA, Melton LJ 3rd, Hench VS, Zinsmeister AR, DiMagno EP. Gallstones, gallbladder cancer, and other gastrointestinal malignancies. An epidemiologic study in Rochester, Minnesota. Ann Intern Med. 1987;107(1):30.
21. Randi G, Frenceschi S, La Vecchia C. Gallbladder cancer worldwide: geographical distribution and risk factors. Int J Cancer. 2006;118(7):1591.

22. Muszynska C, Lundgren L, Lindell G, et al. Predictors of incidental gallbladder cancer in patients undergoing cholecystectomy for benign gallbladder disease: results from a population-based gallstone surgery registry. Surgery. 2017;162(2):256.
23. Hsing AW, Bai Y, Andreotti G, et al. Family history of gallstones and the risk of biliary tract cancer and gallstones: a population-based study in Shanghai, China. Int J Cancer. 2007;121(4):832.
24. Misra S, Chaturvedi A, Misra NC, Sharma ID. Carcinoma of the gallbladder. Lancet Oncol. 2003;4(3):167.
25. Okamoto M, Okamoto H, Kitahara F, et al. Ultrasonographic evidence of association of polyps and stones with gallbladder cancer. Am J Gastroenterol. 1999;94(2):446.
26. Said K, Glaumann H, Bergquist A. Gallbladder disease in patients with primary sclerosing cholangitis. J Hepatol. 2008;48(4):598.
27. Nagaraja V, Eslick GD. Systematic review with meta-analysis: the relationship between chronic Salmonella typhi carrier status and gallbladder cancer. Aliment Pharmacol Ther. 2014 Apr;39(8):745–50.
28. Matsukura N, Yokomuro S, Yamada S, et al. Association between Helicobacter bilis in bile and biliary tract malignancies: *H. bilis* in bile from Japanese and Thai patients with benign and malignant diseases in the biliary tract. Jpn J Cancer Res. 2002;93(7):842.
29. Voyles CR, Smadja C, Shands WC, Blumgart LH. Carcinoma in choledochal cysts. Age-related incidence. Arch Surg. 1983;118(8):986.
30. Elnemr A, Ohta T, Kayahara M, et al. Anomalous pancreaticobiliary ductal junction without bile duct dilatation in gallbladder cancer. Hepato-Gastroenterology. 2001;48(38):382.
31. Yagyu K, Kikuchi S, Obata Y, et al. Cigarette smoking, alcohol drinking and the risk of gallbladder cancer death: a prospective cohort study in Japan. Int J Cancer. 2008;122(4):924.
32. Koshiol J, Gao JT, Dean M, et al. Association of aflatoxin and gallbladder cancer. Gastroenterology. 2017;153(2):488.
33. Chapman RW. Risk factors for biliary tract carcinogenesis. Ann Oncol. 1999;10 Supple 4:308.
34. Rosen CB, Nagorney DM, Wisner RH, Coffey RJ Jr, LaRusso NF. Cholangiocarcinoma complicating primary sclerosing cholangitis. Ann Surg. 1991;213(1):21.
35. Bergquist A, Glaumann H, Persson B, Broome U. Risk factors and clinical presentation of hepatobiliary carcinoma in patients with primary sclerosing cholangitis: a case-control study. Hepatology. 1998;27(2):311.
36. Khan SA, Thomas HC, Davidson BR, Taylor-Robinson SD. Cholangiocarcinoma. Lancet. 2005;366(9493):1303.
37. Scott J, Shousha S, Thomas HC, Sherlock S. Bile duct carcinoma: a late complication of congenital hepatic fibrosis. Case report and review of literature. Am J Gastroenterol. 1980;73(2):113.
38. Lipsett PA, Pitt HA, Colombani PM, Boitnott JK. Cameron JL Choledochal cyst disease. A changing pattern of presentation. Ann Surg. 1994;220(5):644.
39. Shaib YH, El-Serag HB, Davila JA, Morgan R, McGlynn KA. Risk factors of intrahepatic cholangiocarcinoma in the United States: a case-control study. Gastroenterology. 2005;128(3):620.
40. Donato F, Gelatti U, Tagger A, et al. Intrahepatic cholangiocarcinoma and hepatitis C and B virus infection, alcohol intake, and hepatolithiasis: a case-control study in Italy. Cancer Causes Control. 2001;12(10):959.
41. Sorenson HT, Friis S, Olsen JH, et al. Risk of liver and other types of cancer in patients with cirrhosis: a nationwide cohort study in Denmark. Hepatology. 1998;28(4):921.
42. Sahani D, Prasad SR, Tannabe KK, Hahn PF, Mueller PR, Saini S. Thorotrast-induced cholangiocarcinoma: case report. Abdom Imaging. 2003;28(1):72.
43. McGee EE, Jackson SS, Petrick JL, et al. Smoking, alcohol, and biliary tract cancer risk: a pooling project of 26 prospective studies. J Natl Cancer Inst. 2019;111(12):1263.
44. Watanapa P, Watanapa WB. Liver fluke-associated cholangiocarcinoma. Br J Surg. 2002;89(8):962.

45. Jing W, Jin G, Zhou X, et al. Diabetes mellitus and increased risk of cholangiocarcinoma: a meta-analysis. Eur J Cancer Prev. 2021;21(1):24.
46. Welzel TM, Graubard BI, El-Serag HB, et al. Risk factors for intrahepatic and extrahepatic cholangiocarcinoma in the United States: a population-based case-control study. Clin Gastroenterol Hepatol. 2007;5(10):1221.
47. Petrick JL, McMenamin UC, Zhang X, et al. Exogenous hormone use, reproductive factors and risk of intrahepatic cholangiocarcinoma among women: results from cohort studies in the Liver Cancer Pooling Project and the UK Biobank. Br J Cancer. 2020;123(2):316.
48. Nakeeb A, Pitt HA, Sohn TA, et al. Cholangiocarcinoma. A spectrum of intrahepatic, perihilar, and distal tumors. Ann Surg. 1996;224(4):463.
49. Nagorney DM, Donohue JH, Farnell MB, Schleck CD, Ilstrup DM. Outcomes after curative resections of cholangiocarcinoma. Arch Surg. 1993;128(8):871.
50. Blechacz B, Komuta M, Roskams T, Gores GJ. Clinical diagnosis and staging of cholangiocarcinoma. Nat Rev Gastroenterol Hepatol. 2011 Sep;8(9):512–22.
51. Brown KM, Parmar AD, Geller DA. Intrahepatic cholangiocarcinoma. Surg Oncol Clin N Am. 2014;23(2):231.
52. Xynos ID, Sougioltzis S, Zilos A, Evangelou K, Hatzis GS. Hypercalcemia in a patient with cholangiocarcinoma: a case report. Int Arch Med. 2009;2(1):35.
53. Malaguarnera G, Paladina I, Giordano M, Malaguarnera M, Bertino G, Berretta M. Serum markers of intrahepatic cholangiocarcinoma. Dis Markers. 2013;34(4):219.
54. Kim HJ, Kim MH, Myung SJ, et al. A new strategy for the application of CA 19-9 in the differentiation for pancreaticobiliary cancer: analysis using a receiver operating characteristic curve. Am J Gastroenterol. 1999;94(7):1941.
55. Bergquist JR, Ivanics T, Storlie CB, et al. Implications of CA 19-9 elevation for survival, staging, and treatment sequencing in intrahepatic cholangiocarcinoma: a national cohort analysis. J Surg Oncol. 2016;114(4):475.
56. Chung YJ, Choi DW, Choi SH, Heo JS, Kim DH. Prognostic factors following surgical resection of distal bile duct cancer. J Korean Surg Soc. 2013;85(5):212.
57. Patel AH, Harnois DM, Klee GG, LaRusso NF, Gores GJ. The utility of CA 19-9 in the diagnoses of cholangiocarcinoma in patients without primary sclerosing cholangitis. Am J Gastroenterol. 2000;95(1):204.
58. Sinakos E, Saenger AK, Keach J, Kim R, Lindor KD. Many patients with primary sclerosing cholangitis and increased serum levels of carbohydrate antigen 19-9 do not have cholangiocarcinoma. Clin Gastroenterol Hepatol. 2011;9(5):434.
59. Venkatesh PG, Navaneethan U, Shen B, McCullough AJ. Increased serum levels of carbohydrate antigen 19-9 and outcomes in primary sclerosing cholangitis patients without cholangiocarcinoma. Dig Dis Sci. 2013;58(3):850–7.
60. Levy C, Lymp J, Angulo P, Gores GJ, Larusso N, Lindor KD. The value of serum CA 19-9 in predicting cholangiocarcinomas in patients with primary sclerosing cholangitis. Dig Dis Sci. 2005;50(9):1734.
61. Goldaracena N, Gorgen A, Sapisochin G. Current status of liver transplantation for cholangiocarcinoma. Liver Tranpl. 2018;24(2):294–303.
62. Tempero MA, Uchida E, Takasaki H, Burnett DA, Steplewski Z, Pour PM. Relationship of carbohydrate antigen 19-9 and Lewis antigens in pancreatic cancer. Cancer Res. 1987;47(2):5501.
63. Siqueira E, Schoen RE, Silverman W, et al. Detecting cholangiocarcinoma in patients with primary sclerosing cholangitis. Gastrointest Endosc. 2002;56(1):40.
64. Ramage JK, Donaghy A, Farrant JM, Iorns R, Williams R. Serum tumor markers for the diagnosis of cholangiocarcinoma in primary sclerosing cholangitis. Gastroenterology. 1995;108(3):865.
65. Sharma MP, Ahuja V. Aetiological spectrum of obstructive jaundice and diagnostic ability of ultrasonography: a clinician's perspective. Trop Gastroenterol. 1999;20(4):167.
66. Bach AM, Hann LE, Brown KT, et al. Portal vein evaluation with US: comparison to angiography combined with CT arterial portography. Radiology. 1996;201(1):149.

67. Pandey M, Sood BP, Shukla RC, Aryya NC, Singh S, Shukla VK. Carcinoma of the gallbladder: role of sonography in diagnosis and staging. J Clin Ultrasound. 2000;28(5):227.
68. Wibbenmeyer LA, Sharafuddin MJ, Wolverso MK, Heiberg E, Wade TP, Shields JB. Sonographic diagnosis of unsuspected gallbladder cancer: imaging findings in comparison with benign gallbladder conditions. Am J Roentol. 1995;165(5):1169.
69. Bloom CM, Langer B, Wilson SR. Role of US in the detection, characterization, and staging of cholangiocarcinoma. Radiographics. 1999;19(5):1199.
70. Saini S. Imaging of the hepatobiliary tract. N Engl J Med. 1997;336(26):1889.
71. Ohtani T, Shirai Y, Tsukada K, Muto T, Hatakeyama K. Spread of gallbladder carcinoma: CT evaluation with pathologic correlation. Abdom Imaging. 1996;21(3):195.
72. Pilgrim CH, Groeschl RT, Pappas SG, Gamblin TC. An often overlooked diagnosis: imaging features of gallbladder cancer. J Am Coll Surg. 2013 Feb;216(2):333–9.
73. Valls C, Guma A, Puig I, et al. Intrahepatic peripheral cholangiocarcinoma: CT evaluation. Abdom Imaging. 2000;25(5):490.
74. Iavarone M, Piscaglia F, Vavassori S, et al. Contrast enhanced CT-scan to diagnose intrahepatic cholangiocarcinoma in patients with cirrhosis. J Hepatol. 2013;58(6):1188–93.
75. Lee MG, Park KB, Shin YM, et al. Preoperative evaluation of hilar cholangiocarcinoma with contrast-enhanced three-dimensional fast imaging with steady-state precession magnetic resonance angiography: comparison with intraarterial digital subtraction angiography. World J Surg. 2003;27(3):278.
76. Park HS, Lee JM, Choi JY, et al. Preoperative evaluation of bile duct cancer: MRI combined with MR cholangiopancreatography versus MDCT with direct cholangiography. Am J Roentgentol. 2008;190(2):396.
77. Schwartz LH, Black J, Fong Y, et al. Gallbladder carcinoma: findings at MR imaging with MR cholangiopancreatography. J Comput Assist Tomogr. 2002;26(3):405.
78. American Society for Gastrointestinal Endoscopy (ASGE) Standards of Practice Committee. The role of endoscopy in the evaluation and treatment of patients with biliary neoplasia. Gastrointest Endosc. 2013;77(2):167.
79. Sadamoto Y, Kubo H, Harada N, Tanaka M, Eguchi T, Nawata H. Preoperative diagnosis and staging of gallbladder carcinoma by EUS. Gastrointest Endosc. 2003;58(4):536.
80. Wu LM, Jiang XX, Gu HY, et al. Endoscopic ultrasound fine-needle aspiration biopsy in the evaluation of bile duct strictures and gallbladder masses: a systematic review and meta-analysis. Eur J Gastroenterol Hepatol. 2011;23(2):113–20.
81. Abu-Hamda EM, Baron TH. Endoscopic management of cholangiocarcinoma. Semin Liver Dis. 2004;24(2):165.
82. Mohamadnejad M, DeWitt JM, Sherman S, et al. Role of EUS for preoperative evaluation of cholangiocarcinoma: a large single-center experience. Gastrointest Endosc. 2011;73(1):71.
83. Freeman ML, Sielaff TD. A modern approach to malignant hilar biliary obstruction. Rev Gastroenterol Disord. 2003;3(4):187.
84. Mansfield JC, Griffin SM, Wadehra V, Matthewson K. A prospective evaluation of cytology from biliary strictures. Gut. 1997;40(5):671.
85. Ponchon T, Gagnon P, Berger F, et al. Value of endobiliary brush cytology and biopsies for the diagnosis of malignant bile duct stenosis: results of a prospective study. Gastrointest Endosc. 1995;42(6):565.
86. Rabinovitz M, Zajko AB, Hassanein T, et al. Diagnostic value of brush cytology in the diagnosis of bile duct carcinoma: a study of 65 patients with bile duct strictures. Hepatology. 1990;12(4 Pt 1):747.
87. Laurent A, Tayar C, Cherqui D. Cholangiocarcinoma: preoperative biliary drainage (Con). HPB (Oxford). 2008;10(2):126.
88. Nimura Y. Cholangiocarcinoma: preoperative biliary drainage (Pro). HPB (Oxford). 2009;10(2):130.
89. Paik WH, Loganathan N, Hwang JH. Preoperative biliary drainage in hilar cholangiocarcinoma: when and how? World J Gastrointest Endosc. 2014;6(3):68.

90. Kloek JJ, van der Gaag NA, Aziz Y, et al. Endoscopic and percutaneous preoperative biliary drainage in patients with suspected hilar cholangiocarcinoma. J Gastrointest Surg. 2010;14(1):119.
91. Walter T, Ho CS, Horgan AM, et al. Endoscopic or percutaneous biliary drainage for Klatskin tumors? J Vasc Interv Radiol. 2013;24(1):113–21.
92. Su CH, Tsay SH, Wu CC, et al. Factors influencing postoperative morbidity, mortality, and survival after resection for hilar cholangiocarcinoma. Ann Surg. 1996;223(4):384.
93. Liu F, Li Y, Wei Y, Li B. Preoperative biliary drainage before resection for hilar cholangiocarcinoma: whether or not? A systematic review. Dig Dis Sci. 2011;56(3):663.
94. Kennedy TJ, Yopp A, Qin Y, et al. Role of preoperative biliary drainage of liver remnant prior to extended liver resection for hilar cholangiocarcinoma. HPB (Oxford). 2009;11(5):445–51.
95. Takahashi Y, Nagino M, Nishio H, Ebata T, Igami T, Nimura Y. Percutaneous transhepatic biliary drainage catheter tract recurrence in cholangiocarcinoma. Br J Surg. 2010;97(12):1860–6.
96. Sakata J, Shirai Y, Wakai T, Nomura T, Sakata E, Hatakeyama K. Catheter tract implantation metastases associated with percutaneous biliary drainage for extrahepatic cholangiocarcinoma. World J Gastroenterol. 2005;11(44):7024–7.
97. Corvera CU, Blumgart LH, Akhurst T, et al. 18F-fluorodeoxyglucose positron emission tomography influences management decisions in patients with biliary cancer. J Am Coll Surg. 2008;206(1):57.
98. Anderson CD, Rice MH, Pinson CW, Chapman WC, Chari RS, Delbeke D. Fluorodeoxyglucose PET imaging in the evaluation of gallbladder carcinoma and cholangiocarcinoma. J Gastrointest Surg. 2004;8(1):90.
99. Razumilava N, Gores GJ, Lindor KD. Cancer surveillance in patients with primary sclerosing cholangitis. Hepatology. 2011;54(5):1842.
100. Valle JW, Borbath I, Khan SA, et al. Biliary cancer: ESMO Clinical Practice Guidelines for diagnosis, treatment, and follow-up. Ann Oncol. 2016;27(suppl 5):v28.
101. Zhu AX, Pawalik TM, Kooby DA, et al. Gallbladder. In: Amin MB, editor. AJCC cancer staging manual. 8th ed. Chicago: AJCC; 2017. p. 303.
102. Shindoh J, de Aretxabala X, Aloia TA, et al. Tumor location is a strong predictor of tumor progression and survival in T2 gallbladder cancer: an international multicenter study. Ann Surg. 2015;261(4):733.
103. Fong Y, Jarnagin W, Blumgart LH. Gallbladder cancer: comparison of patients presenting initially for definitive operation with those presenting after prior noncurative intervention. Ann Surg. 2000;232(4):557.
104. Society of American Gastrointestinal and Endoscopic Surgeons (SAGES). Guidelines for diagnostic laparoscopy. 2010. https://www.sages.org/publications/guidelines/guidelines-for-diagnostic-laparoscopy.
105. Pelsang RE, Johlin FC. A percutaneous biopsy technique for patients with suspected biliary or pancreatic cancer without a radiographic mass. Abdom Imaging. 1997;22(3):307.
106. Henson DE, Albores-Saavedra J, Corle D. Carcinoma of the gallbladder. Histologic types, stage of disease, grade, and survival rates. Cancer. 1992;70(6):1493.
107. Ethun CG, Postlewait LM, Le N, et al. A novel pathology-based preoperative risk score to predict locoregional residual and distant disease and survival for incidental gallbladder cancer: a 10-institution study from the U.S. Extrahepatic Biliary Malignancy Consortium. Ann Surg Oncol. 2017;24(5):1343.
108. Kim SH, Chong JU, Lim JH, et al. Optimal assessment of lymph node status in gallbladder cancer. Eur J Surg Oncol. 2016;42(2):205.
109. Sakata J, Shirai Y, Wakai T, Ajioka Y, Hatakeyama K. Number of positive lymph nodes independently determines the prognosis after resection in patients with gallbladder carcinoma. Ann Surg Oncol. 2010;17(7):1831.
110. Wen Z, Si A, Yang J, et al. Elevation of CA 19-9 and CEA is associated with poor prognosis in patients with resectable gallbladder carcinoma. HPB (Oxford). 2017;19(11):951.

111. Jarnagin WR, Ruo L, Little SA, et al. Patterns of initial disease recurrence after resection of gallbladder carcinoma and hilar cholangiocarcinoma: implications for adjuvant therapeutic strategies. Cancer. 2003;98(8):1689.
112. Kim WS, Choi DW, You DD, Ho CY, Heo JS, Choi SH. Risk factors influencing recurrence, patterns of recurrence, and the efficacy of adjuvant therapy after radical resection for gallbladder carcinoma. J Gastrointest Surg. 2010 Apr;14(4):679–87.
113. Fong Y, Blumgart LH, Lin E, Fortner JG, Brennan MF. Outcome of treatment for distal bile duct cancer. Br J Surg. 1996;83(12):1712.
114. Klempnauer J, Ridder GJ, von Wasielewski R, Werner M, Weimann A, Pichlmayr R. Resectional surgery of hilar cholangiocarcinoma: a multivariate analysis of prognostic factors. J Clin Oncol. 1994;15(3):947.
115. Rea DJ, Munoz-Jaurez M, Farnell MB, et al. Major hepatic resection for hilar cholangiocarcinoma: analysis of 46 patients. Arch Surg. 2004;139(5):514.
116. Tamandi D, Kaczirek K, Gruenberger B, et al. Lymph node ratio after curative surgery for intrahepatic cholangiocarcinoma. Br J Surg. 2009;96(8):919.
117. Aoba T, Ebata T, Yokoyama Y, et al. Assessment of nodal status for perihilar cholangiocarcinoma: location, number, or ratio of involved nodes. Ann Surg. 2013;257(4):718–25.
118. Hakeem AR, Papoulas M, Menon KV. The role of neoadjuvant chemotherapy or chemoradiotherapy for advanced gallbladder cancer—a systematic review. Eur J Surg Oncol. 2019;45(2):83.
119. Agarwal AK, Kalayarasan R, Javed A, Gupta N, Nag HH. The role of staging laparoscopy in primary gallbladder cancer—an analysis of 409 patients: a prospective study to evaluate the role of staging laparoscopy in the management of gallbladder cancer. Ann Surg. 2013;258(2):318.
120. Weber SM, DeMatteo RP, Fong Y, Blumgart LH, Jarnagin WR. Staging laparoscopy in patients with extrahepatic biliary carcinoma Analysis of 100 patients. Ann Surg. 2002;235(3):392.
121. Callery MP, Strasberg SM, Doherty GM, Soper NJ, Norton JA. Staging laparoscopy with laparoscopic ultrasonography: optimizing resectability in hepatobiliary and pancreatic malignancy. J Am Coll Surg. 1997;185(1):33.
122. Tsao JI, Nimura Y, Kamiya J, et al. Management of hilar cholangiocarcinoma: comparison of an American and a Japanese experience. Ann Surg. 2000;232(2):166.
123. Rajagopalan V, Daines WP, Grossbard ML, Kozuch P. Gallbladder and biliary tract carcinoma: a comprehensive update, Part 1. Oncology (Williston Park). 2004;18(7):889.
124. Ebata T, Nagino M, Kamiya J, Uesaka K, Nagasaka T, Nimura Y. Hepatectomy with portal vein resection for hilar cholangiocarcinoma: audit of 52 consecutive cases. Ann Surg. 2003;238(5):720.
125. Hemming AW, Reed AI, Fujita S, Foley DP, Howard RJ. Surgical management of hilar cholangiocarcinoma. Ann Surg. 2005;241(5):693.
126. Nishio H, Ebata T, Yokohama Y, Igami T, Sugawara G, Nagino M. Gallbladder cancer involving the extrahepatic bile duct is worthy of resection. Ann Surg. 2011;253(5):953.
127. Shirai Y, Yoshida K, Tsukada K, Muto T. Inapparent carcinoma of the gallbladder. An appraisal of a radical second operation after simple cholecystectomy. Ann Surg. 1992;215(4):326.
128. Shirai Y, Yoshida K, Tsukada K, Muto T, Watanabe H. Early carcinoma of the gallbladder. Eur J Surg. 1992;158(10):545.
129. Wakai T, Shirai Y, Yokohama N, Nagakura S, Watanabe H, Hatakeyama K. Early gallbladder carcinoma does not warrant radical resection. Br J Surg. 2001;88(5):675.
130. Abramson MA, Pandharipande P, Ruan D, Gold JS, Whang EE. Radical resection for T1b gallbladder cancer: a decision analysis. HPB (Oxford). 2009;11(8):656.
131. de Aretxabala XA, Roa IS, Burgos LA, Araya JC, Villaseca MA, Silva JA. Curative resection in potentially resectable tumours of the gallbladder. Eur J Surg. 1997;163(6):419.
132. Matsumoto Y, Fujii H, Aoyama H, Yamamoto M, Sugahara K, Suda K. Surgical treatment of primary carcinoma of the gallbladder based on the histologic analysis of 48 surgical specimens. Am J Surg. 1992;163(2):239.

133. Coburn NG, Clearly SP, Tan JC, Law CH. Surgery for gallbladder cancer: a population-based analysis. J Am Coll Surg. 2008;207(3):371–82.
134. Wright BE, Lee CC, Iddings DM, Kavanaugh M, Bilchik AJ. Management of T2 gallbladder cancer: are practice patterns consistent with national recommendations? Am J Surg. 2007;194(6):820–5.
135. Kwon W, Kim H, Han Y, et al. Role of tumour location and surgical extent on prognosis in T2 gallbladder cancer: an international multicentre study. Br J Surg. 2020;107(10):1334.
136. Yamaguchi K, Tsuneyoshi M. Subclinical gallbladder carcinoma. Am J Surg. 1992;163(4):382.
137. Kapoor VK. Incidental gallbladder cancer. Am J Gastroenterol. 2001;96(3):627.
138. D'Angelica M, Dalal KM, DeMatteo RP, Fong Y, Blumgart LH, Jarnagin WR. Analysis of the extent of resection for adenocarcinoma of the gallbladder. Ann Surg Oncol. 2009;16(4):806.
139. Yamamoto M, Onoyama H, Ajiki T, Yamada I, Fujita T, Saitoh Y. Surgical results of operations for carcinoma of the gallbladder. Hepato-Gastroenterology. 1999;46(27):1552.
140. Chijiwa K, Noshiro H, Nakano K, Okido M, Sugitani A, Yamaguchi K, Tanaka M. Role of surgery for gallbladder carcinoma with special reference to lymph node metastases and stage using western and Japanese classification systems. World J Surg. 2000;24(10):1271.
141. Konstantinidis IT, Deshpande V, Genevay M, et al. Trends in presentation and survival for gallbladder cancer during a period of more than 4 decades: a single-institution experience. Arch Surg. 2009;144(5):441.
142. Shih SP, Schulick RD, Cameron JL, et al. Gallbladder cancer: the role of laparoscopy and radical resection. Ann Surg. 2007;245(6):893.
143. Goetze TO, Paolucci V. Benefits of reoperation of T2 and more advanced incidental gallbladder carcinoma: analysis of the German registry. Ann Surg. 2008;247(1):104.
144. Pawlik TM, Gleisner AL, Vigano L, et al. Incidence of finding residual disease for incidental gallbladder carcinoma: implications for re-resection. J Gastrointest Surg. 2007;11(11):1478.
145. Fuks D, Regimbeau JM, Le Treut YP, et al. Incidental gallbladder cancer by the AFC-GBC-2009 Study Group. World J Surg. 2011;35(8):1887.
146. de Savornin Lohman EAJ, van der Geest LG, de Bitter TJJ, et al. Re-resection in incidental gallbladder cancer: survival and the incidence of residual disease. Ann Surg Oncol. 2020;27(4):1132.
147. Ouchi K, Mikuni J, Kakugawa Y, et al. Laparoscopic cholecystectomy for gallbladder carcinoma: results of a Japanese survey of 498 patients. J Hepato-Biliary-Pancreat Surg. 2002;9(2):256.
148. Taner CB, Nagorney DM, Donohue JH. Surgical treatment of gallbladder cancer. J Gastrointest Surg. 2004;8(1):83.
149. de Aretxabala X, Roa I, Burgos L, et al. Gallbladder cancer in Chile. A report on 54 potentially resectable tumors. Cancer. 1992;69(1):60.
150. Bartlett DL, Fong Y, Fortner JG, Brennan MF, Blumgart LH. Long-term results after resection for gallbladder cancer. Implications for staging and management. Ann Surg. 1996;224(5):639.
151. Duffy A, Capanu M, Abou-Alfa GK, et al. Gallbladder cancer (GBC): 10-year experience at Memorial Sloan-Kettering Cancer Centre (MSKCC). J Surg Oncol. 2008;98(7):485.
152. Downing SR, Cadogan KA, Ortega G, et al. Early-stage gallbladder cancer in the Surveillance, epidemiology, and end results database: effect of extended surgical resection. Arch Surg. 2011;146(6):734.
153. Ito H, Ito K, D'Angelica M, et al. Accurate staging for gallbladder cancer: implications for surgical therapy and pathological assessment. Ann Surg. 2011;254(2):320–5.
154. Burke EC, Jarnagin WR, Hochwald SN, Pisters PW, Fong Y, Blumgart LH. Hilar Cholangiocarcinoma: patterns of spread, the importance of hepatic resection for curative operation, and presurgical clinical staging system. Ann Surg. 1998;228(3):385.
155. Sakamoto E, Nimura Y, Hayakwa N, et al. The pattern of infiltration at the proximal border of hilar bile duct carcinoma: a histologic analysis of 62 resected cases. Ann Surg. 1998;227(3):405.
156. Loehrer AP, House MG, Nakeeb A, Kilbane EM, Pitt HA. Cholangiocarcinoma: are North American surgical outcomes optimal? J Am Coll Surg. 2013;216(2):192–200.

157. Merath K, Chen Q, Bagante F, et al. A Multi-Institutional International Analysis of Textbook Outcomes Among Patients Undergoing Curative-Intent Resection of Intrahepatic Cholangiocarcinoma. JAMA Surg. 2019;154(6):e190571.
158. Razumilava N, Gores GJ. Cholangiocarcinoma. Lancet. 2014;383(9935):2168.
159. Spolverato G, Kim Y, Alexandrescu S, et al. Is Hepatic Resection for Large or Multifocal Intrahepatic Cholangiocarcinoma justified? Results from a Multi-Institutional Collaboration. Ann Surg Oncol. 2015;22(7):2218–25.
160. Endo I, Gonen M, Yopp AC, et al. Intrahepatic cholangiocarcinoma: rising frequency, improved survival, and determinants of outcome after resection. Ann Surg. 2008;248(1):84.
161. de Jong MC, Nathan H, Sotiropoulos GC, et al. Intrahepatic cholangiocarcinoma: an international multi-institutional analysis of prognostic factors and lymph node assessment. J Clin Oncol. 2011;29(23):3140–5.
162. Carpizo DR, D'Angelica M. Management and extent of resection for intrahepatic cholangiocarcinoma. Surg Oncol Clin N Am. 2009;18(2):289–305.
163. Paik KY, Jung JC, Heo JS, Choi SH, Choi DW, Kim YI. What prognostic factors are important for resected intrahepatic cholangiocarcinoma? J Gastroenterol Hepatol. 2008;23(5):766.
164. Choi SB, Kim KS, Choi JY, et al. The prognosis and survival outcome of intrahepatic cholangiocarcinoma following surgical resection: association of lymph node metastasis and lymph node dissection with survival. Ann Surg Oncol. 2009;16(11):3048.
165. Weber SM, Jarnagin WR, Klimstra D, DeMatteo RP, Fong Y, Blumgart LH. Intrahepatic cholangiocarcinoma: resectability, recurrence pattern, and outcomes. J Am Coll Surg. 2001;193(4):384.
166. Nimura Y, Kamiya Y, Nagino M, et al. Aggressive surgical treatment of hilar cholangiocarcinoma. J Hepato-Biliary-Pancreat Surg. 1998;5(1):52.
167. Klempnauer J, Ridder GJ, Werner M, Weimann A, Pichlmayr R. What constitutes long-term survival after surgery for hilar cholangiocarcinoma? Cancer. 1997;79(1):26.
168. Hosokawa I, Shimiz H, Yoshidome H, et al. Surgical strategy for hilar cholangiocarcinoma of the left-side predominance: current role of left trisectionectomy. Ann Surg. 2014;259(6):1178–85.
169. Matsumoto N, Ebata T, Yokohama Y, et al. Role of anatomical right hepatic trisectionectomy for perihilar cholangiocarcinoma. Br J Surg. 2014;101(3):261–8.
170. Esaki M, Shimada K, Nara S, et al. Left hepatic trisectionectomy for advanced perihilar cholangiocarcinoma. Br J Surg. 2013;100(6):801–7.
171. Nagino M, Nimura Y, Kamiya J, et al. Segmental liver resections for hilar cholangiocarcinoma. Hepato-Gastroenterology. 1998;45(19):7.
172. Miyazaki M, Ito H, Nakagawa K, et al. Aggressive surgical approaches to hilar cholangiocarcinoma: hepatic or local resection? Surgery. 1998;123(2):131.
173. Kosuge T, Yamamoto J, Shimada K, Yamasaki S, Makuuchi M. Improved surgical results for hilar cholangiocarcinoma with procedures including major hepatic resection. Ann Surg. 1999;230(5):663.
174. Murakami Y, Uemura K, Hayashidani Y, Sudo T, Ohge H, Sueda T. Pancreaticoduodenectomy for distal cholangiocarcinoma: prognostic impact of lymph node metastasis. World J Surg. 2007;31(2):337.
175. Yoshida T, Matsumoto T, Sasaki A, Morii Y, Aramaki M, Kitano S. Prognostic factors after pancreaticoduodenectomy with extended lymphadenectomy for distal bile duct cancer. Arch Surg. 2002;137(1):69.
176. Rea DJ, Heimbach JK, Rosen CB, et al. Liver transplantation with neoadjuvant chemoradiation is more effective than resection for hilar cholangiocarcinoma. Ann Surg. 2005;242(3):451.
177. Sudan D, DeRoover A, Chinnakotla S, et al. Radiochemotherapy and transplantation allow long-term survival for nonresectable hilar cholangiocarcinoma. Am J Transplant. 2002;2(8):774.
178. Brandseater B, Isoniemi H, Broome U, et al. Liver transplantation for primary sclerosing cholangitis; predictors and consequences of hepatobiliary malignancy. J Hepatol. 2004;40(5):815.

179. Goss JA, Shackleton CR, Farmer DG, et al. Orthotopic liver transplantation for primary sclerosing cholangitis. A 12-year single center experience. Ann Surg. 1997;225(5):472.
180. Rosen CB, Heimbach JK, Gores GJ. Surgery for cholangiocarcinoma: the role of liver transplantation. HPB (Oxford). 2008;10(3):186.
181. Rosen CB, Heimbach JK, Gores GJ. Liver transplantation for cholangiocarcinoma. Transpl Int. 2010;23(7):692–7.
182. Gu J, Bai J, Shi X, et al. Efficacy and safety of liver transplantation in patients with cholangiocarcinoma: a systematic review and meta-analysis. Int J Cancer. 2012;130(9):2155.
183. 2021 NCCN Guidelines for Patients: Gallbladder and Bile Duct Cancers. https://www.nccn.org/patients/guidelines/content/PDF/gallandbile-hp-patient.pdf.
184. Organ Procurement and Transplantation Network. Policies. http://optn.transplant.hrsa.gov/policiesAndBylaws/policies.asp.
185. Yokomizo H, Yamane T, Hirata T, Hifumi M, Kawaguchi T, Fukuda S. Surgical treatment of pT2 gallbladder carcinoma: a reevaluation of the therapeutic effect of hepatectomy and extrahepatic bile duct resection based on the long-term outcome. Ann Surg Oncol. 2007;14(4):1366.
186. Oertli D, Herzog U, Tondelli P. Primary carcinoma of the gallbladder: operative experience during a 16 year period. Eur J Surg. 1993;159(8):415.
187. Chijiwa K, Nakano K, Ueda J, et al. Surgical treatment of patients with T2 gallbladder carcinoma invading the subserosal layer. J Am Coll Surg. 2001;192(5):600.
188. Toyonaga T, Chijiwa K, Nakano K, et al. Completion radical surgery after cholecystectomy for accidentally undiagnosed gallbladder carcinoma. World J Surg. 2003;27(3):266.
189. Jayaraman S, Jarnagin WR. Management of gallbladder cancer. Gastroenterol Clin N Am. 2010;39(2):331.
190. Weiland ST, Mahvi DM, Niederhuber JE, Heisey DM, Chicks DS, Rikkers LF. Should suspected early gallbladder cancer be treated laparoscopically? J Gastrointest Surg. 2002;6(1):50.
191. Wullstein C, Woeste G, Barkhausen S, Gross E, Hopt UT. Do complications related to laparoscopic cholecystectomy influence the prognosis of gallbladder cancer? Surg Endosc. 2002;16(5):828.
192. Gall FP, Kockerling F, Scheele J, Schneider C, Hohenberger W. Radical operations for carcinoma of the gallbladder: present status in Germany. World J Surg. 1991;15(3):328.
193. Kosuge T, Sano K, Shimada K, Yamamoto J, Yamasaki S, Makuuchi M. Should the bile duct be preserved or removed in radical surgery for gallbladder cancer? Hepato-Gastroenterology. 1999;46(28):2133.
194. Blumgart LH. Surgery of the liver, biliary tract and pancreas. 4th ed. Philadelphia: Saunders; 2007.
195. Scheingraber S, Justinger C, Stremovskaia T, Weinrich M, Igna D, Shilling MK. The standardized surgical approach improves outcome of gallbladder cancer. World J Surg Oncol. 2007;5:55.
196. Jin LX, Pitt SC, Hall BL, Pitt HA. Aggressive surgical management of gallbladder cancer: at what cost? Surgery. 2013;154(2):266–73.
197. Shimada K, Nara S, Esaki M, Sakamoto Y, Kosuge T, Hiraoka N. Extended right hepatectomy for gallbladder carcinoma involving the hepatic hilum. Br J Surg. 2011;98(1):117–23.
198. Reddy SK, Marroquin CE, Kuo PE, Pappas TN, Clary BM. Extended hepatic resection for gallbladder cancer. Am J Surg. 2007;194(3):355–61.
199. Tsukada K, Hatakeyama K, Kurosaki I, et al. Outcome of radical surgery for carcinoma of the gallbladder according to the TNM stage. Surgery. 1996;120(5):816.
200. Birnbaum DJ, Vigano L, Russolillo N, Langella S, Ferrero A, Capussotti L. Lymph node metastases in patients undergoing surgery for a gallbladder cancer. Extension of the lymph node dissection and prognostic value of the lymph node ratio. Ann Surg Oncol. 2015;22(3):811–8.
201. Steinert R, Nestler G, Sagynaliev E, Muller J, Lippert H, Reymond MA. Laparoscopic cholecystectomy and gallbladder cancer. J Surg Oncol. 2006;93(8):682.

202. Lundberg O, Kristoffersson A. Port site metastases from gallbladder cancer after laparoscopic cholecystectomy. Results of a Swedish survey and review of published reports. Eur J Surg. 1999;165(3):215.
203. Suzuki K, Kimura T, Ogawa H. Long-term prognosis of gallbladder cancer diagnosed after laparoscopic cholecystectomy. Surg Endosc. 2000;14(8):712.
204. Maker AV, Butte JM, Oxenberg J, et al. Is port site resection necessary in the surgical management of gallbladder cancer? Ann Surg Oncol. 2012;19(2):409.
205. Kim SH, Han DH, Choi GH, Choi JS, Kim KS. Recommended minimal number of harvested lymph nodes for intrahepatic cholangiocarcinoma. J Gastrointest Surg. 2021;25(5):1164.
206. Ben-David MA, Griffith KA, Abu-Isa E, et al. External-beam radiotherapy for localized extrahepatic cholangiocarcinoma. Int J Radiat Oncol Biol Phys. 2006;66(3):772.
207. Sasson AR, Hoffman JP, Ross E, et al. Trimodality therapy for advanced gallbladder cancer. Am Surg. 2001;67(3):277.
208. Valle JW, Wasan H, Johnson P, et al. Gemcitabine alone or in combination with cisplatin in patients with advanced or metastatic cholangiocarcinomas or other biliary tract tumours: a multicenter randomized phase II study—the UK ABC-01 study. Br J Cancer. 2009;101(4):621.
209. Valle J, Wasan H, Palmer DH, et al. Cisplatin plus gemcitabine versus gemcitabine for biliary tract cancer. N Engl J Med. 2010;362(14):1273.
210. Yamashita S, Koay EJ, Passot G, et al. Local therapy reduces the risk of liver failure and improves survival in patients with intrahepatic cholangiocarcinoma: a comprehensive analysis of 362 consecutive patients. Cancer. 2017;123(8):1354.
211. Kim YI, Park JW, Kim BH, et al. Outcomes of concurrent chemoradiotherapy versus chemotherapy alone for advanced-stage unresectable intrahepatic cholangiocarcinoma. Radiat Oncol. 2013;8:292.
212. Tao R, Krishnan S, Bhosale PR, et al. Ablative radiotherapy doses lead to a substantial prolongation of survival in patients with inoperable intrahepatic cholangiocarcinoma: a retrospective dose response analysis. J Clin Oncol. 2016;34(3):219–26.
213. Lee J, Yoon WS, Koom WS, Rim CH. Efficacy of stereotactic body radiotherapy for unresectable or recurrent cholangiocarcinoma: a meta-analysis and systematic review. Strahlenther Onkol. 2019;195(2):93.
214. Hong TS, Wo JY, Yeap BY, et al. Multi-institutional phase II study of high-dose hypofractionated proton beam therapy in patients with localized, unresectable hepatocellular carcinoma and intrahepatic cholangiocarcinoma. J Clin Oncol. 2016;34(5):460–8.
215. Edeline J, Touchefeu Y, Guiu B, et al. Radioembolization plus chemotherapy for first-line treatment of locally advanced intrahepatic cholangiocarcinoma: a phase 2 clinical trial. JAMA Oncol. 2020;6(1):51.
216. Shroff RT, Kennedy EB, Bachini M, et al. Adjuvant therapy for resected biliary tract cancer: ASCO clinical practice guideline. J Clin Oncol. 2019;37(12):1015–27.
217. Primrose JN, Fox RP, Palmer DH, et al. Capecitabine compared with observation in resected biliary tract cancer (BILCAP): a randomised, controlled, multicentre, phase 3 study. Lancet Oncol. 2019;20(5):663–75.
218. Ben-Josef E, Guthrie KA, El-Khoueiry AB, et al. SWOG S0809: a phase II intergroup trial of adjuvant capecitabine and gemcitabine followed by radiotherapy and concurrent capecitabine in extrahepatic cholangiocarcinoma. J Clin Oncol. 2015;33(24):2617.
219. Horgan AM, Amir E, Walter T, Knox JJ. Adjuvant therapy in the treatment of biliary tract cancer: a systematic review and meta-analysis. J Clin Oncol. 2012;30(16):1934.
220. Kapoor VK, Pradeep R, Haribhakti SP, et al. Intrahepatic segment III cholangiojejunostomy in advanced carcinoma of the gallbladder. Br J Surg. 1996;83(12):1709.
221. Saluja SS, Gulati M, Garg PK, et al. Endoscopic or percutaneous biliary drainage for gallbladder cancer: a randomized trial and quality of life assessment. Clin Gastroenterol Hepatol. 2008;6(8):944.
222. Sawas T, Al Halabi S, Parsi MA, Vargo JJ. Self-expandable metal stents versus plastic stents for malignant biliary obstruction: a meta-analysis. Gastroinest Endosc. 2015;82(2):256.

223. Lee TH, Kim TH, Moon JH, et al. Bilateral versus unilateral placement of metal stents for inoperable high-grade malignant hilar biliary strictures: a multicenter, prospective, randomized study (with video). Gastrointest Endosc. 2017;86(5):817.
224. Moole H, Jaeger A, Cashman M, et al. Are self-expandable metal stents superior to plastic stents in palliating malignant distal biliary strictures? A meta-analysis and systematic review. Med J Armed Forces India. 2017;73(1):42.
225. Yoon WJ, Ryu JK, Yang KY, et al. A comparison of metal and plastic stents for the relief of jaundice in unresectable malignant biliary obstruction in Korea: an emphasis on cost-effectiveness in a country with a low ERCP cost. Gastrointest Endosc. 2009;70(2):284.
226. Moss AC, Morris E, Leyden J, MacMathuna P. Malignant distal biliary obstruction: a systematic review and meta-analysis of endoscopic and surgical bypass results. Cancer Treat Rev. 2007;33(2):213.
227. Davids PH, Groen AK, Rauws EA, Tytgat GN, Huibregste K. Randomised trial of self-expanding metal stents versus polyethylene stents for distal malignant biliary obstruction. Lancet. 1992;340(8834–8835):1488–92.
228. Sangchan A, Kongkasame W, Pugkhem A, Jenwitheesuk K, Mairiang P. Efficacy of metal and plastic stents in unresectable complex hilar cholangiocarcinoma: a randomized controlled trial. Gastrointest Endosc. 2012;76(1):93.
229. Yoon WJ, Lee JK, Lee KH, et al. A comparison of covered and uncovered Wallstents for the management of distal malignant biliary obstruction. Gastrointest Endosc. 2006;63(7):996.
230. Petersen BT, Kahaleh M, Kozrek RA, et al. A multicenter, prospective study of a new fully covered expandable metal biliary stent for the palliative treatment of malignant bile duct obstruction. Gastroenterol Res Pract. 2013;2013:642428.
231. Patt YZ, Hassan MM, Lozano RD, et al. Phase II trial of cisplatin, interferon alpha-2b, doxorubicin, and 5-fluorouracil for biliary tract cancer. Clin Cancer Res. 2001;7(11):3375.
232. Patt YZ, Hassan MM, Aguayo A, et al. Oral capecitabine for the treatment of hepatocellular carcinoma, cholangiocarcinoma, and gallbladder carcinoma. Cancer. 2004;101(3):578.
233. Tsavaris N, Kosmas C, Gouveris P, et al. Weekly gemcitabine for the treatment of biliary tract and gallbladder cancer. Investig New Drugs. 2002;22(2):193.
234. Malik IA, Aziz Z, Zaidi SH, Sethuraman G. Gemcitabine and Cisplatin is a highly effective combination chemotherapy in patients with advanced cancer of the gallbladder. Am J Clin Oncol. 2003;26(2):174.
235. Meyerhardt JA, Zhu AX, Stuart K, et al. Phase-II study of gemcitabine and cisplatin in patients with metastatic biliary and gallbladder cancer. Dig Dis Sci. 2008;53(2):564.
236. Ducreux M, Rougier P, Fandi A, et al. Effective treatment of advanced biliary tract carcinoma using 5-fluorouracil continuous infusion with cisplatin. Ann Oncol. 1998;9(6):653.
237. Sanz-Altamira PM, Ferrante K, Jenkins RL, Lewis WD, Huberman MS, Stuart KE. A phase II trial of 5-fluorouracil, leucovorin, and carboplatin in patients with unresectable biliary tree carcinoma. Cancer. 1998;82(12):2321.
238. Choi CW, Choi IK, Seo JH, et al. Effects of 5-fluorouracil and leucovorin in the treatment of pancreatic-biliary tract adenocarcinomas. Am J Clin Oncol. 2000;23(4):425.
239. Chen JS, Jan YY, Lin YC, Wang HM, Chang WC, Liau CT. Weekly 24 h infusion of high-dose 5-fluorouracil and leucovorin in patients with biliary tract carcinomas. Anti-Cancer Drugs. 1998;9(5):393.

Oncologic Surgical Emergencies: Spleen 15

Dennis Kim, and Naveen Balan

Highlights

- Oncologic surgical emergencies of the spleen are rare and often result from injury.
- Although a variety of malignant diseases may affect the spleen, splenic rupture is usually due to associated splenomegaly rather than the malignant process itself.
- Management of splenic rupture in the setting of a hematologic or splenic malignancy generally follows the same algorithm as patients with blunt splenic trauma.

15.1 Splenic Surgical Anatomy and Functions

The spleen is the largest collection of lymphoid tissue in the human body, located in the left upper quadrant of the abdomen and usually measuring 7–13 cm in length. It has numerous functions including hematopoiesis of red and white blood cells (WBCs) during gestation; immunologic protection; culling senescent red blood cells; removing inclusions from damaged red blood cells; and serving as a reservoir for platelets. Structurally, it is composed of lymphatic tissue and a dense vascular network surrounded by a fibroelastic capsule (Fig. 15.1) [1].

Within the abdomen, the spleen is suspended by several reflections of peritoneum. The splenorenal ligament, connecting the spleen to the left kidney, is perhaps the most important attachment to the surgeon as the splenic artery and vein course through it. The gastrosplenic ligament connects the spleen to the greater curvature of the stomach and contains the short gastric arteries. The splenophrenic and splenocolic ligaments confer attachments to the left hemidiaphragm and splenic flexure of the colon, respectively (Fig. 15.2).

D. Kim (✉) · N. Balan
Harbor-UCLA, Torrance, CA, USA

A. Tarasconi et al. (eds.), *Oncologic Surgical Emergencies*, Hot Topics in Acute Care Surgery and Trauma, https://doi.org/10.1007/978-3-031-36860-8_15

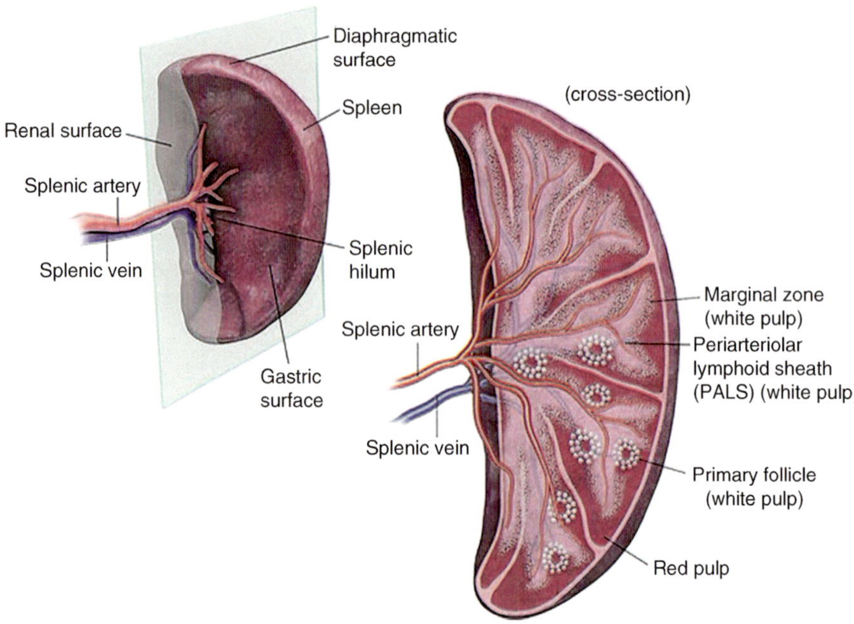

Fig. 15.1 Basic splenic anatomy

The arterial supply to the spleen comes from the tortuous splenic artery, a branch of the celiac trunk. There are two major clinical variations: distributed and magistral. The distributed phenotype involves the splenic artery dividing into smaller branches farther from the splenic hilum, while the magistral type branches close toward the hilum. Several organs lie in close proximity to the spleen: the stomach, pancreas, left kidney, and colon. In the vast majority of patients, the tail of the pancreas terminates within 1 cm from the splenic hilum. Therefore, caution must be taken to ligate the splenic vascular pedicle within 1 cm of the hilum to avoid iatrogenic injury to the tail of the pancreas.

The spleen has four principal physiologic functions: hematopoiesis, reservoir, filtration, and immunologic. Hematopoiesis is a main role of the spleen during early fetal development, serving as one of the main producers of red blood cells. However, this function largely disappears late in fetal life and is assumed by the bone marrow. As a reservoir, the spleen stores nearly one-third of platelets, as is evidenced by the resultant thrombocytopenia from platelet sequestration in the various pathologies that cause splenomegaly and thrombocythemia seen following splenectomy.

Filtration is one of the chief roles of the spleen as it is important in clearing the blood of various damaged or poorly functioning blood elements. As blood enters the red pulp of the spleen, red blood cells encounter reticuloendothelial cells that cull senescent red blood cells, remove dysmorphic red blood cells, and remove cellular inclusions (e.g., Howell-Jolly bodies and Heinz bodies). The immunologic functions of the spleen are essential in preventing bacteremia and infections, particularly for

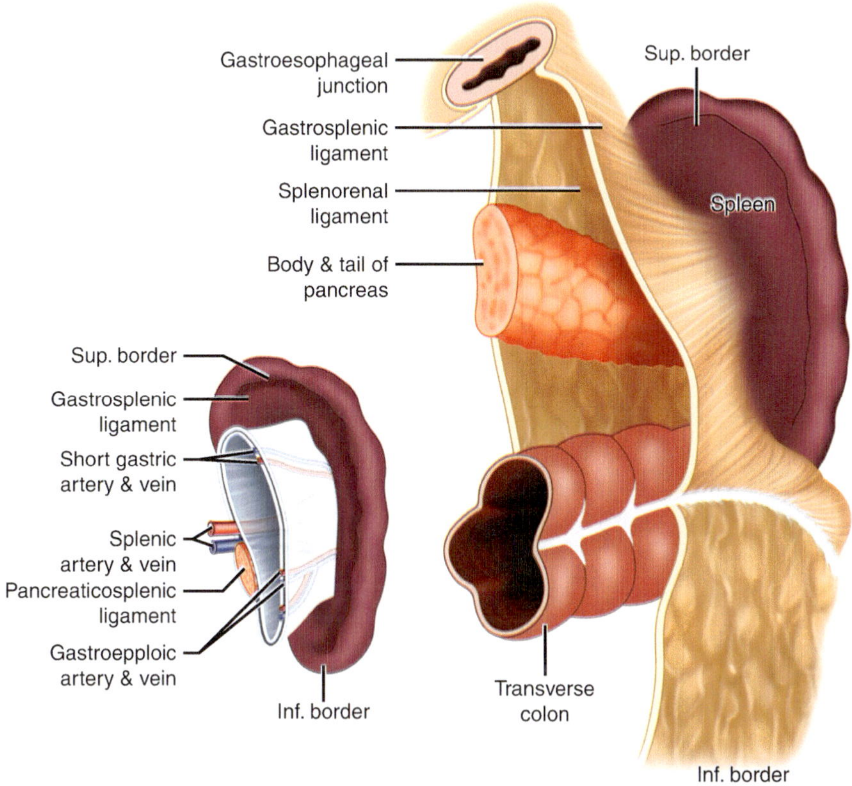

Fig. 15.2 Suspensory ligaments and relation of spleen to surrounding organs

encapsulated bacteria (i.e., *Streptococcus pneumoniae*, *Neisseria meningitidis*, *Haemophilus influenzae*, and Group B Streptococcus). Present in the white pulp of the spleen are the plasma cells which generate large volumes of both IgM and IgG antibodies to aid in opsonization and destruction of microbes.

15.2 Hematologic Malignancies and Splenic Tumors

Various hematopoietic malignancies can cause splenic infiltration with resultant splenomegaly or discrete splenic lesions. Additionally, non-hematologic tumors may also metastasize to the spleen via direct hematogenous spread or peritoneal implants. Nonlymphoid primary tumors are rare. The malignant hematologic disorders most commonly affecting the spleen include leukemias, lymphomas, and myeloproliferative disorders. The varying effects of these hematologic disorders on various blood cell lines may predispose to an increased risk for perioperative morbidity. For example, profound thrombocytopenia may create a high perioperative bleeding risk, whereas low functional WBC counts may increase the risk for surgical site infections.

15.2.1 Leukemias

Leukemias are hematologic cancers caused by malignant transformation of hematopoietic stem cells, which result in displacement and failure of normal bone marrow. Acute leukemias, the most common cancer in children, present rapidly, while chronic leukemias, more common in adults, have a more insidious course [2]. In both malignancies, following bone marrow infiltration, the cancer spreads to the spleen, liver, and lymph nodes. Cases have been reported of patients presenting with atraumatic splenic rupture due to acute lymphoblastic leukemia, acute myeloid leukemia, chronic lymphocytic leukemia, chronic myelogenous leukemia, and chronic myelomonocytic leukemia [3]. Although the exact etiology for splenic rupture due to leukemia is unknown, it has been suggested that hemorrhage originates from either tumor foci, leukostasis, splenic infarction, or dysfunctional hemostasis.

15.2.2 Lymphomas

Lymphomas are hematologic cancers of lymphocytes that preferentially affect the lymph node basins. They are broadly derived into two main categories: Hodgkin's lymphoma and the overwhelmingly more common non-Hodgkin's lymphoma. When lymphomas progress to more advanced stages, they can cause splenomegaly due to the spread of malignant cells. When the splenomegaly reaches a critical point, splenic infarction can occur with subcapsular hemorrhage, which may result in atraumatic splenic rupture. Case reports of atraumatic splenic rupture involve diffuse large B cell lymphoma, T cell lymphoma, and marginal zone lymphoma.

15.2.3 Primary Splenic Malignancy (Angiosarcoma)

Splenic angiosarcoma is a malignant tumor that arises from the vascular endothelium, and, although exceptionally rare, it is the most common primary splenic malignancy. It largely affects young men, and patients often present with advanced disease as initial symptoms of abdominal pain and fatigue are vague and nonspecific. Environmental carcinogens like vinyl chloride monomers and arsenic have historically been implicated in the disease process, but the exact pathophysiology has not been elucidated to this date. Given its late presentation, splenic angiosarcoma usually portends a poor prognosis with less than 20% of patients surviving past 6 months of diagnosis. Splenic angiosarcoma can lead to splenic rupture, likely due to the irregularly arranged, capillary-like vasculature that is a histopathologic hallmark of the neoplasm [4]. In case reports of spontaneous splenic rupture due to splenic angiosarcoma, splenomegaly was a common intraoperative finding.

15.2.4 Secondary Metastatic Disease

Despite the large blood flow to the spleen, splenic metastases are rare and usually associated with widespread disseminated disease. The overall incidence of splenic metastases in autopsy studies varies from 2 to 30%. Melanoma and breast and lung cancers are the most common primary sources for metastatic spread to the spleen. Other less commonly detected metastases originate from the gastric, colon, prostate, ovarian, and endometrial cancers. Atraumatic splenic rupture has been seen in the case of splenic metastases from pancreatic cancer, melanoma, and gestational malignancies.

15.3 Clinical Presentation and Management

Oncologic surgical emergencies of the spleen are rare and usually due to splenic rupture in the setting of splenomegaly [5]. Although hypersplenism is an indication for operative intervention among patients with myeloproliferative disorders, emergent intervention is uncommon and usually indicated only following a course of medical therapy/chemotherapy. Similar to patients with blunt traumatic splenic injury, patients with atraumatic splenic rupture may present along a spectrum from mildly symptomatic without evidence of hemodynamic instability to life-threatening hemorrhagic shock.

In the absence of a traumatic history, abdominal pain is the most common presenting complaint among patients with atraumatic splenic rupture, which may be sudden or acute in onset. Pain may progress to generalized abdominal pain, with or without referred pain to the left shoulder (Kehr's sign) due to irritation of the diaphragm by intraperitoneal blood. Medical history may reveal a history of malignancy; however, in most cases, no underlying diagnosis has been previously made. Use of antithrombotic medications should be queried as well and treated accordingly.

On physical examination, findings include pallor, abdominal distension, and tenderness, and even diffuse peritonitis. Intravenous access should be secured and damage control resuscitation initiated in hemodynamically unstable patients. A Focused Assessment with Sonography for Trauma (FAST) exam may reveal free fluid in the abdomen, and contrast-enhanced computed tomography (CT) with intravenous contrast should be performed in appropriately selected patients to identify the source and severity of bleeding [6, 7] (Fig. 15.3). Where available, viscoelastic assays should be sent.

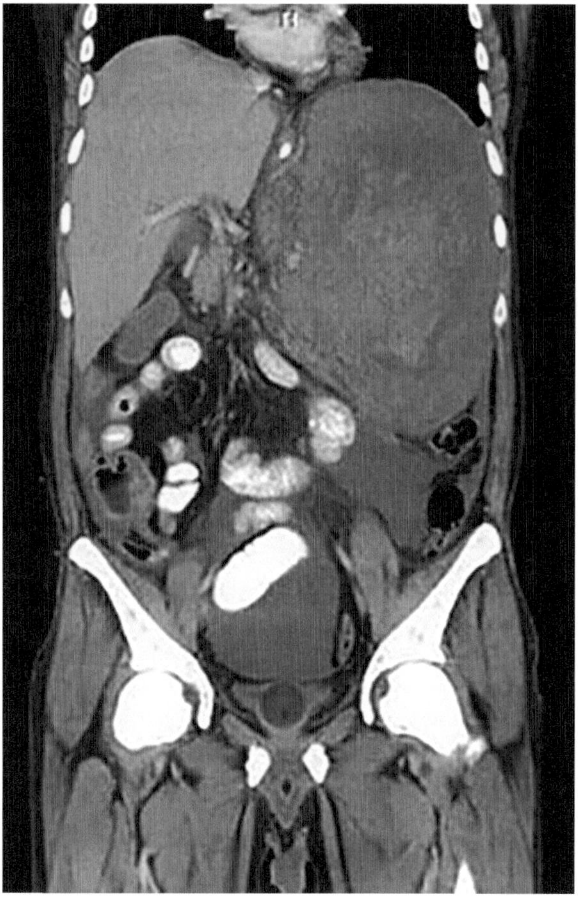

Fig. 15.3 Coronal CT abdomen demonstrating ruptured spleen with hemoperitoneum

15.4 Operative Management

15.4.1 Approach and Techniques

Following diagnosis of a splenic rupture, the approach should be tailored to the patient's physiology and available resources. In the case of stable patients with massive splenomegaly, for example, preoperative angioembolization of the splenic artery may be a reasonable approach at centers with access to angiography followed by laparoscopic or open splenectomy. Patients in hemorrhagic shock should proceed directly to surgery for open splenectomy [8].

15.4.2 Open Splenectomy

Patients should be brought to the operating room and positioned supine on the operating room table with arms extended laterally. Following administration of preoperative antibiotics and a wide prep and drape, a generous midline incision should be made extending to the left of the xyphoid process and the abdomen packed, beginning with the left upper quadrant. Placement of a self-retaining retractor system is strongly encouraged to allow for improved access and exposure to the left upper quadrant. Lap pads may be placed above and behind the spleen in order to bring it to the midline.

For patients with splenomegaly, the splenic artery may be identified running along the posterosuperior aspect of the spleen, isolated and ligated prior to mobilization of the spleen. Otherwise, splenectomy may be carried out in the standard manner. Care should be taken to avoid injury to the pancreatic tail and ensure that the short gastric arteries are well secured. Application of hemostatic adjuncts may be required. Generally, drains are not required following splenectomy; however, in the setting of a hematologic malignancy of the spleen, it may be considered.

15.4.3 Laparoscopic Splenectomy

Laparoscopic splenectomy may also be performed in appropriately selected patients without evidence of hemorrhagic shock. Patients are positioned in right lateral decubitus with the operating surgeon facing the patient (Fig. 15.4). One option for port placement involves a supraumbilical camera port, the assistant aiding in retraction via a lateral port, and the operating surgeon using epigastric and left abdomen working ports (Fig. 15.5). To minimize blood loss, certain laparoscopic considerations must be made. For patients with massive splenomegaly, securing the splenic hilum or splenic artery first is the safest approach. A hand-assisted approach is sometimes required to extract the massively enlarged spleen.

15.4.4 Angioembolization

Splenic artery embolization may be used in isolation or as an adjunct selectively in patients who present with atraumatic splenic rupture—particularly because these patients tend to have poor reserve secondary to reduced or dysfunctional red blood cells and platelets and may therefore be deemed as poor operative candidates. Most patients undergo surgical intervention within 24 h of diagnosis with only 15% of patients treated with conservative management or splenic arterial embolization. Post-procedurally, patients should be closely monitored for ongoing or recurrent bleeding necessitating splenectomy, as well as for complications related to splenic infarction.

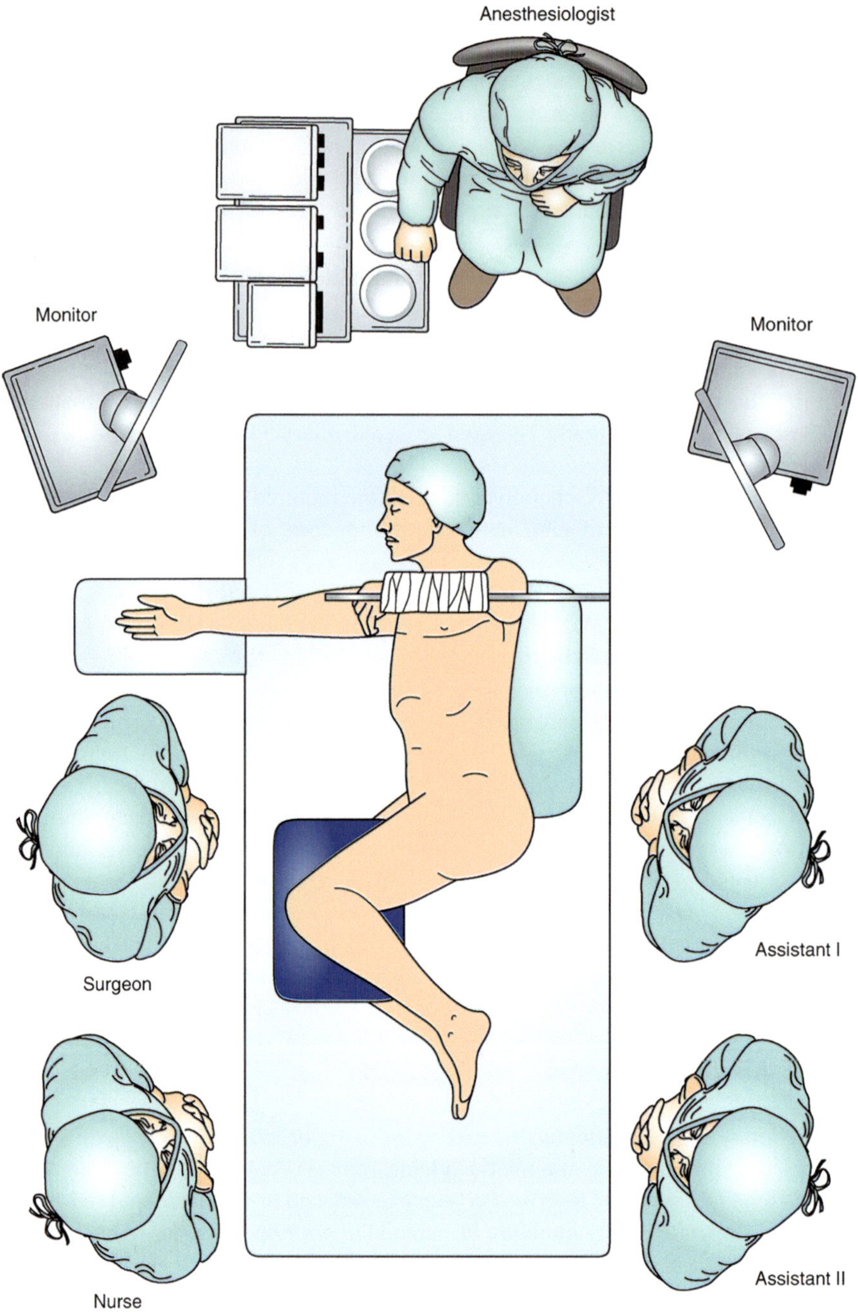

Fig. 15.4 Intraoperative positioning for laparoscopic splenectomy

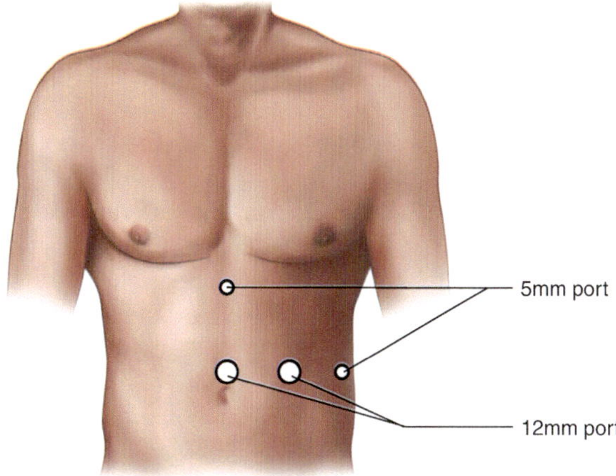

Fig. 15.5 Port placement for laparoscopic splenectomy

15.5 Postoperative Considerations

Patients with atraumatic splenic rupture in the setting of a malignant etiology are at an increased risk for mortality. When compared to other causes, neoplastic etiologies for splenic rupture confer the highest atraumatic splenic rupture-related mortality, as high as 20%. Complications include bleeding, pancreatic leak, and sepsis or overwhelming postsplenectomy infection (OPSI).

Postoperative bleeding usually presents in the immediate postoperative period with vital sign changes, abdominal distension, and worsening anemia. The usual culprit is bleeding from the short gastric vessels along the greater curvature of the stomach, and as such, expeditious operative exploration is mandated.

Pancreatic leak occurs due to stapler or cautery injury to the tail of the pancreas, which lies in close proximity to the splenic hilum. It is usually diagnosed on CT imaging, which shows a fluid collection near the tail of the pancreas which has a high amylase and lipase content. Management of a pancreatic leak involves a stepwise approach including percutaneous drainage of the fluid collection followed by nil per os (NPO) status and, depending on if the output is high, consideration for endoscopic retrograde cholangiopancreatography (ERCP) with sphincterotomy and/or pancreatic duct stent placement in addition to consideration of medical adjuncts such as octreotide (especially if the leak is high output).

It can be challenging to differentiate between the normal postoperative leukocytosis and thrombocytosis that occur following splenectomy from infection or OPSI. Regardless of laboratory values, with clinical signs of sepsis, diagnosis of infection and empiric antibiotics should not be delayed. OPSI, which can occur any time following splenectomy, carries a high mortality rate of 40–50% and risk factors include asplenic patients with hematologic malignancy and immunosuppression. Patients should be advised of the future risk for OPSI and the need for antibiotic prophylaxis and empiric therapy as indicated. Finally, patients should receive postoperative vaccination prior to discharge with outpatient evaluation of appropriate antibody titers to minimize the risk of developing OPSI.

15.6 Conclusions

Overall oncologic splenic emergencies are rare and most commonly due to atraumatic rupture of the spleen in the setting of splenomegaly. Splenectomy is the definitive operation of choice. Select patients may be candidates for splenic artery angioembolization, usually as a preoperative adjunct to either laparoscopic or open splenectomy.

References

1. Townsend CM, Beauchamp RD, Evers BM, Mattox KL, Sabiston DC. The spleen. In: Sabiston textbook of surgery: the biological basis of modern surgical practice. Elsevier; 2021.
2. Bhatnagar N, Qureshi A, Hall G. Leukaemias: a review. Paediatr Child Health. 2017;27(11):489–94.
3. Renzulli P, Hostettler A, Schoepfer AM, Gloor B, Candinas D. Systematic review of atraumatic splenic rupture. Br J Surg. 2009;96(10):1114–21. https://doi.org/10.1002/BJS.6737.
4. Abraham JA, Hornicek FJ, Kaufman AM, et al. Treatment and outcome of 82 patients with angiosarcoma. Ann Surg Oncol. 2007;14(6):1953–67. https://doi.org/10.1245/S10434-006-9335-Y.
5. Aubrey-Bassler FK, Sowers N. 613 cases of splenic rupture without risk factors or previously diagnosed disease: a systematic review. BMC Emerg Med. 2012;12:11. https://doi.org/10.1186/1471-227X-12-11.
6. Alabousi A, Patlas MN, Scaglione M, Romano L, Soto JA. Cross-sectional imaging of nontraumatic emergencies of the spleen. Curr Probl Diagn Radiol. 2014;43(5):254–67. https://doi.org/10.1067/J.CPRADIOL.2014.04.002.
7. Tonolini M, Bianco R. Nontraumatic splenic emergencies: cross-sectional imaging findings and triage. Emerg Radiol. 2013;20(4):323–32. https://doi.org/10.1007/S10140-013-1103-2.
8. Coccolini F, Improta M, Sartelli M, et al. Acute abdomen in the immunocompromised patient: WSES, SIS-E, WSIS, AAST, and GAIS guidelines. World J Emerg Surg. 2021;16(1):1–21. https://doi.org/10.1186/S13017-021-00380-1.

Gynecologic Oncological Surgical Emergencies

16

Pier Andrea De Iaco

16.1 Introduction

Gynecological cancer, which includes cancers of the cervix, ovary, uterus, vulva, vagina, and fallopian tubes, is among the leading causes of cancer-related mortality worldwide. Distribution and frequency vary across regions; cervical carcinoma is more frequent in low-income countries; on the contrary, endometrial cancer is highly represented in high-income countries.

The incidence of cervical cancer cases has increased over the past few years; cervical cancer is the fourth most frequently diagnosed cancer and the fourth leading cause of cancer death in women, with an estimated 604,000 new cases (cumulative risk of 1.39%) and 342,000 global deaths in 2020 [1].

Instead, cancer of the corpus uteri is the sixth most common neoplasm in women worldwide, with 417,000 new cases (2.2%) in 2020 (cumulative risk 1.05%) and 97,000 deaths in 2020 [2].

Vulvar cancer is a rare gynecologic malignancy and has a world incidence of more than 45,000 new diagnoses in 2020 and more than 17,000 deaths worldwide in 2020. Ninety percent of vulvar cancers are predominantly squamous cell carcinomas (SCCs), which can arise through human papillomavirus (HPV)-dependent and HPV-independent pathways [3].

Vaginal cancer constitutes only 1–2% of all female genital tract malignancies and only 10% of all vaginal malignant neoplasms. In 2020, the global incidence of vaginal neoplasms reached about 17,000 cases (with a cumulative risk of 0.09%). Diagnosis of a primary vaginal cancer is rare because most lesions are metastasis from another primary site. Although cancer of the vagina is more common in postmenopausal women, an increased diagnosis in young women has been reported,

P. A. De Iaco (✉)
Division of Oncologic Gynecology, IRCCS Azienda Ospedaliero Universitaria di Bologna, Bologna, Italy
e-mail: pierandrea.deiaco@unibo.it

A. Tarasconi et al. (eds.), *Oncologic Surgical Emergencies*, Hot Topics in Acute Care Surgery and Trauma, https://doi.org/10.1007/978-3-031-36860-8_16

especially in countries with a high HIV prevalence (e.g., African countries) and persistence of high-risk HPV infection [4].

In 2020, ovarian cancer world incidence was 313,959 (1.6%) with a cumulative risk of about 0.73% and a number of deaths reaching 207,252 (2.1%). Although ovarian cancer may occur at any age, it is more common in patients that are older than 50 years. Prognosis is typically determined by the cancer stage and grade. Epithelial ovarian cancer is the most common type of ovarian cancer, and because of absence of symptoms and screening, 70% of cases are diagnosed at stage III or IV, and it is associated with a poor prognosis [2, 5, 6].

Advanced gynecologic malignancies are known to have a poor prognosis, due to local invasion in adjacent organs. Surgery is often difficult to perform, and for this reason, an interdisciplinary management is the best option. In case of advanced disease, the risk of emergency conditions may be higher due to the disease or as a consequence of specific treatments.

An oncologic emergency is defined as an acute, potentially life-threatening condition in a cancer patient that has developed, directly or indirectly, as a result of the malignant disease or cancer treatment. To determine which procedures should be undertaken or avoided, it is essential that the surgeon is informed on the performance status of the patient, cancer stage and prognosis, (need for) future cancer treatment, and the patient's wishes regarding aggressive interventions and treatment at the end of life [7].

Indications for surgery are classified as elective/nonurgent, semi-urgent, and urgent/emergent.

The conditions of surgical emergency usually include bowel perforation, malignant bowel obstruction, hemorrhage, and urinary obstruction. Yet, uncommon emergencies in gynecologic oncology are numerous and will be discussed in this chapter.

16.2 Bowel Perforation

Patients with gynecologic malignancies are especially susceptible to bowel injury. Intestinal perforation is generally an emergent condition associated with high mortality.

Tumor invasion of the bowel is common in advanced-stage gynecological cancers (especially ovarian cancer) and in case of peritoneal carcinosis; this condition can evolve in perforation. It can be associated with large bowel obstruction presenting with acute abdomen and radiological findings of pneumoperitoneum. Also, treatments for advanced disease can determine an intestinal perforation. Radiation is frequently planned in patients with cervical cancer (also in the early stages of the disease) and can potentially cause radiation-related bowel complications. Fortunately, grade 4 or worse complication of the small intestine from irradiation for gynecologic malignancy by Radiation Therapy Oncology Group/European Organization for Research and Treatment of Cancer (RTOG/EORTC) scoring system is uncommon. The incidence of such injuries has been reported to be 2.4–8.6% of patients, and signs of peritonitis may be equivocal or even absent [8].

Late effects of irradiation determine mucosal ulceration that may be complicated by stenosis, obstruction, or hemorrhage with occasionally subsequent peritonitis. The mesentery is usually foreshortened and edematous, which contributes to disturbances of intestinal motility. Late-stage complications may appear from a few months to 20 years or more after RT [9].

Also, infusive treatments may lead to intestinal perforation. Bevacizumab is associated with a higher perforation rate in patients with ovarian cancer than in those with other cancer types (e.g., colorectal, pancreatic, non-small cell lung, breast cancer). Patients at major risk of perforation are usually heavily pretreated, with peritoneal carcinomatosis, and have a history of either prior or concurrent bowel obstruction; these factors are all known to increase the risk of bowel perforation [10]. Administration of bevacizumab further increases the susceptibility for bowel perforation by promoting tumor regression/necrosis or compromising the structure and function of the gastrointestinal vasculature, including onset of microemboli [11–13].

Immediate surgery is often necessary in the event of bowel injury except when the leak is walled off; in this case, conservative treatment with careful observation may be justified. However, patients with gynecologic cancers are often at an advanced age with high disease extension and frequently have concurrent comorbidities. Life expectancy may already be limited due to an extensive cancer burden that has been treated with multiple chemotherapy regimens [14].

The most important determinant of survival in these patients is the amount of cancer burden present at the time of perforation.

Bowel perforation and pneumatosis intestinalis carry severe prognosis in patients with gynecologic cancers. Although surgical management is performed in patients with free intestinal leak, overall prognosis is poor and conservative management should be considered [15].

Surgery is generally performed by laparotomic route; after thorough and careful assessment of all abdominal quadrants and intestinal loops, the perforation is identified. In case of bowel perforation, a partial colectomy is performed, the distal colon is closed, and an end colostomy is prepared. In case of ileal loop perforation, the possibility of resection and anastomosis should be evaluated, but in most cases, the safest procedure is to divert the intestine by means of a double-barrel ileostomy.

16.3 Bowel Obstruction

Patients with gynecological cancer are at a higher risk of developing gastrointestinal complications.

Malignant bowel obstruction (MBO) is a complication particularly frequent in patients with gynecological cancer and occurs in 5–35% of all patients with ovarian cancers. In 20% of patients with gynecologic malignancy, MBO may be the initial presentation, but, in most cases, MBO is a feature of advanced or recurrent disease associated with a poor prognosis. In 3–11% of uterine cancer patients, MBO is an end-of-life condition [16].

MBO can be caused by extrinsic pressure at multiple sites in the gastrointestinal tract due to tumor direct extension or its metastatic spread. Direct invasion or intraperitoneal seeding is the main mechanism of spread in ovarian cancer, while cervical cancer frequently spreads by direct invasion or lymphatic extension. In 76% of patients, the bowel obstruction is multifocal; in 13% of cases, the small bowel is involved; and in 8% of patients, the site of obstruction is the large bowel (Fig. 16.1) [17–19].

There are also some nonmalignant bowel obstructions that occur in up to 23% of patients with ovarian cancers. Injury induced by pelvic irradiation for cervical or endometrial cancers and postoperative intraperitoneal adhesions are more frequent. Intestinal obstruction can also be favored by opioid use and electrolyte imbalances. Ogilvie's syndrome, consisting of acute dilation of the colon in the absence of mechanical obstruction typically caused by surgical interventions or by drugs that inhibit colonic motility, is an important differential diagnosis to make as it resolves conservatively and does not need a surgical approach [20].

The partial or total blockage of the intestine causes pain, constipation, distension, and/or vomiting.

The diagnosis is clinical, and it is confirmed by radiological imaging demonstrating fluid levels.

In the management of bowel obstruction, the symptom control is the main goal in patients with limited life expectancy [21].

In most patients, the bowel obstruction is incomplete and the symptoms are chronic; thus, in most cases, bowel obstruction is not really urgent, although its complications are the main cause of death in patients with gynecological cancer. Management of these serious complications is a difficult clinical challenge, and it is useful to consider the nature of the obstruction, the disease status, and the patient physical condition. It is not clear which patients should be treated aggressively because the resolution of symptoms is not certain and obstruction might relapse [22].

Individualized decisions should be made with a multidisciplinary team involving oncologists, surgeons, and palliative caregivers to ensure the best management [23].

Clinical observation and supporting management with fasting, intravenous fluids, and insertion of a nasogastric tube constitute the initial approach. Medical management depends on clinical status and includes steroids, drugs for enemas, and

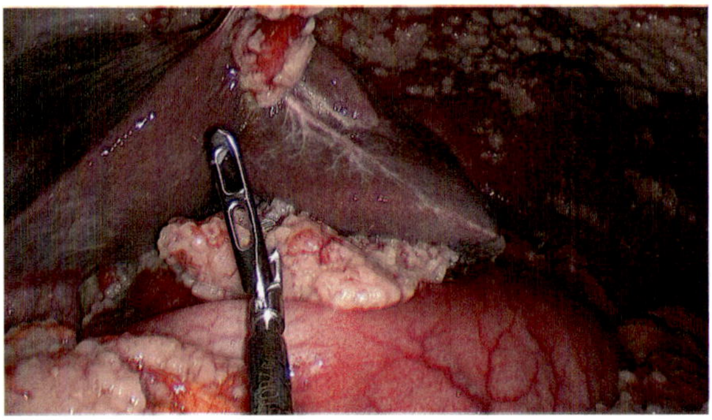

Fig. 16.1 Ovarian cancer carcinosis; small and large nodules cover large peritoneal and gastrointestinal surfaces. Normal gastrointestinal function is frequently impaired

pain control. Other treatments like total parenteral nutrition and chemotherapy might be considered [24].

An effective surgical treatment depends on the different etiology factors and different anatomical sites involved. In patients with relapsing ovarian cancer, surgery is associated with high rates of morbidity and mortality; therefore, its role is controversial. There is not much evidence that guides clinical decision-making.

Previous surgery, radiotherapy/chemotherapy, free interval after treatment (TFI), multiple sites of disease, ascites, and serum albumin levels are possible factors to predict successful surgery palliation.

In patients with large ascites, acute abdomen, chemoresistance, and short TFI, the surgical approach appears to be less effective [21].

In some conditions, metallic stents inserted under radiologic or endoscopic guidance might be an alternative for patients excluded from surgery. In these patients, chemotherapy appears not to be effective for the control of symptoms.

A particularly difficult case is intestinal obstruction in a patient with a newly diagnosed advanced ovarian neoplasia. Malignant ovarian cancer that spreads in the peritoneum covers large peritoneal areas with neoplastic nodules that alter organ function; in particular, the presence of numerous tumor nodules covering long loops of the small intestine and its meso can alter the normal progression of intestinal contents. Moreover, the presence of significant amounts of ascites with consequent hydro-electrolyte imbalances and albumin and protein losses leads to intestinal obstruction that worsens the general clinical condition. In this case, emergency surgery should be reduced to a minimum, as the prompt start of chemotherapy might allow regression of the disease, a marked decrease in ascitic fluid, and rapid recovery of intestinal function [25, 26].

On the other hand, in patients with benign causes of bowel obstruction such as irradiation or postsurgical adhesion, surgery is usually effective. A radiological study is necessary, generally, CT associated with Gastrografin per os, for more precise diagnosis of intestinal obstruction; moreover, Gastrografin has prokinetic intestinal action. If symptoms fail to resolve after conservative therapy, surgery must be performed to improve the patient's symptoms and intestinal function and obtain hydro-saline balance [27].

16.4 Vaginal Bleeding

Vaginal bleeding is a common problem in gynecological cancer patients related to multiple causes as local tumor invasion, tumor angiogenesis, systemic effects of the cancer, or anticancer treatments.

Vaginal bleeding commonly occurs in gynecological cancer including vaginal, vulvar, cervical, and endometrial cancer at diagnosis, mostly in advanced disease cases, and can be potentially life-threatening.

Malignant cervical cancer in its early stages is responsible for minor genital bleeding; postcoital bleeding may be frequently observed, due to the fragility of the neoplastic cervix. In more advanced cases, the neoplasm increases in size, involves the entire cervix, and may cause profuse bleeding. In fact, locally advanced cervical cancer may present with uncontrollable vaginal bleeding in up to 70% of cases. At diagnosis, in non-Western countries, more than two-thirds of patients present with advanced cervical disease (FIGO stage IB2-IVA). In this scenario, approximately 6% of patients will die of unstoppable cervicovaginal bleeding, especially in countries with a low level of sanitary assistance [28].

The maneuver to be performed in case of copious bleeding due to cervical neoplasia is vaginal packing, which consists of placing long gauze pads in the vagina to fill completely the vagina, compress the external surface of the cervix, and stop bleeding. Gauzes in the vagina lead to compression of the urethra, so a bladder catheter must be left in place. Meanwhile, hemoderivatives are administered, as well as tranexamic acid. Generally, gauzes are removed after 24–48 h [29, 30].

After growing within the cervix, cervical cancer expands to infiltrate vagina, parametrium, and subsequently bladder and rectum. Hemorrhage from infiltration and progressive rupture of the uterine artery may occur. In this case, at gynecological examination, the cervix is completely replaced by necrotic tissue, often ulcerated, and excavated. In such advanced cases, which are not uncommon in a population not screened for cancer, the situation may be severe, as bleeding may be very profuse and vaginal tamponade may be ineffective. The patient should be adequately treated with fluids, blood transfusion, and fresh plasma. A useful maneuver is the uterine artery embolization: the procedure requires the patient to be in stable condition, not in shock state, and an interventional radiology service to be available. Interventional radiologist must have adequate expertise for endo-arterial embolization procedures (liver embolization, oncology, etc.). The uterine artery embolization procedure is performed under radiological guidance; with a vascular percutaneous femoral artery approach, uterine arteries are selectively cannulated and embolized using mechanical devices such as coils, sclerosing agents, or polymerizing agents (polyvinyl alcohol particles and trisacryl gelatin microspheres). Uterine artery embolization is successful in 70% of cases; certainly, the size of the tumor, the involvement of surrounding organs, and the extent of bleeding are factors that influence success. Uterine or iliac artery embolization may be an important tool in controlling massive hemorrhage due to gynecologic neoplasms, since it provides an exact visualization of the bleeding vessel and allows minimally invasive direct therapy to achieve hemostasis. Compared with surgical ligation, this procedure lowers the number of blood transfusions and surgical complications in almost all cases and may be preferred [31, 32].

Historically, the other surgical method to control hemorrhage is surgical ligation of the hypogastric artery; the procedure causes an 85% decrease in blood flow from the bleeding area [29, 33].

In 1893, Howard Kelly performed the bilateral hypogastric artery ligation at Johns Hopkins Hospital, to control an intraoperative hemorrhage during a hysterectomy for uterine cancer [34]. This method leads to a decrease in the blood pressure of the pelvic area in 85% of the cases [35]. Surgery may be risky as the hypogastric vein is located under the artery; therefore, accurate dissection of external and internal iliac arteries and veins is warranted before ligating the hypogastric artery

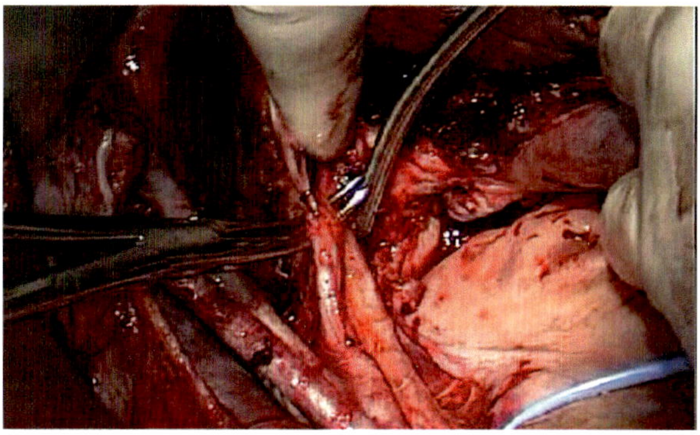

Fig. 16.2 Internal iliac artery closure; the procedure has to carefully cleavage external iliac artery, external iliac vein, and internal iliac vein; the procedure warrants reduced pelvic perfusion to obtain hemostasis in difficult procedures

downward to the gluteal artery (Fig. 16.2). However, in case of severe pelvic hemorrhages (due to multiple bleeding sources) that are difficult to control, it has been shown that hypogastric artery ligation alone is not enough and might require concomitant ligation of the infundibulopelvic, round, and uterosacral ligament veins. Concomitant hypogastric artery embolization, by direct injection of an embolic material below the level of ligation on the hypogastric artery, can be considered in case of uncontrolled severe hemorrhage [36].

Sometimes, bleeding of an advanced cervical tumor fails to be completely controlled as described above. If patients are hemodynamically stable, radiation therapy to palliate bleeding can be effective within 24–48 h of the delivery of the first dose. Radiation treatment regimens for palliation of bleeding include various strategies such as single treatments of 8–10 Gray (Gy), intermediate courses of 4–8 Gy given in 3–5 treatments, or longer courses of 30–45 Gy in 10–15 treatments. No treatment scheme has been proven more effective, but one randomized trial suggests that side effects are less likely with shorter treatment courses [37]. Large 10 Gy, monthly radiation fractions with misonidazole have been investigated for palliation of advanced pelvic malignancies. Although approximately 40% of patients achieved complete or partial response, the study was a small stage I/II trial, and the rate of gastrointestinal complications was considered unacceptably high [38].

Another important consideration is whether the patient has a history of prior radiation to the same anatomic site. Re-irradiation may be an option if the benefits outweigh the risks, but care must be taken to respect the constraints of critical normal tissues [39].

Endometrial cancer is characterized by the occurrence of abnormal uterine bleeding (AUB) and is noted in about 90% of patients. It is often minor and occurs in pre-menopausal patients in the intermenstrual phase or in menopausal patients without any premonitory signs. Usually, these symptoms lead the woman to seek medical advice and the disease is diagnosed at early stage. Sometimes, however, the rapid growth of the tumor or the patient's delay in seeking counselling leads to the presence of a large endometrial mass with significant vaginal bleeding. In this case, bleeding is often associated with abdominal pain, as the accumulation of blood in the uterus causes contractions of the bowel with cramping pain [40]. Treatment of major bleeding provides for fluids and hemoderivatives, and tranexamic acid. If treatments fail, the choice must be made between urgent hemostatic radiotherapy and hysterectomy. The decision must be made taking into account the patient's age, general clinical conditions, spread of the disease, and possibility of waiting. Certainly, a surgical operation to remove the uterus requires a patient in good general condition, with an acceptable anesthesiological risk and with a reduced spread of disease, while the choice of hemostatic radiotherapy should be reserved for older patients, with comorbidities and with advanced disease [41].

Uterine sarcomas can cause continuous, uncontrollable bleeding. Rarely, the first presentation may be hemoperitoneum. Leiomyosarcomas are characterized by a poor prognosis; 5-year survival rate is more than 76% for women with stage I disease confined to the uterus, and 60% for women with stage II disease. Patients with metastatic disease present survival rates of 10–15% at 5 years. In the presence of uterine sarcomas with severe bleeding, conservative management (use of tranexamic acid, vaginal packing, arterial embolization) is often unsatisfactory. The result is usually achieved by emergency removal of the uterus. The uterus is greatly increased in volume, and becomes soft, often with cancer spread to adjacent organs. Surgery should primarily aim to remove the uterus, although an attempt at radicalization, i.e., ablation of residual neoplastic tissue on other abdominal organs, should be considered [42].

Ovarian cancer may present with vaginal bleeding, but emergency hemorrhagic conditions that need a surgical approach are usually rare and derive from perioperative complications or advanced-stage metastasis [43, 44].

16.5 Hemoperitoneum

Hemoperitoneum is an uncommon complication of ovarian neoplasms. Few cases of massive bleeding are described in literature (for example due to ovarian malignant cyst rupture) that needed an invasive approach [45, 46].

Specific histologic ovarian tumors may be more at risk of bleeding than others. Malignant germ cell tumors of the ovary account for approximately 5% of all ovarian malignancies, and age of presentation is 19–21 years. They are frequently unilateral and extremely chemosensitive. In case of advanced stage with abdominal involvement, intra-abdominal hemorrhage, bowel occlusion or urinary tract invasion, and hydroureteronephrosis can be observed [47].

Among germ cell tumors (yolk sac tumor, teratoma, embryonal carcinoma, choriocarcinoma), choriocarcinoma presents the highest risk of bleeding. Non-gestational ovarian choriocarcinoma (NGOC) accounts for <1% of ovarian germ cell tumors. Abdominal hemorrhage in choriocarcinoma can occur from the primary site or from metastasis. The tumor bleeds because of its high vascularity, as the vessels are highly fragile as in gestational trophoblastic disease. Choriocarcinoma is characterized by rapid proliferation, invasiveness, and vascularity and outgrows its blood supply with subsequent necrosis of tumor. Choriocarcinoma cells directly invade, erode, and destroy blood vessels. It is also believed that some products of tumor cells induce blood vessel damage without direct invasion. Metastases to regional lymph nodes, as well as hematogenous spread to lung, liver, and brain, occur at an early stage and are at risk of bleeding [48]. Of interest is a rare complication, the "choriocarcinoma syndrome" resulting from massive tumor lysis after chemotherapy [49]. The choriocarcinoma syndrome is characterized by cytokine release enhanced by chemotherapy, inducing alveolar hemorrhage that can lead to acute respiratory failure (ARDS) and death [50]. Considering the usually young age of patients, the high chemosensitivity of these tumors, and the consistent probability of healing even with advance disease, a surgical approach in case of severe bleeding is highly recommended. Another rare cause of hemoperitoneum is tubal rupture due to tubaric localization of metastasis or primary tumor [51].

Bleeding risk can also be exacerbated by oncological therapies such as bevacizumab that is widely used in the treatment of cancers including advanced epithelial ovarian, fallopian tube, and cervical cancer [52]. By binding to vascular endothelial cell growth factor (VEGF), a key promoter of vasculogenesis and angiogenesis, bevacizumab prevents the latter from binding to its receptors, Flt-1 (VEGFR-1) and KDR (VEGFR-2), on the surface of the endothelial cells. The VEGF activity block arrests tumor vascularization, thus preventing cancer growth. In case of emergency surgery, bevacizumab should be interrupted prior to surgery and careful intraoperative hemostasis should be obtained [53, 54].

16.6 Ovarian Torsion

Ovarian torsion is a rare emergency condition in women. Early diagnosis is necessary to preserve the function of the ovaries and prevent severe morbidity. Ovarian torsion refers to complete or partial rotation of the adnexa with subsequent ischemia. It can affect females of all ages. Ovarian torsion occurs in around 2–15% of patients with surgically treated adnexal masses. Ovarian torsion is more likely to occur with a benign than a malignant tumor. The incidence of ovarian torsion with ovarian malignancy was less than 2% in reported case series [55].

Ovarian tumors are often cystic and sometimes increase very rapidly in size. Torsion depends on the mobility and weight of the tumor, as well as on the length of the ovarian pedicle. Clinical signs include a palpable abdominal mass, acute lower abdominal pain, vomiting, and shock. The treatment is surgical. Through a laparoscopic or laparotomic approach, detorsion of the mass is the first maneuver, followed by the decision to remove the ovarian cyst or the entire ovary in case of irreversible ischemia [56–58].

16.7 Hematometra

Patients, often of older age, may be referred for emergency because of pelvic pain, a sense of weight, and abdominal distension due to distension of the uterine cavity, even of significant size, for liquid collection that is drained through the cervical canal. In fact, the presence of severe stenosis of the cervical canal, associated with a slowly growing endometrial neoplastic process, may result in the appearance of serous, hematic, or frankly purulent material within the endometrial cavity. The patient is usually apyretic, not severely distressed, and complains of compression symptoms on nearby organs (pollakiuria, bladder, and rectal tenesmus). The patient may present some rare purulent vaginal discharge or none. The diagnosis is made by ultrasonography, which shows a mid-pelvic mass that is identified as the uterus, often with thinned walls, distended by anechogenic or hypoechogenic fluid, referable to serum, blood, or pus. The diagnosis is confirmed by probing the cervix. Cautious dilation of the cervical canal should be carried out, sometimes under ultrasound guidance, and the fluid is drained. Dilation of the cervical canal is followed by endometrial biopsy to verify the presence of endometrial neoplastic cells [59].

16.8 Urinary Obstruction

Access to the emergency department can be caused by recent onset of lumbosacral pain; CT images may show significant unilateral hydronephrosis. Causes of unilateral hydronephrosis include gynecological tumors: cervical cancer when infiltrating the para-uterine tissues (parameters) may close the ureter and cause hydronephrosis. Ureteral obstruction is reported in 11–44% of cervical carcinoma patients [60, 61].

Sometimes, this condition sets in slowly; sometimes, the rapid distension of the renal basins causes pain. Generally, hydronephrosis due to local spread of cervical cancer is also associated with involvement of the para-uterine nerve and vessels, so that patients complain of vaginal bleeding, chronic pelvic pain with reported "vaginal" and "rectal" pain, widespread lower limb pain, and lower limb edema.

Hydronephrosis should be quickly resolved to avoid impairment of renal function. The choice of urinary drainage depends on the patient's clinical condition, the possibility of performing endoscopic drainage, and the characteristics of the ureteral stenosis; ureteral stent placement by cystoscopy or percutaneous drainage with nephrostomy is the procedure of choice [61].

Advanced endometrial carcinoma may also cause unilateral hydronephrosis in 12–20% of cases; this may be induced by a large metastatic pelvic lymph node that may compress or infiltrate the nearby ureter. These are generally stenoses situated high in the pelvis. Rarely, direct spread of an endometrial tumor through the uterine serosa reaches the surrounding tissues and causes ureteral stricture. The diagnosis of the genital origin of the stenosis has to be made by clinical and radiological examinations.

Ovarian cancer rarely causes ureteral obstruction, generally associated with large pelvic masses or retroperitoneal diffusion [61, 62].

Radiation therapy can cause urologic complications. External radiotherapy for cervical and endometrial cancer includes in the radiation field bladder and distal ureters. Usually, the onset of ureteric strictures is slow, and rarely these adverse events (e.g., ureteric stenosis) can be considered a surgical emergency [63].

16.9 Complicated Ascites

Ovarian cancer is characterized by insidious growth, without accompanying symptoms, and therefore diagnosis is late in 85% of cases. Tumor spread within the abdomen results in the appearance of carcinomatous nodules on the peritoneal surfaces and the development of a diffuse abdominal effusion. Abdominal distension due to ascites may be the first manifestation of the disease, and the patient may be referred to an emergency department for difficulty in movement, difficulty in eating, diffuse abdominal pain, and weight loss or gain. Clinical examination shows a severely distended abdomen, generally associated with a hard, fixed, painful pelvic mass. Complementary imaging includes pelvic sonography and thoracic-abdomino-pelvic CT scan. Evacuative paracentesis can therefore be considered with the aim of reducing abdominal tension and analyzing the fluid with cytological examination [64]. The procedure is generally performed in an outpatient clinic. Aspiration of the ascitic fluid improves the condition of the patient and allows cytological investigation. The fluid generally relapses within a week. The procedure is generally associated with low risk of complications, as fine needle perforation of intestinal loops and bladder has no consequences. The occurrence of an intra-abdominal or abdominal wall infection requires antibiotic therapy and possibly hospitalization [65].

16.10 Conclusion

Management of gynecologic oncologic emergencies is a difficult challenge. The base for a sensitive approach to emergency cases is multidisciplinarity, as general surgeon, urologist, gynecologist, intervention radiologist, and internal medicine specialist should collaborate to find the best solution.

In any case, the necessity of quick decision-making should not be made at the expense of the patient's quality of life.

References

1. Buskwofie A, David-West G, Clare CA. A review of cervical cancer: incidence and disparities. J Natl Med Assoc. 2020;112(2):229–32.
2. Sung H, Ferlay J, Siegel RL, Laversanne M, Soerjomataram I, Jemal A, Bray F. Global cancer statistics 2020: GLOBOCAN estimates of incidence and mortality worldwide for 36 cancers in 185 countries. CA Cancer J Clin. 2021;71(3):209–49.
3. Koh WJ, Greer BE, Abu-Rustum NR, Campos SM, Cho KR, Chon HS, Chu C, Cohn D, Crispens MA, Dizon DS, Dorigo O, Eifel PJ, Fisher CM, Frederick P, Gaffney DK, Han E, Higgins S, Huh WK, Lurain JR 3rd, Mariani A, Mutch D, Nagel C, Nekhlyudov L, Fader

AN, Remmenga SW, Reynolds RK, Tillmanns T, Ueda S, Valea FA, Wyse E, Yashar CM, McMillian N, Scavone J. Vulvar cancer, version 1.2017, NCCN clinical practice guidelines in oncology. J Natl Compr Cancer Netw. 2017;15(1):92–120.
4. Adams TS, Rogers LJ, Cuello MA. Cancer of the vagina: 2021 update. Int J Gynaecol Obstet. 2021;155(Suppl 1):19–27.
5. Roett MA, Evans P. Ovarian cancer: an overview. Am Fam Physician. 2009;80(6):609–16.
6. Yi M, Li T, Niu M, et al. Epidemiological trends of women's cancers from 1990 to 2019 at the global, regional, and national levels: a population-based study. Biomark Res. 2021;9:55.
7. Bosscher MR, van Leeuwen BL, Hoekstra HJ. Surgical emergencies in oncology. Cancer Treat Rev. 2014;40(8):1028–36.
8. Ramirez PT, Levenback C, Burke TW, Eifel P, Wolf JK, Gershenson DM. Sigmoid perforation following radiation therapy in patients with cervical cancer. Gynecol Oncol. 2001;82(1):150–5.
9. Yamashita H, Nakagawa K, Tago M, Igaki H, Shiraishi K, Nakamura N, Sasano N, Yamakawa S, Ohtomo K. Small bowel perforation without tumor recurrence after radiotherapy for cervical carcinoma: report of seven cases. J Obstet Gynaecol Res. 2006;32(2):235–42.
10. Richardson DL, Backes FJ, Hurt JD, Seamon LG, Copeland LJ, Fowler JM, Cohn DE, O'Malley DM. Which factors predict bowel complications in patients with recurrent epithelial ovarian cancer being treated with bevacizumab? Gynecol Oncol. 2010;118:47–51.
11. Sasaki A, Harano K, Kogawa T, Matsubara N, Naito Y, Hosono A, Mukai H, Yoshino T, Mukohara T. Intestinal perforation due to neutropenic enterocolitis in a patient treated with bevacizumab for ovarian cancer. Case Rep Oncol Med. 2020;2020:7231358.
12. Hapani S, Chu D, Wu S. Risk of gastrointestinal perforation in patients with cancer treated with bevacizumab: a meta-analysis. Lancet Oncol. 2009;10:559–68.
13. Cannistra SA, Matulonis UA, Penson RT, Hambleton J, Dupont J, Mackey H, Douglas J, Burger RA, Armstrong D, Wenham R, McGuire W. Phase II study of bevacizumab in patients with platinum-resistant ovarian cancer or peritoneal serous cancer. J Clin Oncol. 2007;25:5180–6.
14. Garg G, Massad LS, Pourabolghasem S, Zhou G, Powell MA, Thaker PH, Hagemann AR, Wilkinson-Ryan I, Mutch DG. Intestinal perforation in gynecologic oncology: do all patients benefit from surgical management? Gynecol Oncol. 2013;129(3):538–43.
15. Garg G, Pourbolghasem S, Zhou G, Powell MA, Thaker PH, Hagemann AR, Wilkinson-Ryan I, Massad LS, Mutch DG. Factors influencing survival in gynecologic oncology patients diagnosed with intestinal perforation and pneumatosis intestinalis. Cancer Res. 2013;73(8 Supplement):1378.
16. Tuca A, Guell E, Martinez-Losada E, Codorniu N. Malignant bowel obstruction in advanced cancer patients: epidemiology, management, and factors influencing spontaneous resolution. Cancer Manag Res. 2012;4:159–69.
17. Bais JMJ, Schilthuis MS, Slors JFM, et al. Intestinal obstruction in patients with advanced ovarian cancer. Int J Gynecol Cancer. 1995;5:346–50.
18. Camignani CP, Sugarbaker TA, Bromley CM, et al. Intraperitoneal cancer dissemination: mechanisms of the patterns of spread. Cancer Metastasis Rev. 2003;22:465–72.
19. Dvoretsky PM, Richards KA, Angel C, et al. Distribution of disease at autopsy in 100 women with ovarian cancer. Human Pathol. 1988;19:57–63.
20. Jatoi A, Podratz KC, Gill P, Hartmann LC. Pathophysiology and palliation of inoperable bowel obstruction in patients with ovarian cancer. J Support Oncol. 2004;2:323–37.
21. Kucukmetin A, Naik R, Galaal K, Bryant A, Dickinson HO. Palliative surgery versus medical management for bowel obstruction in ovarian cancer. Cochrane Database Syst Rev. 2010;2010(7):CD007792.
22. Kolomainen DF, Barton DP. Surgical management of bowel obstruction in gynaecological malignancies. Curr Opin Support Palliat Care. 2011;5(1):55–9.
23. Feuer DJ, Broadley KE, Shepherd JH, et al. Systematic review of surgery in malignant bowel obstruction in advanced gynecological and gastrointestinal cancer. Gynecol Oncol. 1999;75:313–22.

24. Tunca JC, Buchler DA, Mack EA, Ruzicka FF, Crowley JJ, Carr WF. The management of ovarian-cancer-caused bowel obstruction. Gynecol Oncol. 1981;12(2 Pt 1):186–92.
25. Paul Olson TJ, Pinkerton C, Brasel KJ, Schwarze ML. Palliative surgery for malignant bowel obstruction from Carcinomatosis: a systematic review. JAMA Surg. 2014;149:383.
26. Jin M, Shen F, Li M, Chen Y. Palliative treatment for bowel obstruction in ovarian cancer: a meta-analysis. Arch Gynecol Obstet. 2020;302:241–8.
27. Armbrust R, Chekerov R, Sander S, Biebl M, Chopra S, Krell J, Rinne N, Nixon K, Fotopoulou C, Sehouli J. Surgery due to mechanical bowel obstruction in relapsed ovarian cancer: clinical and surgical results of a bicentric analysis of 87 patients. Arch Gynecol Obstet. 2021;305(4):963–8. https://doi.org/10.1007/s00404-021-06237-x.
28. Shrivastava S, Mahantshetty U, Engineer R, et al. Treatment and outcome in cancer cervix patients treated between 1979 and 1994: a single institutional experience. J Cancer Res Ther. 2013;9:672–9.
29. Eleje GU, Eke AC, Igberase GO, et al. Palliative interventions for controlling vaginal bleeding in advanced cervical cancer. Cochrane Database Syst Rev. 2015;5:CD011000.
30. Yanazume Y, Douzono H, Yanazume S, Iio K, Kojima N, Mukaihara K, et al. Clinical usefulness of Mohs' paste for genital bleeding from the uterine cervix or vaginal stump in gynecologic cancer. J Palliat Med. 2013;16(2):193–7.
31. Pisco JM, Martins JM, Correia MG. Internal iliac artery: embolization to control hemorrhage from pelvic neoplasms. Radiology. 1989;172:337–9.
32. Çaypınar SS, Güraslan H, Şentürk B, Cengiz H, Yaşar L. Salvage therapy in acute life-threatening vaginal bleeding of cervical cancer: hypogastric artery embolization. Taiwan J Obstet Gynecol. 2016;55(4):607–8.
33. Siegel P, Mengert WF. Internal iliac artery ligation in obstetrics and gynecology. JAMA. 1961;178:1059–62.
34. Kelly H. Ligation of both internal iliac arteries for hemorrhage in hysterectomy for carcinoma uteri. Bull John Hopkins Hosp. 1984;5:53.
35. Chitragari G, Schlosser FJ, Ochoa Chaar CI, Sumpio BE. Consequences of hypogastric artery ligation, embolization, or coverage. J Vasc Surg. 2015;62(5):1340–7.el.
36. Popovici LR, Ciulcu A, Dorobat B, Dumitraşcu M, Horhoianu VV, Cirstoiu M. Therapeutic approaches in pelvic bleeding of neoplastic origin. J Med Life. 2014;7(3):391–5.
37. Johnstone C, Rich SE. Bleeding in cancer patients and its treatment: a review. Ann Palliat Med. 2018;7(2):265–73.
38. Spanos WJ Jr, Wasserman T, Meoz R, et al. Palliation of advanced pelvic malignant disease with large fraction pelvic radiation and misonidazole: final report of RTOG phase I/II study. Int J Radiat Oncol Biol Phys. 1987;13:1479–82.
39. Yan J, Milosevic M, Fyles A, et al. A hypofractionated radiotherapy regimen (0-7-21) for advanced gynaecological cancer patients. Clin Oncol (R Coll Radiol). 2011;23:476–81.
40. Morice P, Leary A, Creutzberg C, Abu-Rustum N, Darai E. Endometrial cancer. Lancet. 2016;387(10023):1094–108.
41. Concin N, Matias-Guiu X, Vergote I, Cibula D, Mirza MR, Marnitz S, Ledermann J, Bosse T, Chargari C, Fagotti A, Fotopoulou C, Martin AG, Lax S, Lorusso D, Marth C, Morice P, Nout RA, O'Donnell D, Querleu D, Raspollini MR, Sehouli J, Sturdza A, Taylor A, Westermann A, Wimberger P, Colombo N, Planchamp F, Creutzberg CL. ESGO/ESTRO/ESP guidelines for the management of patients with endometrial carcinoma. Radiother Oncol. 2021;154:327–53.
42. Roberts ME, Aynardi JT, Chu CS. Uterine leiomyosarcoma: a review of the literature and update on management options. Gynecol Oncol. 2018;151(3):562–72.
43. Bankhead CR, Kehoe ST, Austoker J. Symptoms associated with diagnosis of ovarian cancer: a systematic review. BJOG. 2005;112(7):857–65.
44. Urbano-Ruiz A, Soares JM Jr, da Motta EV, Granuzzo P, Julião CC, Baracat EC. When to perform palliative surgery in the treatment of ovarian cancer: a brief review. Eur J Gynaecol Oncol. 2013;34(6):532–4.

45. Casal Rodriguez AX, Sanchez Trigo S, Ferreira Gonzalez L, Brage GS. Hemoperitoneum due to spontaneous rupture of ovarian adenocarcinoma. Emerg Radiol. 2011;18(3):267–9.
46. Lee WL, Yuan CC, Lai CR, Wang PH. Hemoperitoneum is an initial presentation of recurrent granulosa cell tumors of the ovary. Jpn J Clin Oncol. 1999;29(10):509–12.
47. Principles and Practice of Oncology 11th edition (July 2018): by Vincent T. Devita (Editor), Samuel Hellman, Steven A. Rosenberg (Editor) By Lippincott Williams & Wilkins Publishers.
48. Zon RT, Nichols C, Einhorn LH. Management strategies and outcomes of germ cell tumor patients with very high human chorionic gonadotropin levels. J Clin Oncol. 1998;16: 1294–7.
49. Peng H, Li L, Bi Y. Successful management of nongestational ovarian choriocarcinoma complicated with choriocarcinoma syndrome: a case report and a literature review. Curr Probl Cancer. 2020;44(4):100539.
50. Rejlekova K, Cursano MC, De Giorgi U, Mego M. Severe complications in testicular germ cell tumors: the Choriocarcinoma syndrome. Front Endocrinol (Lausanne). 2019;10:218.
51. Gupta R, Jenison EL. A rare case of carcinosarcoma of the fallopian tube presenting with torsion, rupture and hemoperitoneum. Gynecol Oncol Case Rep. 2011;2(1):4–5.
52. Hapani S, Sher A, Chu D, Wu S. Increased risk of serious hemorrhage with bevacizumab in cancer patients: a meta-analysis. Oncology. 2010;79(1–2):27–38.
53. Iwasa-Inoue N, Nomura H, Kataoka F, Chiyoda T, Yoshihama T, Nanki Y, Sakai K, Kobayashi Y, Yamagami W, Morisada T, Hirasawa A, Aoki D. Prospective feasibility study of neoadjuvant dose-dense paclitaxel plus carboplatin with bevacizumab therapy followed by interval debulking surgery for advanced ovarian, fallopian tube, and primary peritoneal cancer patients. Int J Clin Oncol. 2021;27(2):441–7.
54. Turco LC, Ferrandina G, Vargiu V, Cappuccio S, Fagotti A, Sallustio G, Scambia G, Cosentino F. Extreme complications related to bevacizumab use in the treatment of ovarian cancer: a case series from a III level referral Centre and review of the literature. Ann Transl Med. 2020;8(24):1687.
55. Huang C, Hong MK, Ding DC. A review of ovary torsion. Ci Ji Yi Xue Za Zhi. 2017;29(3): 143–7.
56. Lee CH, Raman S, Sivanesaratnam V. Torsion of ovarian tumors: a clinicopathological study. Int J Gynaecol Obstet. 1989;28(1):21–5.
57. Bah A, Diakite I, Maiga A, Sidibe BY, Konaté M, Saye Z, Kelly B, Koné T, Konate S, Doumbia AA, Traore B, Karembe B, Diakite ML, Traoré AA, Diarra A, Mangane MI, Almeimoune AH, Dembélé BT, Traoré A, Kanté L, Togo AP. Torsion of ovarian tumor in the elderly: about a case. Surg Sci. 2020;11:69–73.
58. Toba N, Takahashi T, Ota K, Takanashi A, Iizawa Y, Endo Y, Furukawa S, Soeda S, Watanabe T, Mizunuma H, Fujimori K, Takeichi K. Malignant transformation arising from mature cystic teratoma of the ovary presenting as ovarian torsion: a case report and literature review. Fukushima J Med Sci. 2020;66(1):44–52.
59. Salakos N, Bakalianou K, Deligeoroglou E, Kondi-Pafiti A, Papadias K, Creatsas G. Endometrial carcinoma presenting as hematometra: clinicopathological study of a rare case and literature review. Eur J Gynaecol Oncol. 2007;28(3):239–40.
60. Patel K, Foster NR, Kumar A, et al. Hydronephrosis in patients with cervical cancer: an assessment of morbidity and survival. Support Care Cancer. 2015;23:1303–9.
61. Perri T, Meller E, Ben-Baruch G, Inbar Y, Apter S, Heyman L, Dotan Z, Korach J. Palliative urinary diversion in patients with malignant ureteric obstruction due to gynaecological cancer. BMJ Support Palliat Care. 2012;12(e6):e855–61.
62. Geisler JP, Perry RW, Ayres GM, Holland TF 3rd, Melton ME, Geisler HE. Ovarian cancer causing upper and lower urinary tract obstruction. Eur J Gynaecol Oncol. 1994;15(5): 343–4.

63. Wit E, Horenblas S. Urological complications after treatment of cervical cancer. Nat Rev Urol. 2014;11:110–7.
64. Kietpeerakool C, Rattanakanokchai S, Jampathong N, Srisomboon J, Lumbiganon P. Management of drainage for malignant ascites in gynaecological cancer. Cochrane Database Syst Rev. 2019;12(12):CD007794.
65. Meyer L, Suidan R, Sun C, Westin S, Coleman RL, Mills GB. The management of malignant ascites and impact on quality of life outcomes in women with ovarian cancer. Expert Rev Qual Life Cancer Care. 2016;1(3):231–8.

Kidney

17

Amanda Hambrecht, Natalie Escobar, William Huang, Ann Lee, and Cherisse Berry

17.1 Introduction

While there are nuanced complications associated with specific malignancies, oncologic emergencies for the acute care surgeon fall into several discrete categories: hemorrhage, obstruction, and perforation. We will discuss surgical emergencies associated with the collecting system and tumors of the kidney as well as complications secondary to treatment therapies for metastatic renal cell carcinoma with which general surgeons should be familiar.

17.2 Parenchymal and Collecting System Emergencies

First described by Carl Wunderlich in 1856, Wunderlich syndrome is defined as nontraumatic spontaneous hemorrhage of the kidney into the subcapsular and perinephric spaces [1, 2]. Significant retroperitoneal hemorrhage can present as

A. Hambrecht · C. Berry (✉)
Division of Acute Care Surgery, Department of Surgery, New York University Grossman School of Medicine, New York, NY, USA
e-mail: Amanda.Hambrecht@med.usc.edu; Cherisse.Berry@nyulangone.org

N. Escobar
New York University Grossman School of Medicine, New York, NY, USA
e-mail: Natalie.Escobar@ucsf.edu

W. Huang
Department of Urology, New York University Grossman School of Medicine, New York, NY, USA
e-mail: William.Huang@nyulangone.org

A. Lee
Division of Surgical Oncology, Department of Surgery, New York University Grossman School of Medicine, Health+Hospitals/Bellevue Hospital, New York, NY, USA
e-mail: Ann.Lee2@nyulangone.org

A. Tarasconi et al. (eds.), *Oncologic Surgical Emergencies*, Hot Topics in Acute Care Surgery and Trauma, https://doi.org/10.1007/978-3-031-36860-8_17

hypovolemic shock without abdominal pain and be difficult to diagnose, leading to increased morbidity and mortality [1–3]. Wunderlich syndrome classically presents as Lenk's triad: acute flank or abdominal pain, hypovolemic shock, and a palpable flank mass on physical exam. Hemodynamically significant hematuria is also often present [2, 3]. The acute management of these patients is similar to that of hemorrhagic shock from other etiologies and should include large-bore intravenous access, type and cross, volume resuscitation with transfusion of blood products, and emergent cross-sectional imaging if hemodynamically stable.

There are multiple etiologies of Wunderlich syndrome; however, the most common cause is renal neoplasms, which are responsible for up to 65% of Wunderlich cases [2–4]. Both benign and malignant neoplasms can cause Wunderlich syndrome, with renal angiomyolipoma (AML) as the most common benign etiology and renal cell carcinoma as the most common malignant etiology [2, 4]. Though extremely rare, other renal neoplasms such as Wilms' tumor, fibromas, oncocytomas, sarcomas, or metastases can also cause spontaneous perirenal hemorrhage [2, 4].

Angiomyolipomas are composed of smooth muscle cells, adipocytes, and epithelioid cells that are clonally proliferated around blood vessels. These tumors are more common in females and are typically found when patients are in their fourth or fifth decades of life [1, 5]. AMLs can be sporadic, diagnosed incidentally on imaging or autopsy in up to 2% of the population [6, 7]; however, they are more commonly associated with tuberous sclerosis complex (TSC) or pulmonary lymphangioleiomyomatosis (LAM) [2]. Studies have shown that AMLs are found in up to 60% of patients with TSC or LAM [8, 9].

Although AMLs are largely asymptomatic, hemorrhagic rupture is the primary presentation in up to 25% of patients [2]. However, not all AMLs will rupture, and the risk of Wunderlich syndrome secondary to tumor rupture is directly proportional to the size of both the tumor and the aneurysm within the tumor [2, 10, 11]. Current guidelines recommend prophylactic embolization or nephron-sparing surgery to remove tumors >4 cm or those with aneurysms >5 mm, as these have increased risk of hemorrhage [10, 12]. Surgical intervention is also recommended for patients with persistent symptoms such as flank pain or hematuria.

Renal cell carcinoma (RCC) is the second most common neoplastic etiology of Wunderlich syndrome [2, 3, 13]. RCC is twice as likely to be found in males and is most commonly diagnosed in the sixth or seventh decade of life [14]. There are multiple subtypes of renal cell carcinoma, including clear cell, papillary, and chromophobe variations. The most common subtype that leads to perirenal hemorrhage, or Wunderlich syndrome, is clear cell [2, 15].

Spontaneous hemorrhage is much more rare in renal cell carcinomas compared to AMLs; however, it can still be potentially lethal and requires urgent intervention [2, 16]. Patients with clear cell renal carcinoma whose tumors are large, grow rapidly, and invade into renal vasculature are more prone to spontaneous hemorrhage [1, 2, 17]. If possible, patients should be stabilized with embolization, with surgery largely dependent on the cancer stage and overall clinical state of the patient, including their performance status.

Patients with autosomal dominant polycystic kidney disease (ADPKD) are predisposed to Wunderlich syndrome due to both the increased incidence of cyst rupture and renal cell carcinoma. ADPKD is much more common than both AML and RCC, with an incidence of 1 in 1000; however, it is estimated that almost half of the patients with ADPKD will have no symptoms or complications [18]. Patients with polycystic kidney disease without end-stage renal disease requiring dialysis have a 1.77 increased risk of developing RCC compared to the general population [19]. Multiple case studies have documented that rupture of cysts in patients with ADPKD can cause hemorrhage resulting in shock or peritonitis if the cyst ruptures secondary to infection [2, 20–22].

Total nephrectomy carries a significant risk of developing chronic kidney disease. Therefore, the treatment approach selected should be the one that optimizes kidney function as much as possible, preferably nephron-sparing heminephrectomy or embolization [7, 12, 23]. Embolization is used for tumors that are centrally located and have large feeding vessels, making a successful heminephrectomy unlikely, and has been shown to reduce tumor size and occlude tumor aneurysms [2, 24, 25]. A total nephrectomy should be reserved for patients who cannot undergo heminephrectomy due to risk of hemorrhage and multiple failed embolizations, or for patients who have a tumor thrombus in the renal vein, inferior vena cava, or right atrium [7, 12, 13]. When patients with Wunderlich syndrome present with life-threatening shock secondary to hemorrhage, embolization is the preferred initial intervention, if the patient is stable enough to undergo the procedure, as it can decrease active bleeding and allow for a less radical surgical intervention later on [2, 12–14].

In addition to hemodynamic compromise, massive hematuria can also lead to acute urinary retention due to blood clot obstruction in the bladder neck or urethra. Hematuria from hemorrhage into the collecting system will develop into a blood clot when the amount of blood in the bladder overwhelms the ability of the urinary urokinase to prevent clot formation. Clot retention requires prompt intervention to relieve the obstruction and is a true urologic emergency [26–28]. Placement of a large three-way urethral catheter, typically 22 French or larger, allows for continuous bladder irrigation (CBI) with 0.9% normal saline to prevent new clot formation. If the urine is unable to be cleared with CBI, the patient may need cystoscopy and removal of intravesical clots in the operating room.

17.3 Ureteral Obstruction

Ureteral obstruction is a common urologic emergency necessitating operative intervention. Ureteral obstruction is most often due to stones but can also be caused by blood clots or tumors. Decompression in the form of a ureteral stent or percutaneous drainage from a nephrostomy tube is needed in the setting of infection, acute worsening of renal function, uncontrollable pain, and obstruction of both kidneys or in patients with a solitary functioning kidney [26]. Patients who are immunosuppressed, such as those on chemotherapy and antirejection medications or those who are diabetic or pregnant, should also undergo stenting or drainage.

17.4 Bowel-Related Emergencies

Malignancy of the kidney is the sixth most common cancer among men and ninth most common cancer among women in the United States [29]. While the 5-year survival rate for localized disease is >90%, approximately one-third of patients with renal cell carcinoma will develop metastases [30, 31]. Common metastatic sites include lung, liver, bone, brain, and adrenal gland, although case reports have described metastases to the small bowel, colon, and peritoneum [32–34]. Metastatic disease to the small bowel has presented as bowel obstruction with intussusception, gastrointestinal bleeding, or both [35–40].

As discussed above, the initial management of a gastrointestinal bleed should focus on maintaining an active type and cross and stabilizing the patient with transfusion of blood products and minimal crystalloid intravenous fluids as needed. For bleeding metastases, identifying the location of the bleed, with either upper endoscopy, capsule endoscopy, or angiography, is an important step in the diagnostic workup. Both a diagnostic and therapeutic intervention and selective angiographic embolization can identify and control intestinal hemorrhage prior to an operation, which typically includes a segmental bowel resection (Fig. 17.1). Although the most

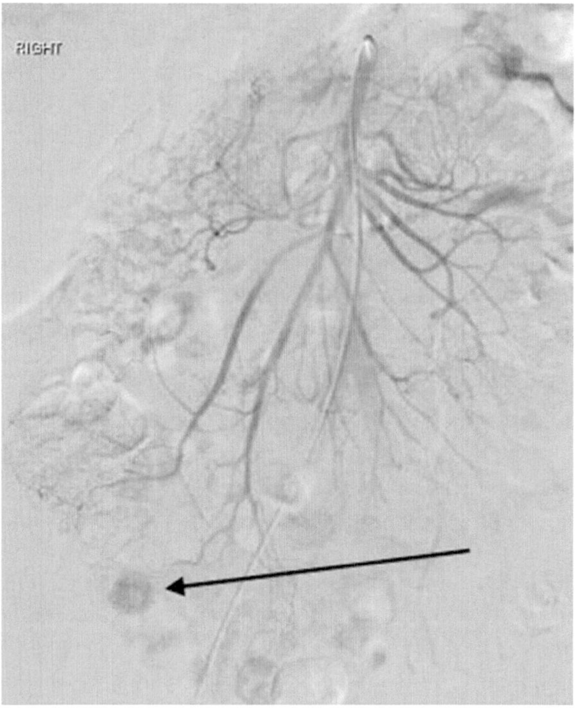

Fig. 17.1 Mesenteric angiogram with ovoid, hyper-enhancing lesion (arrow), likely in the small bowel, supplied by branches of the ileocolic artery. Obtained with permission from Mueller JL, Guyer RA, Adler JT, Mullen JT. Metastatic renal cell carcinoma to the small bowel: three cases of GI bleeding and a literature review. CEN Case Rep, 2018; 7(1): 39–43

common causes of lower gastrointestinal bleeding are angiodysplasia and diverticulosis, the acute care surgeon should maintain a high level of suspicion for a bleeding metastasis in patients with a history of renal cell carcinoma.

Metastases to the bowel or the peritoneum can result in a small bowel obstruction. If there is a single point of obstruction and there are no concerning peritoneal signs or hemodynamic instability, an initial period of nonoperative management is reasonable not only to allow for the possibility of resolution with nasogastric tube decompression alone, but also to have a multidisciplinary discussion regarding cancer prognosis, treatment options, and goals of care. Similar to small bowel obstructions from other causes, if the patient is unstable, there is evidence of a closed-loop obstruction, or the patient does not improve with decompression alone, surgical exploration is warranted. If resection of the affected area is not feasible due to the extent of disease, other considerations include intestinal bypass and a venting gastrostomy tube.

With the development of targeted molecular therapy and immunotherapy, there are more available treatment options for metastatic disease. The National Comprehensive Cancer Network (NCCN) has several first-line recommendations for tyrosine kinase inhibitors and monoclonal antibodies in treating stage IV or relapsed clear cell kidney cancer, including sunitinib and pazopanib [41]. Potent vascular endothelial growth factor (VEGF) inhibitors, sunitinib and pazopanib, decrease angiogenesis and have shown survival benefits in patients with metastatic RCC. The most common gastrointestinal side effects of VEGF inhibitors include nausea, vomiting, and diarrhea. However, both sunitinib and pazopanib have a rare risk of gastrointestinal perforation, with case reports of small bowel and colon perforation [42, 43]. These perforations were fatal in 0.3% of cases [44]. These patients can present with signs of septic shock and diffuse peritonitis on physical examination, necessitating surgical exploration with emergency laparotomy.

17.5 Conclusion

Surgical emergencies related to kidney tumors can present as hemorrhage, obstruction, or perforation. General surgeons should be knowledgeable about the potential for life-threatening retroperitoneal hemorrhage or hemodynamically significant hematuria from tumor rupture, with the potential for acute urinary retention or ureteral obstruction secondary to clots, as well as gastrointestinal bleeding or obstruction from metastases or bowel perforation related to chemotherapy side effects. Prompt evaluation and treatment are indicated in each emergent presentation, requiring urinary decompression in the cases of collecting system obstruction and angioembolization and/or surgery for patients presenting with bleeding.

References

1. McDougal WS, Kursh ED, Persky L. Spontaneous rupture of the kidney with perirenal hematoma. J Urol. 1975;114(2):181–4.
2. Katabathina VS, Katre R, Prasad SR, Surabhi VR, Shanbhogue AK, Sunnapwar A. Wunderlich syndrome: cross-sectional imaging review. J Comput Assist Tomogr. 2011;35(4):425–33.
3. Albi G, del Campo L, Tagarro D. Wünderlich's syndrome: causes, diagnosis and radiological management. Clin Radiol. 2002;57(9):840–5.
4. Zhang JQ, Fielding JR, Zou KH. Etiology of spontaneous perirenal hemorrhage: a meta-analysis. J Urol. 2002;167(4):1593–6.
5. Rule AD, Sasiwimonphan K, Lieske JC, Keddis MT, Torres VE, Vrtiska TJ. Characteristics of renal cystic and solid lesions based on contrast-enhanced computed tomography of potential kidney donors. Am J Kidney Dis. 2012;59(5):611–8.
6. Hajdu SI, Foote FW Jr. Angiomyolipoma of the kidney: report of 27 cases and review of the literature. J Urol. 1969;102(4):396–401.
7. Nelson CP, Sanda MG. Contemporary diagnosis and management of renal angiomyolipoma. J Urol. 2002;168(4 Pt 1):1315–25.
8. Rakowski SK, Winterkorn EB, Paul E, Steele DJ, Halpern EF, Thiele EA. Renal manifestations of tuberous sclerosis complex: incidence, prognosis, and predictive factors. Kidney Int. 2006;70(10):1777–82.
9. Bernstein SM, Newell JD Jr, Adamczyk D, Mortenson RL, King TE Jr, Lynch DA. How common are renal angiomyolipomas in patients with pulmonary. Am J Respir Crit Care Med. 1995;152(6):2138–43.
10. Yamakado K, Tanaka N, Nakagawa T, Kobayashi S, Yanagawa M, Takeda K. Renal angiomyolipoma: relationships between tumor size, aneurysm formation, and rupture. Radiol. 2002;225(1):78–82.
11. Eble JN. Angiomyolipoma of kidney. Semin Diagn Pathol. 1998;15(1):21–40.
12. Oesterling JE, Fishman EK, Goldman SM, Marshall FF. The management of renal angiomyolipoma. J Urol. 1986;135(6):1121–4.
13. Simkins A, Maiti A, Cherian SV. Wunderlich Syndrome. Am J Med. 2017;130(5):e217–8.
14. Siegel RL, Miller KD, Fuchs HE, Jemal A. Cancer statistics, 2021. CA Cancer J Clin. 2021;71(1):7–33.
15. Cheville JC, Lohse CM, Zincke H, Weaver AL, Blute ML. Comparisons of outcome and prognostic features among histologic subtypes of renal cell carcinoma. Am J Surg Pathol. 2003;27(5):612–24.
16. Watanabe S, Hama Y, Kaji T, Kimura F, Kosuda S. Pre-operative embolization for spontaneous rupture of renal cell carcinoma. Ulster Med J. 2005;74(1):66–7.
17. Mydlo JH, Kaplan J, Thelmo W, Macchia RJ. Spontaneous renal hemorrhage associated with renal tumors. Clin Imaging. 1997;21(4):287–9.
18. Davies F, Coles GA, Harper PS, Williams AJ, Evans C, Cochlin D. Polycystic kidney disease re-evaluated: a population-based study. Q J Med. 1991;79(290):477–85.
19. Yu TM, Chuang YW, Yu MC, et al. Risk of cancer in patients with polycystic kidney disease: a propensity-score matched analysis of a nationwide, population-based cohort study. Lancet Oncol. 2016;17(10):1419–25.
20. Hammami M, Guirat A, Ksibi H, Azzaza M, Rekik N, Beyrouti MI. Intraperitoneal rupture of renal cyst in autosomal dominant polycystic kidney disease. N Am J Med Sci. 2010;2(5):238–40.
21. Yaman İ, Sağlam İ, Kurt K. Acute abdomen and hemorrhagic shock caused by spontaneous rupture of renal cyst in autosomal dominant polycystic kidney disease. Ulus Cerrahi Derg. 2013;29(1):45–7.
22. Reiter WJ, Haitel A, Heinz-Peer G, Pycha A, Marberger M. Spontaneous nontraumatic rupture of a contracted kidney with subcapsular and perirenal hematoma in a patient receiving chronic hemodialysis. Urology. 1997;50(5):781–3.

23. Heidenreich A, Hegele A, Varga Z, von Knobloch R, Hofmann R. Nephron-sparing surgery for renal angiomyolipoma. Eur Urol. 2002;41(3):267–73.
24. Lenton J, Kessel D, Watkinson AF. Embolization of renal angiomyolipoma: immediate complications and long-term outcomes. Clin Radiol. 2008;63(8):864–70.
25. Williams JM, Racadio JM, Johnson ND, Donnelly LF, Bissler JJ. Embolization of renal angiomyolipomata in patients with tuberous sclerosis complex. Am J Kidney Dis. 2006;47(1):95–102.
26. Kieran K, Yates J, Kaplan D, and Kohn T. Urologic emergencies. American Urological Association. 2021. https://www.auanet.org/education/auauniversity/for-medical-students/medical-students-curriculum/medical-student-curriculum/urologic-emergencies.
27. Dungerwalla M, Davies N, Perera M, Papa N. Manual bladder washouts for urinary clot retention: a survey of knowledge among healthcare workers. Can J Urol. 2015;22:9083–8.
28. Aydin C, Senturk A, Akkoc A, Topaktas R, Aydin ZP, Ekici M. Clot retention: our experiences with a simple new technique of evacuation with a thoracic catheter. Cureus. 2019;11:e4329.
29. Sachdeva K, Jana BRP, Curti B, Abel EJ. Renal cell carcinoma. Medscape. 2021. https://emedicine.medscape.com/article/281340-overview.
30. Flanigan RC, Campbell SC, Clark JI, Picken MM. Metastatic renal cell carcinoma. Curr Treat Options in Oncol. 2003;4(5):385–90.
31. Surveillance Epidemiology and End Results. SEER stat fact sheets. National Cancer Institute; 2021. http://seer.cancer/gov/statfacts/html/kidrp.html.
32. Vo E, Palacio CH, Omino R, Link RE, Sada Y, Avo A. Solitary colon metastasis from renal cell carcinoma nine years after nephrectomy: a case report. Int J Surg Case Rep. 2016;27:55–8.
33. Park HJ, Kim HJ, Park SH, Lee JS, Kim AY, Ha HK. Gastrointestinal involvement of recurrent renal cell carcinoma: CT findings and clinicopathologic features. Korean J Radiol. 2017;18:452–60.
34. Gonçalves MO, Benidir T, Erbano BO, Jung JE, de Almeida LM. Peritoneal metastases from renal cell carcinoma: images in urology. Can Urol Assoc J. 2014;8(5–6):E391–2.
35. Bellio G, Mis TC, Kaso G, Dattola R, Casagranda B, Bortul M. Small bowel intussusception from renal cell carcinoma metastasis: a case report and review of the literature. J Med Case Rep. 2016;10(222):222. https://doi.org/10.1186/s13256-016-0998-0.
36. Mishra S, Hazra SP, Priyadarshi V, et al. Synchronous jejunal metastasis presenting as intussusception in a case of advanced RCC: a rare presentation. Indian J Surg. 2015;77(1):59–61.
37. Eo WK, Kim GY, Choi SII. A case of multiple intussusceptions in the small intestine caused by metastatic renal cell carcinoma. Cancer Res Treat. 2008;40(2):97–9.
38. Hedge RG, Gowda HK, Agrawal RD, et al. Renal cell carcinoma presenting as small bowel obstruction secondary to metastatic ileal intussusception. Radiol Case. 2014;8(4):25–31.
39. Mueller JL, Guyer RA, Adler JT, Mullen JT. Metastatic renal cell carcinoma to the small bowel: three cases of GI bleeding and a literature review. CEN Case Rep. 2018;7(1):39–43.
40. Sadler GJ, Anderson MR, Moss MS, Wilson PG. Metastases from renal cell carcinoma presenting as gastrointestinal bleeding: two case reports and a review of the literature. BMC Gastroenterol. 2007;7(4). https://doi.org/10.1186/1471-230X-7-4.
41. National Comprehensive Cancer Network. NCCN clinical practice guidelines in oncology. Kidney Cancer NCCN. 2021. http://www.nccn.org/professionals/physician_gls/pdf/kidney.pdf. Accessed 3 Feb 2021.
42. Vorient [prescribing information]. East Hanover, NJ: Novartis Pharmaceuticals Corp; 2017.
43. Sutent [prescribing information]. New York, NY: Pfizer Medical; 2011.
44. Akoluk A, Douedi S, Dattadeen J, Grille V, Kaufman E, Liu E, Parer G, Nahum K. Colonic perforation associated with necrotizing fasciitis in a patient receiving tyrosine kinase inhibitor (pazopanib) for recurrent retroperitoneal renal cell carcinoma. J Curr Surg. 2020;10(3):54–8.

Urologic Emergencies in Oncology Patients

18

Lily Kong and Fernando J. Kim

18.1 Introduction

Ureteral obstruction is seen in advanced stages of both genitourinary and non-genitourinary cancers. Clinical presentation can vary based on the mechanism of obstruction. Management is also patient and provider specific and typically involves a multidisciplinary approach.

18.2 Ureteral Obstruction

Malignant ureteral obstruction (MUO) is a complication of a wide range of cancers, including genitourinary cancers such as bladder or prostate cancer and non-genitourinary cancers including lymphoma, colorectal, uterine, cervical, ovarian, and breast cancer. MUO affects patients with more advanced stages of cancer and is associated with a high rate of morbidity in many cancers. A prospective study showed that the median range for survival in all cancer patients after urinary diversion was 144 days; survival rates at 1, 6, and 12 months were 80%, 42%, and 21%, respectively [1]. Recognition and expeditious management of ureteral obstruction are crucial to preserve optimal renal function.

18.2.1 Epidemiology

Between 3 and 16% of patients treated for advanced prostate cancer can develop MUO from local tumor spread [2]. In cervical cancer, ureteral obstruction can occur

L. Kong · F. J. Kim (✉)
Division of Urology, Department of Surgery, Denver Health Medical Center and University of Colorado, Denver, CO, USA
e-mail: lily.kong@cuanschutz.edu

A. Tarasconi et al. (eds.), *Oncologic Surgical Emergencies*, Hot Topics in Acute Care Surgery and Trauma, https://doi.org/10.1007/978-3-031-36860-8_18

in up to 11% of patients [3]. The overall incidence of MUO is unknown, although one source suggests that ureteral obstruction may occur in up to one-third of patients with primary or metastatic pelvic malignancies [4, 5].

18.2.2 Etiology

Among the cancers causing MUO, the most common include prostate, cervical (Fig. 18.1), and bladder cancers. Other cancers that less frequently cause MUO include colorectal, gastrointestinal, ovarian, and uterine cancers [1, 6].

18.2.3 Pathophysiology

MUO occurs most commonly from direct tumor invasion by ureter infiltration, extrinsic ureteral compression from large tumors, or retroperitoneal/pelvic lymphadenopathy. Direct metastasis can cause MUO, but less commonly so. Obstruction can also be a sequelae of cancer treatment, e.g., secondary to retroperitoneal fibrosis from surgery, chemotherapy, or radiotherapy [7].

The most common mechanism of upper urinary tract obstruction in prostate cancer is direct invasion of the tumor to the ureter [8]. In prostate cancer, malignant bilateral ureteral obstruction can also be seen. In these cases, the mechanism of

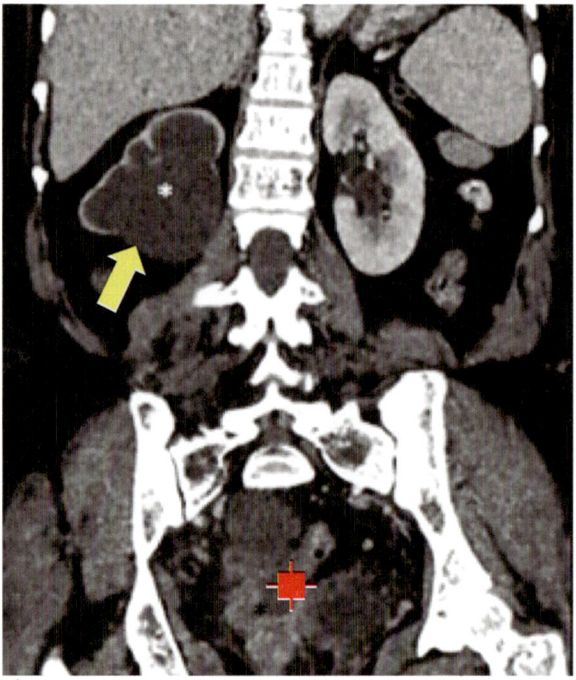

Fig. 18.1 Coronal view of abdominal computed tomography demonstrating right-sided hydronephrosis (yellow arrow) in the setting of advanced cervical cancer (red asterisk)

obstruction is often invasion of the bladder trigone and ureteral orifices causing upper urinary tract obstruction and, less frequently, obstruction of the lower one-third of the ureter from local spread or impaired drainage secondary to retroperitoneal lymph node metastases [9]. In very rare cases, prostate cancer can metastasize to the ureters, with fewer than 100 cases of this phenomenon reported in literature [5].

Lupu et al. described the main variables in MUO that are likely to change as MUO progresses: glomerular filtration rate (GFR), renal blood flow (RBF), and ureteral pressure (UP). These variables change in stages, which are different depending on whether the patient has unilateral obstruction or bilateral obstruction [5]. In unilateral obstruction, animal experiments have demonstrated a triphasic pattern:

1. First phase (1–2 h after obstruction):
   (a) RBF increases, UP is high, GFR is maintained (due to an increase in RBF)
   (b) Facilitated by afferent arteriole vasodilation
2. Second phase (3–4 h after obstruction)
   (a) RBF decreases, UP continues to decrease, GFR decreases (due to decrease in RBF)
   (b) Facilitated by efferent arteriole vasoconstriction
3. Third phase (5 h after obstruction)
   (a) Both RBF and UP decrease, GFR decreases
   (b) Facilitated by efferent and afferent arteriole vasoconstriction [5, 10]

In bilateral obstruction, the phases are less distinct. In the first 90 min after obstruction, RBF increases and then slowly decreases and UP increases, remaining elevated for a longer time than unilateral obstruction due to persistent afferent vasodilation [10]. There is also a post-obstructive phase that is more commonly seen in bilateral obstruction than unilateral obstruction. In this stage, the obstruction causes large retention of osmolar substances such as sodium, urea, and water, which may lead to significant diuresis [5].

18.2.4 Clinical Presentation

Because MUO can be due to several primary cancers, clinical presentations may differ from patient to patient. Patients can present with vague symptoms, including pain and fever. Presentation also differs with the level of the obstruction.

18.2.4.1 Lower Urinary Tract Obstruction

In lower urinary tract obstruction (LUTO), patients may experience urinary urgency, frequency, nocturia, incontinence, decreased urinary stream, hesitancy, post-void dribbling, and a sensation of inadequate emptying. Patients may also have suprapubic pain or a palpable bladder if urinary retention is present. Infection can also occur, leading to dysuria [5]. LUTO will be discussed further in the next section on bladder outlet obstruction.

18.2.4.2 Acute Upper Urinary Tract Obstruction

Acute upper urinary tract obstruction manifests as a colicky abdominal pain that often radiates to the iliac fossa. The pain can be dull or sharp, and intermittent or persistent. Nausea and vomiting are common associated symptoms. Patients with complete bilateral upper urinary tract obstruction can present with anuria [5].

18.2.4.3 Chronic Upper Urinary Tract Obstruction

Chronic upper urinary tract obstruction can be a result of compression from an enlarging pelvic malignancy. Patients may present with vague, dull abdominal pain that is less severe than that of acute upper urinary tract obstruction, most likely due to gradual distention of the renal pelvis. Chronic obstruction can eventually cause symptoms related to electrolyte abnormalities and changes in volume status [10].

18.2.5 Evaluation

Initial workup includes taking a thorough patient history and physical examination. Basic laboratory studies should be obtained, including serum electrolytes and urinalysis [5, 10]. There are multiple imaging modalities that may be used to aid in the diagnosis of MUO, which are presented below.

18.2.5.1 Renal Ultrasonography

Renal ultrasound is an appropriate first-line imaging modality for detecting hydronephrosis, which may be present in patients with MUO. Bedside ultrasound in the ED has been shown to have a reported sensitivity of 72–87% and specificity of 73–83% for detection of unilateral hydronephrosis compared to CT [11, 12]. Ultrasound has many advantages over other imaging modalities, including lack of ionizing radiation; safety in pregnancy, pediatric populations, and patients with renal insufficiency; and cost. However, ultrasound has a distinct disadvantage in that it can only determine anatomic dilatation of the urinary tract and cannot assess any functional obstructions [5, 10].

18.2.5.2 Nuclear Medicine Renography

Nuclear medicine renography uses radioisotopes, typically technetium diethylenetriaminepentaacetic acid (Tc-99m DTPA) and technetium mercaptoacetyltriglycine (Tc-99m MAG), to determine renal function [5, 10]. Tc-99m DTPA is freely filtered and neither secreted nor reabsorbed; Tc-99m MAG is eliminated by the proximal tubules without reabsorption [10]. Diuresis renography, in which the study is combined with the use of diuretics, commonly furosemide, can help distinguish between obstruction and prolonged renal drainage [13, 14]. Furosemide is administered intravenously to increase urine flow rate; in obstruction, washout of the radioisotope remains slow even with the administration of furosemide and can build up proximal to the obstruction [13]. This study allows providers to measure relative renal function and has very low radiation exposure [14].

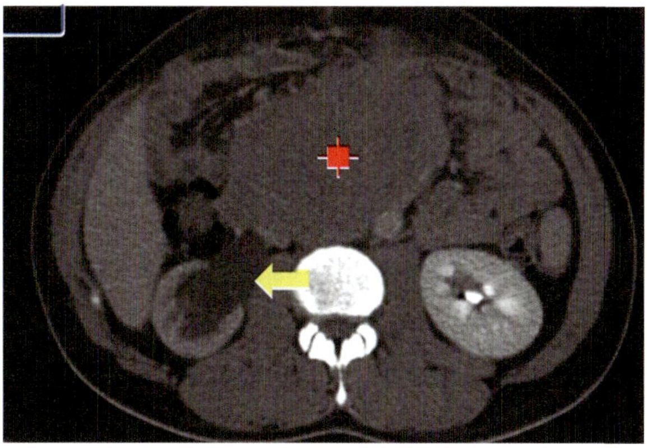

Fig. 18.2 Axial view computed tomography demonstrating right-sided hydronephrosis (yellow arrow) with a retroperitoneal mass (red asterisk)

18.2.5.3 Computed Tomography and Magnetic Resonance Imaging

Computed tomography (CT) (Fig. 18.2) has become the preferred imaging modality for assessing the urinary tract. CT has a 95% sensitivity and 98% specificity in detecting ureteral stone disease [5]. CT urography can be especially useful in evaluating for ureteral obstruction as it can visualize the renal system in three phases—non-contrast, nephrogenic, and excretory. In the non-contrast phase, CT urography can detect stones and other calcifications, and it can detect filling defects in the excretory phase [5].

Magnetic resonance imaging (MRI) can provide similar information as CT, but without ionizing radiation. It may be a safer option in pregnant patients, pediatric patients, and those at risk for contrast-induced nephropathy, i.e., patients with renal insufficiency [5, 10].

18.2.5.4 Urodynamics

Urodynamics testing assesses patterns of bladder filling, urine storage, and emptying. Though it is not often used in the diagnosis of ureteral obstruction, it can be useful if initial workup and diagnostic testing are equivocal or insufficient [10].

18.2.6 Management

There are currently no guidelines for the management of MUO given the varied etiologies of MUO. Because MUO typically presents in patients with advanced-stage cancer, management has evolved into a multidisciplinary approach involving urologists, oncologists, palliative care physicians, general medicine physicians, and interventional radiologists [6]. Management can vary widely depending on the etiology and individual practice and can be curative or palliative. In this chapter, we review common courses of management for ureteral obstruction in general while being cognizant that treatment can differ by patient. Careful consideration should be given to the risks and benefits of each treatment.

18.2.6.1 Ureteral Stents

Ureteral stents are often first-line treatments in ureteral obstruction as a method of decompression, as they can bypass the narrowed portion of the ureter to allow effective drainage of the affected kidney(s) [10]. Advancements in technique and technology have increased the success rate of stents to 73–95% compared to 50% in older studies; however, the success rate varies based on other presenting factors. For instance, grade 4 hydronephrosis, multiple areas of ureteral narrowing, and altered anatomy of the ureteral orifices and trigone are all factors that are predictive of stent failure. Long-term failure rates of stents have been reported to be anywhere between 11 and 44%, although failure rates as high as 58% have been reported for conventional polymeric stents [7, 15].

Classically, ureteral stenting used double-pigtail polymeric stents, but newer options have also emerged. Tandem ureteral stenting, in which two double-pigtail stents are used in the same ureter to relieve obstruction, is a relatively newer technique [7]. Conceptually, this method is thought to be advantageous compared to single stents because the space between the stents and ureteral wall allows for additional drainage capacity [15]. One study found that stent patency was significantly better in tandem ureteral stenting compared to single ureteral stenting (mean patency time of 176.7 days versus 214.7, $p = 0.022$) [15]. Overall survival was similar in both groups; however, the increased patency time for tandem ureteral stenting may require fewer stent exchanges and thus has potential for improved quality of life.

Metallic stents are another option for ureteral stents as they require less frequent exchanges (one stent exchange every 12 months). However, even with the development of newer metallic stents, they are associated with higher failure rates and complications. As such, they are typically used as second-line therapy after single or tandem ureteral stenting has failed [7]. The most widely utilized metallic ureteral stents are Resonance, Uventa, and Allium.

Ureteral stents have the advantage of internal decompression, so there is a lower risk for dislodgement and no need for external appliances, such as with nephrostomy tubes [7]. However, ureteral stents are not without complications; patients can experience lower urinary tract symptoms, somatic pain, encrustation, ureteral perforation, pyelonephritis, stent migration or fracture, hematuria, and, rarely, arterio-ureteral fistula causing significant hematuria [16]. Stents may also not be able to be placed in patients with extensive pelvic disease [1]. Additionally, patients with MUO have higher rates of encrustation compared to patients with benign obstruction [7].

18.2.6.2 Percutaneous Nephrostomy Tubes

Percutaneous nephrostomy (PCN) tubes are another method used to drain the kidneys in ureteral obstruction. A catheter is placed directly into the renal pelvis through the patient's back. PCN tubes can be used for urgent decompression or as alternate therapy if patients have failed ureteral stents and need chronic decompression [10]. One advantage PCN tubes have over ureteral stents is that placement of PCN tubes can be carried out using local anesthesia instead of general anesthesia [7, 10]. Because PCN tubes involve external tubes and drainage bags, complications may arise related to these appliances. Tube blockage, leakage, and dislodgement of the PCN tube are common, and additional tube changes are required in up to 83% of patients with PCN tubes [16]. Other complications include pyelonephritis, hematuria, and hospital readmission [1]. PCN tubes also need to be exchanged every 6–12 weeks [10].

18.2.6.3 Surgical Management

If initial treatment options for MUO are not effective, surgical management exists for such refractory cases. Surgical treatment options include ureterolysis and ureteral reimplantation to restore urinary flow. However, ureteral reimplantation may not be an option for patients with pelvic malignancies that have grown in a way that makes reimplantation nonoptimal or patients who have had radiation therapy with resulting poor bladder tissue quality [10].

18.3 Bladder Outlet Obstruction

In this section, we will examine bladder outlet obstruction (BOO) in the setting of malignancy. BOO is an umbrella term that encompasses posterior urethral stenosis (PUS), which describes a narrowing from the distal bladder neck to the proximal bulbar urethra, and vesicourethral anastomotic stenosis (VUAS), which occurs at the anastomosis site after prostatectomy [17]. For the most part, this type of obstruction is common in prostate cancer (Fig. 18.3) and the treatment of prostate cancer but can occur as a result of other cancers as well.

18.3.1 Epidemiology

The incidence of BOO in the setting of prostate cancer treatment varies as pathogenesis differs by type of treatment. Five to ten percent of patients with radical

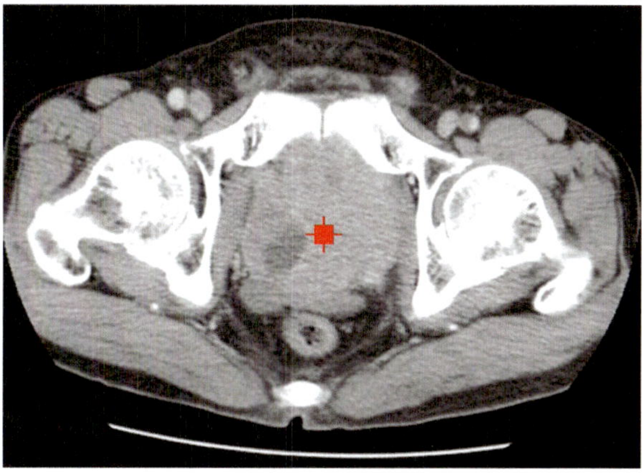

Fig. 18.3 Axial view computed tomography of advanced prostate cancer (red asterisk) causing bladder outlet obstruction (not pictured)

prostatectomy can have PUS and 1–13% after external beam radiotherapy, with a greater rate after combination therapy [18]. One study reported that, by 10 years after prostate cancer therapy, 20–38% of elderly men have surgery for BOO [19]. One obstacle to estimating the incidence of BOO in general is that many studies only investigate patients who have received treatment, which likely underestimates true incidence [17].

18.3.2 Etiology

In patients with male anatomy, bladder outlet obstruction is most linked to the treatment of prostate cancer. Malignant causes of bladder outlet obstruction in patients with female anatomy include urethral, vaginal, and cervical cancers [20]. There have also been a few reported cases of acute urinary retention from bladder obstruction caused by uterine tumors [21].

18.3.3 Pathophysiology

BOO in the setting of cancer is strongly associated with pelvic cancer treatment, especially radical prostatectomy and radiation therapy. Its pathogenesis is thought to be related to several factors, such as prior bladder neck or prostate procedures, surgical approaches, severe hemorrhage, prior radiotherapy, and surgeon experience. A variety of patient factors may also contribute to its pathogenesis, including preexisting medical conditions such as cardiovascular disease, diabetes mellitus, and hypertension; smoking; BMI; and age [17].

Studies have offered several causes for BOO after radical prostatectomy, including urine leak at the anastomosis site, intraoperative hemorrhage, and mucosal eversion [17]. Radiation therapy can cause BOO through target tissue injury via two mechanisms: (1) induction of apoptosis and (2) inhibition of mitosis associated with the generation of highly reactive oxygen species that can damage DNA, RNA, and cell membranes [22]. The long-term effects of this tissue injury cause scarring and fibrosis, which leads to urethral stenosis [17]. Alternative and adjuvant therapies for prostate cancer, such as cryoablation and high-intensity focused ultrasound (HIFU), can also cause BOO. These therapies utilize local coagulative necrosis that can lead to fibrosis and, thus, BOO [17].

18.3.4 Clinical Presentation

Bladder outlet obstruction most commonly presents with lower urinary tract symptoms (LUTSs). These symptoms may be obstructive, irritative, or a combination of both. Obstructive symptoms include urinary hesitancy, decreased urinary stream, post-void dribbling, and a sensation of incomplete bladder emptying. Irritative symptoms include urinary urgency, urinary frequency, dysuria, and nocturia.

Patients may also present without any of the above symptoms but have urinary retention [20]. Complications such as persistent hematuria, high residual urine volume, and bladder stones may also be present [23].

18.3.5 Evaluation

Like ureteral obstruction, evaluation should begin with a thorough history that reviews lower urinary symptoms, prior history of pelvic cancer, pelvic radiation, and prior treatment for urinary symptoms [17]. Dmochowski suggests that evaluation is gender specific, as etiologies can differ based on anatomy [20].

18.3.5.1 Female Anatomy

In patients with female anatomy, a physical exam may reveal pelvic organ prolapse and urethral hypermobility [20]. Typically, a combination of urodynamic and non-urodynamic testing can aid in making a diagnosis. Non-urodynamic testing includes a post-void residual (PVR), cystoscopy, voiding cystourethrogram (VCUG), and, occasionally, MRI of the bladder outlet and urethra [20].

PVR can be done via urethral catheterization or portable ultrasound, which is becoming increasingly popular due to accessibility and ease of use. Urethral catheterization is the standard, with a reported 100% specificity and sensitivity for estimating PVR [24]. However, it can cause patient discomfort and trauma to the urethra; additionally, catheters can increase the risk of urinary tract infections (UTIs). A recent study comparing the use of portable bladder scanner with catheters for measuring PVR in women with pelvic organ prolapse showed no significant difference between the two but found that stage III/IV prolapse was associated with increased error in the bladder scanner ($p = 0.03$) [25]. However, another study done in men with LUTS showed that PVR obtained by catheter was significantly higher than ultrasound measurement ($p < 0.05$) [24].

Cystoscopy can provide a visual assessment of the urethra and bladder, as well as identify urethral abnormalities and foreign bodies within the urinary. VCUG, a fluoroscopic procedure in which the bladder is filled with a contrast agent and X-rays are taken as the patient voids, can be helpful in identifying specific areas of obstruction [20].

MRI of the urethra is the gold standard for assessment of extrinsic and intrinsic urethral pathology, including extrinsic lesions that may be causing BOO in patients with female anatomy [20].

18.3.5.2 Male Anatomy

Diagnosis of BOO in patients with male anatomy can include lab studies, PVR, urine flow rate measurement, validated questionnaires, cystoscopy, other imaging, and urodynamic studies.

Lab studies include urinalysis, urine culture, PSA to rule out persistent or recurrent cancer, and renal function tests if clinically indicated [18].

The utility of urodynamic studies (UDSs) in the diagnosis of BOO is a debated topic. While considered the gold standard by some, there have been recent studies that argue that it should be used only in certain situations. UDSs reproduce patient symptoms and make precise measurements, and the results have been proven to be reproducible [26]. However, the European Association of Urology guidelines only advise UDS for patients who have failed invasive treatment, patients between the ages of 50 and 80, and patients with low voided volumes or high PVR measurements [27]. The UPSTREAM trial concluded that UDS did not reduce the number of surgeries for BOO compared to routine care (urine flow rate measurement, bladder diaries, and validated questionnaires) and thus did not support the routine use of UDS in the evaluation of men considering prostate surgery for LUTS [28].

Urine flow rate measurements are standardized, with a flow of less than 10 mm/s being consistent with obstruction. However, diminished flow rate can also be a result of poor detrusor contractility. Additionally, a normal flow rate does not rule out obstruction [17]. Thus, urine flow rate measurements should not be used alone to diagnose BOO and should be used in combination with other tests.

Validated questionnaires include the International Prostate System Score (IPSS) and the AUA Urinary Symptom Index (AUA-7).

Cystoscopy can evaluate the degree of stricture present within the urethra and assess other urethral pathologies [17, 18].

Further imaging is performed if previous tests cannot accurately identify the degree and location of the stenosis. Retrograde urethrography and VCUG imaging can be used if cystourethroscopy cannot be performed. Prostate imaging can show abscesses, calcifications, and cancer recurrence. CT or MRI may be performed if the disease is thought to be more extensive [18].

18.3.6 Management

Management of BOO can differ based on individual presentation and other patient factors, as well as the etiology of the obstruction. This section will describe management of BOO as a result of prostate cancer therapy using the Société Internationale d'Urologie/International Consultation on Urologic Disease guidelines on PUS after prostate cancer treatment.

18.3.6.1 Management After Radiation Therapy

External beam radiation therapy (EBRT) commonly involves the membranous or bulbar urethra. Treatment options include endoscopic dilation and endoscopic internal urethrotomy, in which an incision is made to relieve the stricture; however, recurrence rates are high with these procedures. Forty-nine percent required second-line endoscopic therapy within 16 months and 9% needed additional intermittent self-catheterization or urethroplasty as third-line therapy [29]. Success rates for urethroplasty after failure of endoscopic approaches are between 73 and 90% [18]. Excision and primary anastomosis have also been proven to be successful.

18.3.6.2 Management of Post-radical Prostatectomy Vesicourethral Anastomotic Strictures

Definitive management is endourologic or open surgical management. Initial management for early postoperative stenoses is urethral dilation, but for stenoses that fail dilation or occur later, a stepwise approach is suggested. Low-energy incision is attempted first, followed by transurethral electrosurgical incision [18]. For severe cases of stenoses, open surgical reconstruction may be necessary, which may require temporary suprapubic cystostomy or long-term suprapubic drainage [18].

For patients with metastatic prostate cancer and resulting BOO who have failed medications or do not want long-term catheter use, palliative transurethral resection of the prostate (TURP) can be performed. It is controversial whether palliative TURP may accelerate tumor progression [23].

References

1. Cordeiro MD, Coelho RF, Chade DC, Pessoa RR, Chaib MS, Colombo-Júnior JR, et al. A prognostic model for survival after palliative urinary diversion for malignant ureteric obstruction: a prospective study of 208 patients. BJU Int. 2016;117(2):266–71. https://doi.org/10.1111/bju.12963.
2. Nariculam J, Murphy DG, Jenner C, Sellars N, Gwyther S, Gordon SG, et al. Nephrostomy insertion for patients with bilateral ureteric obstruction caused by prostate cancer. Br J Radiol. 2009;82(979):571–6. https://doi.org/10.1259/bjr/38306763.
3. Goldfarb RA, Fan Y, Jarosek S, Elliott SP. The burden of chronic ureteral stenting in cervical cancer survivors. Int Braz J Urol. 2017;43(1):104–11. https://doi.org/10.1590/s1677-5538.Ibju.2016.0667.
4. Kumar A, Mynderse L, Patel K, Grudem M, Bakkum-Gamez J, Longenbach S, et al. Ureteral obstruction in cancer patients: a qualitative study. Psychooncology. 2016;25(5):605–9. https://doi.org/10.1002/pon.3889.
5. Lupu S, Brinza A, Socea B, Marcu D, Peride I, Stănescu A, et al. A brief review of the literature on the malignant ureteral obstruction. J Mind Med Sci. 2018;5:189–94. https://doi.org/10.22543/7674.52.P189194.
6. Prentice J, Amer T, Tasleem A, Aboumarzouk O. Malignant ureteric obstruction decompression: how much gain for how much pain? A narrative review. J R Soc Med. 2018;111(4):125–35. https://doi.org/10.1177/0141076818766725.
7. Tabib C, Nethala D, Kozel Z, Okeke Z. Management and treatment options when facing malignant ureteral obstruction. Int J Urol. 2020;27(7):591–8. https://doi.org/10.1111/iju.14235.
8. Roy S, Ambelil M, Ayala G, Buja LM. Prostate adenocarcinoma metastasis to the bilateral ureters: a rare but potentially important finding. Ann Clin Lab Sci. 2016;46(4):425–7.
9. Kass-Iliyya A, Okeke A, Gibson M. The baby pacifier sign: bilateral ureteric obstruction secondary to prostate cancer. J Clin Urol. 2022;15(2):173–5. https://doi.org/10.1177/2051415820927810.
10. Zhu G, Rais-Bahrami S. Diagnosis and management of obstructive uropathy in the setting of advanced pelvic malignancies. J Nephrol Res. 2015;1(3). https://doi.org/10.17554/j.issn.2410-0579.2015.01.21.
11. Leo MM, Langlois BK, Pare JR, Mitchell P, Linden J, Nelson KP, et al. Ultrasound vs. computed tomography for severity of hydronephrosis and its importance in renal colic. West J Emerg Med. 2017;18(4):559–68. https://doi.org/10.5811/westjem.2017.04.33119.
12. Riddell J, Case A, Wopat R, Beckham S, Lucas M, McClung CD, et al. Sensitivity of emergency bedside ultrasound to detect hydronephrosis in patients with computed tomography-proven

stones. West J Emerg Med. 2014;15(1):96–100. https://doi.org/10.5811/westjem.2013.9.15874.

13. Bäck A-K, Savvopoulos C, Geijer H. Timing of diuretics in diuresis renography. Clin Transl Imaging. 2022;10(1):37–43. https://doi.org/10.1007/s40336-021-00461-w.
14. Tartaglione G, Townsend DM, Bassi PF, Delgado Bolton RC, Giammarile F, Rubello D. Diuresis renography in equivocal urinary tract obstruction. A historical perspective. Biomed Pharmacother. 2019;116:108981. https://doi.org/10.1016/j.biopha.2019.108981.
15. Liu K-L, Lee B-C, Ye J-D, Chang Y-H, Chang C-C, Huang K-H, et al. Comparison of single and tandem ureteral stenting for malignant ureteral obstruction: a prospective study of 104 patients. Eur Radiol. 2019;29(2):628–35. https://doi.org/10.1007/s00330-018-5560-6.
16. Hsu L, Li H, Pucheril D, Hansen M, Littleton R, Peabody J, et al. Use of percutaneous nephrostomy and ureteral stenting in management of ureteral obstruction. World J Nephrol. 2016;5(2):172–81. https://doi.org/10.5527/wjn.v5.i2.172.
17. Martins FE, Holm HV, Lumen N. Devastated bladder outlet in pelvic cancer survivors: issues on surgical reconstruction and quality of life. J Clin Med. 2021;10(21):4920. https://doi.org/10.3390/jcm10214920.
18. Herschorn S, Elliott S, Coburn M, Wessells H, Zinman L. SIU/ICUD consultation on urethral strictures: posterior urethral stenosis after treatment of prostate cancer. Urology. 2014;83(3, Supplement):S59–70. https://doi.org/10.1016/j.urology.2013.08.036.
19. Liberman D, Jarosek S, Virnig BA, Chu H, Elliott SP. The patient burden of bladder outlet obstruction after prostate cancer treatment. J Urol. 2016;195(5):1459–63. https://doi.org/10.1016/j.juro.2015.11.072.
20. Dmochowski RR. Bladder outlet obstruction: etiology and evaluation. Rev Urol. 2005;7 Suppl 6(Suppl 6):S3–s13.
21. Huang Y-W, Fan Y-H, Lin AT-L, Chen K-K. The clinical characteristics of uterine tumor-related bladder outlet obstruction. Int Urogynecol J. 2012;23(1):105–10. https://doi.org/10.1007/s00192-011-1545-6.
22. Citrin D, Cotrim AP, Hyodo F, Baum BJ, Krishna MC, Mitchell JB. Radioprotectors and Mitigators of radiation-induced Normal tissue injury. Oncologist. 2010;15(4):360–71. https://doi.org/10.1634/theoncologist.2009-S104.
23. Fang K, Song P, Zhang J, Yang L, Liu P, Lu N, et al. The impact of palliative transurethral resection of the prostate on the prognosis of patients with bladder outlet obstruction and metastatic prostate cancer: a population-matched study. Front Surg. 2021;8:726534. https://doi.org/10.3389/fsurg.2021.726534.
24. Abdelwahab HA, Abdalla HM, Sherief MH, Ibrahim MB, Shamaa MA. The reliability and reproducibility of ultrasonography for measuring the residual urine volume in men with lower urinary tract symptoms. Arab J Urol. 2014;12(4):285–9. https://doi.org/10.1016/j.aju.2014.10.002.
25. Theisen JG, Deveneau NE, Agrawal A, Kinman C, Gaskins J, Meriwether K, et al. The accuracy of portable ultrasound bladder scanner measurements of Postvoid residual volume in women with pelvic organ prolapse. Female Pelvic Med Reconstr Surg. 2019;25(5):388–91. https://doi.org/10.1097/spv.0000000000000565.
26. Rademakers K, Drake MJ, Gammie A, Djurhuus JC, Rosier PFWM, Abrams P, et al. Male bladder outlet obstruction: time to re-evaluate the definition and reconsider our diagnostic pathway? ICI-RS 2015. Neurourol Urodyn. 2017;36(4):894–901. https://doi.org/10.1002/nau.23178.
27. Gratzke C, Bachmann A, Descazeaud A, Drake MJ, Madersbacher S, Mamoulakis C, et al. EAU guidelines on the assessment of non-neurogenic male lower urinary tract symptoms including benign prostatic obstruction. Eur Urol. 2015;67(6):1099–109. Epub 20150119. https://doi.org/10.1016/j.eururo.2014.12.038.
28. Lewis AL, Young GJ, Selman LE, Rice C, Clement C, Ochieng CA, et al. Urodynamics tests for the diagnosis and management of bladder outlet obstruction in men: the UPSTREAM non-inferiority RCT. Health Technol Assess. 2020;24(42):1–122. https://doi.org/10.3310/hta24420.

29. Sullivan L, Williams SG, Tai KH, Foroudi F, Cleeve L, Duchesne GM. Urethral stricture following high dose rate brachytherapy for prostate cancer. Radiother Oncol. 2009;91(2):232–6. https://doi.org/10.1016/j.radonc.2008.11.013.

Peritoneal Carcinomatosis

19

De Stefano Francesca, Paola Fugazzola,
Cobianchi Lorenzo, Dominioni Tommaso,
Tomasoni Matteo, Viganò Jacopo, and Ansaloni Luca

19.1 Peritoneal Carcinomatosis: Overview

Several gastrointestinal, gynecological, and peritoneal tumors have the potential to disseminate in the peritoneal cavity. In peritoneal carcinomatosis (PC), multiple tumor deposits of variable dimensions adhere on visceral and parietal peritoneal surfaces [1]. PC is the most common site of metastasis in gastric cancer and the second most common site of colorectal cancer (CRC) metastases. About 30% of patients with gastric cancer, 10% of colon cancers, and 3% of rectal cancers present with peritoneal dissemination at diagnosis. Up to 50% of patients with gastric cancer and 30–40% of patients with CRC will develop PC after a potentially curative surgical treatment [2, 3]. Finally, about 60% of diagnosed epithelial ovarian cancers are at stage FIGO III, which implies peritoneal involvement [4].

PC decreases overall survival in oncologic patients and poorly responds to systemic chemotherapy. In the last years, many international guidelines have recommended a multimodal treatment, including systemic chemotherapy, cytoreductive surgery (CRS), and hyperthermic intraperitoneal chemotherapy (HIPEC), as the first-line treatment in selected cases of gastrointestinal, gynecological, and peritoneal tumors with PC. At the base of this novel approach, there is the reinterpretation of peritoneal carcinomatosis as a disease localized to the peritoneal cavity, an innovative concept developed in the late 1990s [5]. The two parameters affecting the prognosis of patients potentially benefiting from CRS and HIPEC are the volume of peritoneal dissemination and the possibility to reach a complete cytoreduction. The former can be estimated by calculating the peritoneal carcinomatosis index (PCI); the latter is identified by the completeness cytoreduction score (CCS) [6].

D. S. Francesca · P. Fugazzola (✉) · C. Lorenzo · D. Tommaso · T. Matteo · V. Jacopo
A. Luca
Department of General Surgery I, IRCCS San Matteo Hospital, Pavia, Italy
e-mail: lorenzo.cobianchi@unipv.it; t.dominioni@smatteo.pv.it; m.tomasoni@smatteo.pv.it; j.vigano@smatteo.pv.it; luca.ansaloni@unipv.it

A. Tarasconi et al. (eds.), *Oncologic Surgical Emergencies*, Hot Topics in Acute Care Surgery and Trauma, https://doi.org/10.1007/978-3-031-36860-8_19

19.2 The Role of the Acute Care Surgeon (ACS) in Patients with Peritoneal Carcinomatosis

PC can lead to surgical emergencies, e.g., bowel occlusion or perforation, and it often puts the surgeon in front of intraoperative pictures of complex management, especially in an emergency setting. The 10–28% of patients with recurrent CRC and the 20–50% of patients with recurrent ovarian cancer will present with bowel obstruction alone. These patients have a very poor prognosis, with a mean survival ranging from 3 to 8 months, and currently no established, evidence-based guideline exists for their surgical management [7]. Surgeons and radiologists often fail to diagnose PC during preoperative imaging, due to its unspecific signs, and then, it is often an intraoperative finding. Furthermore, patients with peritoneal metastases are often frail due to malnutrition, immunosuppression, and chemotherapy toxicity. Therefore, in the emergency setting, the surgeon should be aware of the best surgical approaches in case of preoperative or intraoperative detection of PC.

PC can lead to actual time-dependent surgical emergencies, e.g., gastrointestinal perforations, volvulus, or strangulation, or less urgent, but perhaps more difficult-to-manage, pictures that often require surgery, e.g., malignant bowel obstruction (MBO).

Surgical palliation should be considered in situations where the patients are not actively dying, and reversal of enteral failure could make therapeutic options viable. Treatment goals should be centered on relief of peritonitis, infection, vomiting, and pain; enabling oral intake; and allowing the patient to return to the care setting of their choice, if feasible, offering an improvement in survival. In the past, PC was seen as a terminal incurable condition, while nowadays a multimodal approach including systemic chemotherapy and CRS and HIPEC can offer these patients a significant prolongation of survival (Fig. 19.1).

In 2014, van Oudheusden et al. retrospectively analyzed all patients referring to their center with synchronous PC of CRC within 8 years of activity. The aim of this study was to investigate the feasibility of CRS + HIPEC in CRC patients who previously underwent emergency surgery with the presence of PC. According to their data, CRS + HIPEC should be offered also to patients in whom PC was diagnosed during emergency surgery. Postoperative morbidities, operative outcomes, and postoperative survival in these patients are similar compared with patients with PC diagnosed in elective setting [8].

Managing these patients, the ACS should consider these new therapeutical approaches and not think at them as a priori terminally ill. For these reasons, after the resolution of the acute pathology, the ACS should address the patient to a specialized center for PC treatment.

When PC is detected intraoperatively, it is paramount that the initial surgery is as sparing as possible, trying not to excessively damage peritoneal surfaces and to avoid intraperitoneal release of growth factors, especially in case of perforated bowel. This is because once a tumor is perforated, tumor cells are released in the peritoneal cavity increasing the tumor burden on the peritoneal surfaces. Furthermore, these patients are likely to undergo subsequent oncological surgery

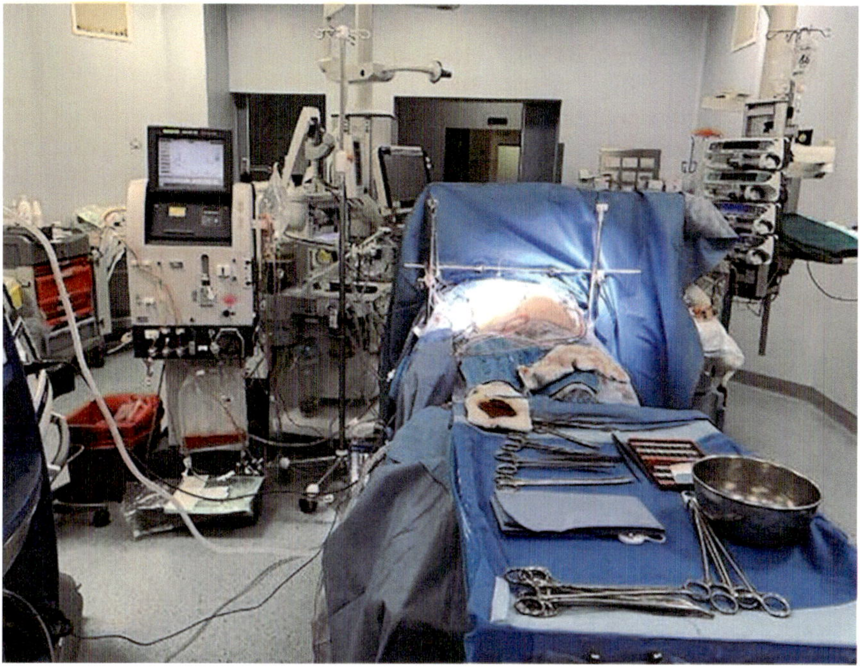

Fig. 19.1 HIPEC setting in operating room; on the right side of the patient, the HIPEC machine

and bowel resection, and then the ACS during emergency surgery should minimize the bowel resections and save as much bowel as possible, to avoid an immediate or future short bowel syndrome.

After resolution of the acute pathology (occlusion or perforation), accurate exploration and PCI calculation, with biopsies of peritoneal tumor deposits, should be performed. The aim of the surgical approach should always be to solve the acute problem reducing at most the possible postoperative complications due to extensive surgical resection. Once the patient has recovered from the postoperative period, CRS + HIPEC could be considered in an elective setting, when feasible, in order to increase overall survival of these patients.

In these patients, the ACS should always consider the nutritional aspect. They are often undernourished, for the effect of advanced cancer and of chemotherapies. A parenteral or, if possible, enteral nutritional support in the perioperative period is paramount, and a specialist nutritional assessment should be done. Nutritional supplement and immunonutrition could be considered too.

19.3 Diagnosis

Due to its 24-h availability and speed of execution, computer tomography (CT) scan is the gold standard for surgical emergencies related to PC. With multidetector CT, a spatial resolution of 1 mm can be achieved and CT can reach a sensitivity of 83% and specificity of 86% for peritoneal metastases. However, CT scan has many limits in the diagnosis of PC. The sensitivity of CT dramatically decreases with smaller peritoneal tumors. Many authors reported a CT sensitivity of only 11–28% for lesions <0.5 cm. When lesions are placed in areas where the contrast between the tumor and surrounding tissues is subtle or when they are large but thin plaque-like lesions, even larger implants may be missed on a CT scan [9]. Chua et al. [10] reported a 21–25% sensitivity of the CT scan for PC in the small intestinal regions.

Four key goals of a CT scan in this situation are the following [11]:

- Diagnose PC.
- Confirm the mechanical obstruction.
- Recognize a surgical emergency, such as a strangulation, perforation, or volvulus, that requires surgery even in palliative care.
- Look for a noncancerous reason of the obstruction. CT scans can be used to identify the three primary causes of noncancerous obstructions, which are adhesions, hernias, and eventration from prior surgery. Noncancerous obstructions affect 15% of patients with a known PC.

19.4 Malignant Bowel Obstruction (MBO) Due to Peritoneal Carcinomatosis

MBO is a common condition in patients with advanced abdominal cancer with PC. Patients present significant discomfort related to the progression of the disease and symptoms related to bowel obstruction due to PC and ascites. Nausea, vomiting, and diffuse abdominal pain are the most common acute symptoms that lead the patient to refer to the emergency department. Conservative treatment is preferred at first, with supportive care, antiemetics, analgesic drugs, and nasogastric decompression. Nevertheless, this noninvasive approach can be unsuccessful in terms of symptom relief. There is no consensus on the best treatment in case of MBO not amenable to medical therapy. In the acute setting, saving the patient's life remains the main goal for the surgeon, but the only possible tool to increase long-term survival of these patients is to enable them to continue their oncological path as soon as possible. While bowel obstruction occurring due to dominant disease in the large intestine presents with a single site of obstruction, bowel obstruction from PC usually presents with multiple sites of disease, making stent-based strategies futile and the surgical approach more complex (Fig. 19.2).

Surgical palliation can significantly improve the quality of life of these patients, but it is associated with a high morbidity rate, due to inanition and cachexia. Factors affecting the decision-making can be divided into two groups (Fig. 19.3):

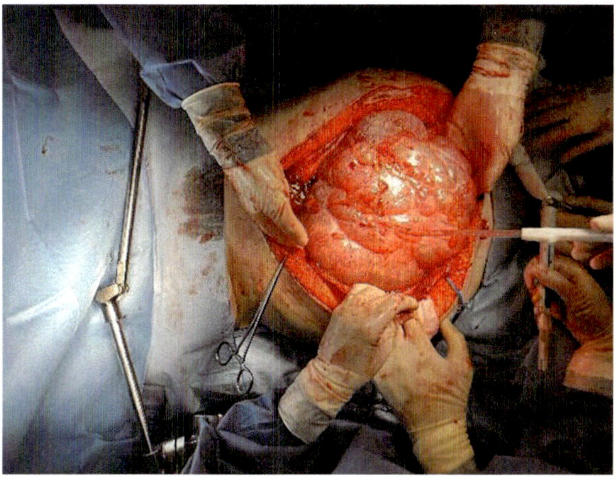

Fig. 19.2 Malignant bowel occlusion due to advanced peritoneal carcinomatosis

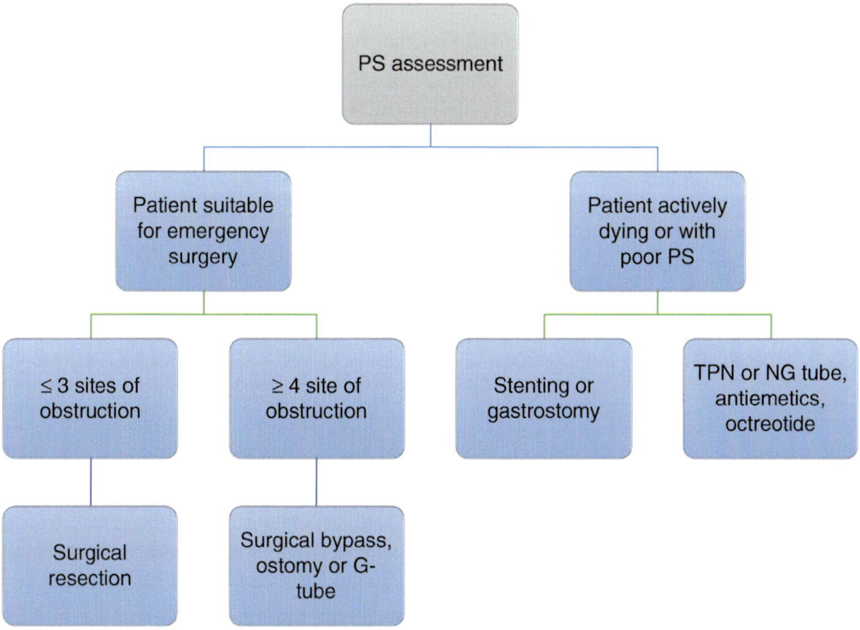

Fig. 19.3 Algorithm for management of malignant bowel obstruction. *PS* performance status; *TPN* total parenteral nutrition; *NG* nasogastric. (Modified from Shariat-Madar et al. [12])

patient-related factors and technical factors. Tumor origin, performance status, nutritional status, comorbidities, previous chemotherapy and radiotherapy, potential future therapeutic options, psychological status, and social support are the patient-related aspects. Technical considerations include the location and quantity of sites of obstruction, the extent of the malignancy, and the length of the preservable bowel [12].

19.4.1 Surgical Palliation

Surgical palliation should be taken into consideration in patients who have low peritoneal disease burden, low-grade histology, and satisfactory performance status. The best surgical choices are typically resection, bypass, and colostomy because cytoreduction techniques are infrequently practical [7]. Resection, however, gives the best results in terms of obstructive symptom alleviation and survival, particularly if there are three or fewer intestinal obstruction sites, according to certain research [7, 12]. Furthermore, because an anastomosis must be made in both circumstances with the potential for an anastomotic leakage, the technical difficulties of bypass and resection are identical. The most terrifying side effect of palliative surgery is the recurrence of malignant obstruction, and resection has been shown to have a lower re-obstruction rate than bypass. Several studies have shown that ostomy (both colostomy and ileostomy) can remove obstruction and increase survival [12]. In the choice between ileostomy and colostomy, colostomy leads to lower output of liquids and stools are less irritating for skin. Some reviews [7, 12] support the use of colostomy rather than bypass because it is associated with longer survival.

It is paramount to inform candidates of surgery about the probability of successful palliation, as well as the possibility of postoperative complications and death. Patients should be aware that they could spend the most part of their remaining life at hospital. Indeed, the median hospital stay after surgery is longer than in patients receiving conservative treatments; considering the short life expectancy, this risk must be explained.

19.4.2 Nonsurgical Palliation

Poor surgical candidates may benefit from venting gastrostomy tube or stenting (Fig. 19.4).

When a single obstruction is found in the gastroduodenal tract or in the large bowel in patients with a poor performance status, stenting should be used. More than 80% of patients reported technical success in stent positioning, and in more than 75% of cases, clinical improvement with symptom relief was seen. Perforation, stent migration, or reocclusion are the three main complications. When compared to surgical methods, stenting is connected with a shorter hospital stay and fewer pain. Several sites of obstruction or presence of obstruction in the distal jejunum are the main factors limiting the effectiveness of bowel stenting. Hence, a surgical procedure or a drainage gastrostomy could be considered in these situations. In order to restore oral intake, gastrostomies may be particularly helpful for upper GI obstructions that cause vomiting and nausea [7, 12].

Medical care using complete parenteral nourishment or nasogastric tubes is able to effectively manage symptoms in patients who have low performance status or who are actively dying. While anticholinergics can help with the treatment of colicky pain, opioids and antiemetics can both effectively reduce pain and vomiting.

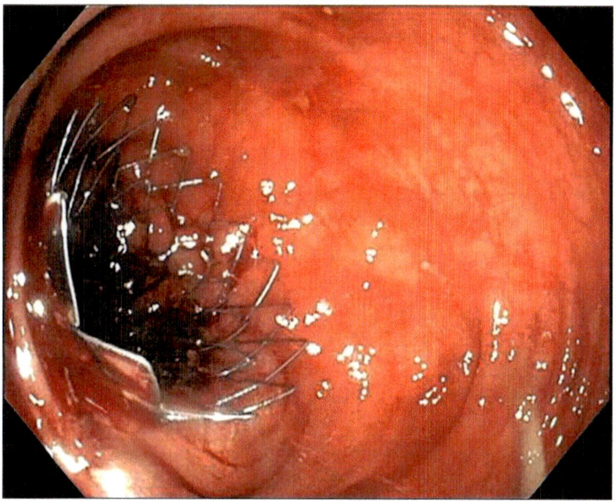

Fig. 19.4 Self-expandable metal stent placed to solve occlusion

Somatostatin analogues are also useful for treating vomiting, nausea, and pain [7, 12]. Yet, choosing not to operate and to halt treatment, particularly in an emergency situation, is a difficult choice. Although different authors in the literature addressed this issue comparing a conservative approach or endoscopic stenting with palliative surgery, it is difficult to obtain a consensus on the topic, due to its technical and ethical implications. Even if some authors recommend surgical palliation, when possible, to prolong survival, other authors argue that the survival benefit from palliative surgery is minimal, while postoperative complications, hospital readmission due to recurrence of symptoms, and long hospital stay are significant and often force patients to spend most of their remaining life in the hospital setting. Furthermore, most of them die in the hospital or in a hospice directly following discharge [13]. Therefore, it is paramount to inform the patient and the relatives about the possible implications of a surgical intervention in terms of adverse events and long-term survival.

19.5 Other Surgical Emergencies in Patients with PC

Other surgical emergencies in patients with PC are perforation, volvulus, and strangulation. These conditions are time dependent and need an emergency surgical intervention, even in the context of palliative care. When these situations occur, the initial surgery should be directed to the treatment of perforation and peritonitis or of the ischemic bowel tract, even, if necessary, with a damage control surgery. If the PC is an intraoperative finding and if appropriate, a biopsy sampling and a PCI evaluation should be obtained. Direct anastomosis or use of stomas should be analyzed case by case, according to the patient's general condition. However, the nutritional and general consequences of a high ileostomy should always be considered in these patients, whose general conditions at the end of the acute phase will be decisive for the subsequent oncological path and the therapeutic possibilities. In the postoperative setting, detailed staging can be completed, histological confirmation can be obtained, and the patient should be addressed to the most appropriate treatment plan according to tumor stage and general conditions. In case of confirmed PC, the patient should be sent to a referral center in order to evaluate a possible cytoreductive surgery.

19.6 Conclusions

It is not uncommon to encounter patients affected by PC in the emergency setting. This represents a challenge for the ACS, because the treatment of choice is not standardized and multiple aspects should be taken into consideration. Not only the survival of the patient in the acute setting, but also the oncological long-term outcome has to be addressed as the goal of the chosen treatment. In the past, peritoneal carcinomatosis was seen as a terminal incurable condition, while nowadays, multimodal approaches including systemic chemotherapy and CRS and HIPEC can offer these patients a significant prolongation of survival. Therefore, the ACS should consider these new therapeutical approaches and not think at these patients as a priori terminally ill. The aim of the surgical approach should be to solve the acute pathology, minimizing the possible postoperative acute and long-term complications due to extensive surgical resection and, after the resolution of the acute phase, address the patient to a specialized center for PC treatment.

In patients that have poor performance status or are actively dying, a palliative medical therapy should be offered to relieve symptoms.

Moreover, a case-by-case discussion is paramount in a multidisciplinary team, not only for curative purposes, but also in case of end-of-life treatments. Adequate information to the patient on his state of health and on the risks associated with possible surgery and the involvement of the patient and relatives in the therapeutic choices are essential.

In conclusion, the ACS has the responsibility to not only offer each patient the best damage control treatment available, but also include the patient in the most appropriate long-term oncological path, in case of either a new diagnosis or a known terminal condition.

References

1. van Baal JO, Van de Vijver KK, Nieuwland R, van Noorden CJ, van Driel WJ, Sturk A, et al. The histophysiology and pathophysiology of the peritoneum. Tissue Cell. 2017;49(1):95–105.
2. Manzanedo I, Pereira F, Rihuete Caro C, Pérez-Viejo E, Serrano Á, Gutiérrez Calvo A, et al. Cytoreductive Surgery and Hyperthermic Intraperitoneal Chemotherapy (HIPEC) for gastric cancer with peritoneal Carcinomatosis: multicenter study of Spanish Group of Peritoneal Oncologic Surgery (GECOP). Ann Surg Oncol. 2019;26(8):2615–21.
3. Davis CH, Alexander HR Jr. What is the current role of Hyperthermic intraperitoneal chemotherapy in colorectal cancer? Adv Surg. 2021;55:159–74.

4. Coccolini F, Fugazzola P, Montori G, Ansaloni L, Chiarugi M. Intraperitoneal chemotherapy for ovarian cancer with peritoneal metastases, systematic review of the literature and focused personal experience. J Gastrointest Oncol. 2021;12(Suppl 1):S144–81. https://doi.org/10.21037/jgo-2020-06.
5. Yonemura Y, Canbay E, Li Y, Coccolini F, Glehen O, Sugarbaker PH, et al. A comprehensive treatment for peritoneal metastases from gastric cancer with curative intent. Eur J Surg Oncol. 2016;42(8):1123–31.
6. González-Moreno S, Kusamura S, Baratti D, Deraco M. Postoperative residual disease evaluation in the locoregional treatment of peritoneal surface malignancy. J Surg Oncol. 2008;98(4):237–41.
7. Shariat-Madar B, Jayakrishnan TT, Gamblin TC, Turaga KK. Surgical management of bowel obstruction in patients with peritoneal carcinomatosis. J Surg Oncol. 2014;110(6):666–9.
8. van Oudheusden TR, Braam HJ, Nienhuijs SW, Wiezer MJ, van Ramshorst B, Luyer MD, et al. Cytoreduction and hyperthermic intraperitoneal chemotherapy: a feasible and effective option for colorectal cancer patients after emergency surgery in the presence of peritoneal carcinomatosis. Ann Surg Oncol. 2014;21(8):2621–6.
9. Low RN, et al. Peritoneal MRI in patients undergoing cytoreductive surgery and HIPEC: history, clinical applications, and implementation. Eur J Surg Oncol. 2021;47(1):65–74. https://doi.org/10.1016/j.ejso.2019.02.030.
10. Chua TC, Al-Zahrani A, Saxena A, Glenn D, Liauw W, Zhao J, et al. Determining the association between preoperative computed tomography findings and post-operative outcomes after cytoreductive surgery and perioperative intraperitoneal chemotherapy for pseudomyxoma peritonei. Ann Surg Oncol. 2011;18:1582e9.
11. Laval G, Marcelin-Benazech B, Guirimand F, Chauvenet L, Copel L, Durand A, Francois E, Gabolde M, Mariani P, Rebischung C, Servois V, Terrebonne E, Arvieux C, French Society for Palliative Care; French Society for Digestive Surgery; French Society for Gastroenterology; French Association for Supportive Care in Oncology; French Society for Digestive Cancer. Recommendations for bowel obstruction with peritoneal carcinomatosis. J Pain Symptom Manag. 2014;48(1):75–91. https://doi.org/10.1016/j.jpainsymman.2013.08.022. Epub 2014 May 4.
12. Santangelo ML, Grifasi C, Criscitiello C, Giuliano M, Calogero A, Dodaro C, et al. Bowel obstruction and peritoneal carcinomatosis in the elderly. A systematic review. Aging Clin Exp Res. 2017;29(Suppl 1):73–8.
13. de Boer NL, Hagemans JAW, Schultze BTA, Brandt-Kerkhof ARM, Madsen EVE, Verhoef C, et al. Acute malignant obstruction in patients with peritoneal carcinomatosis: the role of palliative surgery. Eur J Surg Oncol. 2019;45(3):389–93.

Miscellaneous Rare Malignancies: Intra-abdominal Lymphomas

20

Alessandro Gemini, Barza Afzal, Amr Elserafy, Lucia Lazzereschi, Antonio Matarangolo, and Giovanni Domenico Tebala

20.1 Introduction

Malignant lymphomas are a group of neoplasms derived from the basic cells of the lymphoid tissue in any of their developmental stages. When they primarily affect the lymphoid tissue of the lymph nodes, lymphomas are called "nodal." When they primarily affect the non-lymph node lymphoid tissue, they are called "extranodal." A further classification of lymphomas is based on their clinical course: aggressive forms are distinguished from subclinical ones. The aggressive forms have a rapid course (such as most lymphomas involving T-lymphocytes). Indolent lymphomas, on the other hand, occur slowly and progressively (e.g., B-lymphocyte neoplasms). Historically, the World Health Organization (WHO) classified lymphomas into two main categories: Hodgkin's lymphomas and non-Hodgkin's lymphomas. Hodgkin's lymphoma (HL) is a lymphoproliferative disease characterized by the presence of Reed-Sternberg cells. Reed-Sternberg cells represent 1% of the HL cell population. The other key feature of LH is the presence of an abundant inflammatory infiltrate surrounding the neoplastic cells [1]. Non-Hodgkin's lymphomas (NHLs) are a heterogenous group of lymphoproliferative malignancies that are much less predictable than Hodgkin's lymphomas and have a far greater predilection to disseminate

A. Gemini
Department of Digestive and Emergency Surgery, S. Maria Hospital Trust, Terni, Italy
e-mail: a.gemini@aospterni.it

B. Afzal · A. Elserafy · L. Lazzereschi · A. Matarangolo
Surgical Emergency Unit, Oxford University Hospitals NHS Foundation Trust, Oxford, UK
e-mail: lucia.lazzereschi1@nhs.net

G. D. Tebala (✉)
Department of Digestive and Emergency Surgery, S. Maria Hospital Trust, Terni, Italy

Surgical Emergency Unit, Oxford University Hospitals NHS Foundation Trust, Oxford, UK
e-mail: Giovanni.Tebala@ouh.nhs.uk

A. Tarasconi et al. (eds.), *Oncologic Surgical Emergencies*, Hot Topics in Acute Care Surgery and Trauma, https://doi.org/10.1007/978-3-031-36860-8_20

to extranodal locations. Nearly 25% of NHLs arise in extranodal sites, and in many of these cases, there is both extranodal and nodal involvement [2].

The latest revision of the WHO lymphoma classification is from 2017 and includes more than 80 different entities. These differ from each other in morphology, immunophenotype, molecular profile, genetic mutations, clinical characteristics, and type of cellular derivation [3].

Non-Hodgkin's lymphomas are divided into B-cell neoplasm and T- and NK-cell neoplasm. Hodgkin's lymphomas are divided into two main subgroups: nodular lymphocyte predominance Hodgkin's lymphoma and classical Hodgkin's lymphoma. These main groups are further divided into various categories [4]. Classification of lymphomas is beyond the scope of this chapter; therefore, we suggest the reader to refer to more specialized publications [4].

The gastrointestinal tract (GI) is the extranodal site most frequently affected by lymphoma (5–20% of all cases [5]). However, primary gastrointestinal lymphomas (PGILs) are rare tumors. In fact, they represent only 1–4% of all gastrointestinal neoplasms [6]. The exact incidence is hard to determine, but it has been estimated to affect 1 in 100,000 individuals per year [7], although time-trend analyses have demonstrated an increase of 2.7% per annum of incidence for gastric (6.3%) and small bowel diseases (5.9%) [8]. Gastrointestinal lymphomas are usually secondary to diffuse lymph nodal forms, representing 5–20% of NHLs [5, 6, 9]. The clinical criteria distinguishing these two groups of neoplasms (primary and secondary forms) were first proposed by Dawson in 1961 [10]. These criteria are (I) absence of peripheral lymphadenopathy at the time of presentation, (II) lack of enlarged mediastinal lymph nodes, (III) normal total and differential white blood cell count, (IV) predominance of bowel lesion at the time of laparotomy with only lymph nodes obviously affected in the immediate vicinity, and (V) no lymphomatous involvement of liver and spleen. The most frequent site for gastrointestinal lymphomas (GILs) is the stomach (60–75% of all cases), followed by the small intestine, ileum, cecum, colon, and rectum [11].

Histopathologically, almost 90% of gastrointestinal lymphomas are non-Hodgkin's lymphomas, whose majority affect the B line, while T-cell lymphomas and Hodgkin's lymphomas are rare [12]. Two of the most prevalent diagnoses are diffuse large B-cell lymphoma (DLBCL) and mucosa associated lymphoid tissue lymphoma (MALT lymphoma) [11–13].

Immunoproliferative small intestinal disease (IPSID) is a variant of MALT lymphoma that arises in the small bowel. Peripheral T-cell lymphomas are less common and typically associated with poor prognosis. Other histological subtypes are less commonly observed, among them being follicular lymphoma (FL), mantle cell lymphoma (MCL), Burkitt's lymphoma (BL), and enteropathy-associated T-cell lymphoma (EATL). Finally, the GI tract is frequently the site of post-transplant lymphoproliferative diseases (PTLDs) [12]. Moreover, it has been noted that some histological subtypes arise in specific segments of the gastrointestinal tract, such as mucosa-associated lymphoid tissue (MALT) in the stomach; mantle cell lymphoma (MCL) in terminal ileum, jejunum, and colon; enteropathy-associated T-cell lymphoma (EATL) in jejunum; and follicular lymphoma (FL) in duodenum [6]. However, multifocality is more common in MALT lymphoma and follicular lymphoma [14].

20.2 Pathogenesis

Complex pathogenetic mechanisms are involved in lymphomagenesis, and their understanding impacts the disease classification and has significant implications for diagnosis and management. Thanks to the integration of immunologic advances and monoclonal antibody technology, it has been possible to mesh molecular diagnostics in hemopathology, leading to the identification of chromosomal translocations underlying the pathogenesis of lymphomas. In fact, most of the large subclasses of B- and T-cell lymphomas have been characterized at the genomic level [15].

Known risk factors for lymphoma include hereditary traits, chronic infection, and immunosuppression. Chronic infection might lead to lymphomagenesis through direct viral effects, or due to the chronic stimulation of the immune system.

A strong association between chronic *H. pylori* infection and gastric MALT lymphoma has been demonstrated in 80–90% of cases [16–18]. Chronic *H. pylori* infection provides the antigenic stimulus, resulting in clonal expansion of lymphoid cells leading to the evolution of MALT lymphoma. Immunoproliferative small intestinal disease (IPSID) is a variant form of MALT lymphoma that occurs in the small intestine. As for the *H. pylori* in MALT lymphoma, Lecuit et al. demonstrated *C. jejuni* as a possible stimulus for this proliferation [19]. Epstein-Barr virus (EBV) infection has been cited as a pathogenetic factor in various forms of gastrointestinal lymphoma. For example, in Burkitt's lymphoma, three clinical variants are distinguished: the endemic forms which are generally related to infection, the sporadic forms which are related to infection in only 30% of cases, and the forms associated with immunodeficiency. However, in addition to Burkitt's lymphoma, other gastrointestinal lymphomas are also associated with EBV infection: the Epstein-Barr virus-positive diffuse large B-cell lymphoma (EBV-positive DLBCL) of the elderly; the lymphomatoid granulomatosis (LG); and the extranodal NK/T-cell lymphomas, nasal type (ENKTL). Furthermore, human immunodeficiency virus (HIV) infection is often associated with plasmablastic lymphoma (PBL); human T-lymphotropic virus type 1 (HTLV-1) is related to adult T-cell leukemia/lymphoma; human herpesvirus 8 (HHV8) is associated with primary effusion lymphoma; and hepatitis C virus (HCV) is related to splenic and extranodal marginal zone lymphoma.

The chronic stimulation of the immune system in autoimmune diseases may increase the risk of lymphoma, giving rise to dysregulated clone of B cells. Specifically, diffuse large B-cell lymphomas (DLBCLs) and marginal zone lymphomas are both associated with rheumatoid arthritis and Sjogren syndrome, while enteropathy-associated T-cell lymphoma (EATL) is linked to celiac sprue.

Furthermore, immunosuppression plays a critical role as well, representing a clear risk for the development of Hodgkin's and non-Hodgkin's lymphomas, as can be seen in the increased incidence of these diseases in patients infected by human immunodeficiency virus (HIV) as well as patients on immunosuppressive treatment following solid-organ transplantation.

Therefore, it seems clear that stress factors, be they inflammatory, infectious, or toxic, interact with the host genetic makeup in a complex way leading to lymphomagenesis. There is a hereditary risk too, given the fact that odds of developing Hodgkin's lymphoma are increased for first-degree relatives of probands, and further increased for siblings of probands. This is also true for non-Hodgkin's lymphoma, although patterns of heritability vary by subtype. Nowadays, however, no specific genetic testing is available, and screening for family members is not routine [20].

20.3 Staging

The stage and histologic grade of the disease are the most clinically important independent prognostic factors [21]. There are various different staging systems for the classification of gastrointestinal lymphoma. One of the most widely used is the nonspecific Ann Arbor classification modified by Musshoff et al. [6], which considers four stages; stage I is for cases with a single lymphatic organ or extranodal localization; stage II is for cases with multiple sites on the same side of the diaphragm; stage III entails cases with nodal involvement on both sides of the diaphragm; and stage IV is for disseminated disease. Rohatiner and colleagues in 1994 proposed the Lugano system [22], which deals only with gastrointestinal lymphomas. It classifies gastrointestinal lymphomas into four stages. Stage I is for lymphomas confined to the gastrointestinal tract, with Ia for mucosal-submucosal-only involvement and Ib for tumors infiltrating beyond the submucosa. Stage II is for cases of local (IIa) or distant (IIb) nodal involvement beyond the primary gastrointestinal site and cases with infiltration of adjacent organs (IIE). Stage III covers disseminated disease and cases with involvement on both sides of the diaphragm. The modified Ann Arbor classification is very useful for prognosis but has been accompanied by the Paris staging system, which can differentiate the manifestations of distant lymphoma according to the organ involved and further subdivides the involvement of the lymph nodes. This is of great use for gastrointestinal lymphomas [10]. The International Prognostic Index (IPI) was initially formulated to assess the clinical risk in patients with diffuse large-cell lymphoma (DLCL). To date, it is one of the most widely used systems for risk stratification of nearly all NHL subtypes [10].

20.4 Diagnosis

Gastrointestinal lymphoma is a disease encountered by the surgeon in both the elective and emergency setting. The diagnosis therefore depends on the clinical conditions of the patient. The necessary investigations are determined on the basis of the patient's presenting symptoms and may include blood tests, endoscopic examinations, CT-scan, and PET-scan. Accurate diagnosis and staging of gastrointestinal lymphomas are essential for establishing the appropriate treatment in this diverse group of malignancies. Obviously, blood tests are part of the diagnostic and the staging process in patients with suspected gastrointestinal lymphoma. These must be taken both in the elective and in the emergency setting and should include blood cells count with leukocyte formula and biochemical test including LDH, β2-microglobulin, and serum protein electrophoresis. Other serological examinations should be performed when indicated on the basis of the type of lymphoma identified, to document specific infections or autoimmune diseases. When feasible, endoscopy can be a valuable diagnostic technique in gastrointestinal lymphomas and can show a wide variety of presentations: from enlarged lymph nodes and lymphoid follicles, which can sometimes appear reactive, through polyps, to infiltrative and necrotic lesions [11]. In the esophagus, stomach, duodenum, and colon, the diagnosis of gastrointestinal lymphoma can be made on endoscopic biopsies and definitive subtyping of the lymphoma is possible with the use of additional immunological markers. Endoscopic biopsy diagnosis allows disease staging and intervention planning. The small intestine can be explored endoscopically using double- and even single-balloon enteroscopy [23, 24]. Another option for the study of the small intestine is capsule endoscopy, which can highlight the presence of abnormal mucosal patterns [25]. The diagnosis of gastric lymphoma can be established on biopsies in over 95% of cases [26, 27], but it is important that an adequate number of biopsy samples are performed both on abnormal mucosa and on macroscopically normal mucosa. In fact, it should be remembered that surgery, especially in gastric lymphoma, always plays a second-choice role, and therefore the histological diagnosis depends above all on endoscopic biopsies. Symptoms and signs of gastrointestinal lymphomas are often nonspecific, such as dyspepsia, weight loss, abdominal pain, change in bowel habits, and/or bleeding. In the stomach, endoscopic features can simulate benign disease. The diagnosis of gastric lymphoma is therefore often not clinically suspected. A second endoscopic examination is recommended using a mapping protocol with 8–12 biopsies from involved sites and additional biopsies from the antrum, body, and fundus not involved. Biopsies should also be performed to detect the presence of *H. pylori* [28, 29]. From the histological examination of the biopsy, numerous information can be obtained, such as on the immunophenotype, including the presence of t(11; 18), which in MALT gastric lymphoma is associated with forms that are not responsive to the eradication of *H. pylori* and in more advanced stages of the disease [30]. As highlighted, since most gastric MALT lymphomas are associated with chronic infection with *H. pylori* and in a minority with *Helicobacter heilmannii*, the presence of these pathogens must be carefully investigated by endoscopically examining the gastric mucosa not involved in the lymphoma. The recommendation is to use histology (modified HE and Giemsa staining) and invasive culture or molecular tests [31]. Bone marrow aspirate with biopsy is part of the staging of lymphoma as is the peripheral blood test for monoclonal cells. However, bone marrow involvement is rare in gastric and in MALT lymphoma, while it is more common in nodal lymphomas and splenic marginal zone B-cell lymphoma [31–33]. A contrast-enhanced CT scan is the fundamental investigation in patients who are hospitalized as urgently for acute abdomen. In urgency, in addition to suspecting lymphoma, it allows to diagnose the presence of an intestinal perforation or obstruction. In election, it is a necessary exam for staging the patient; the neck, the chest, and the abdomen including the pelvis should be examined. Staging in many lymphomas also includes 18F-fluorodeoxyglucose positron-emission tomography (FDG PET), especially in DLBCL, follicular lymphoma, and mantle cell lymphoma [34, 35]. Further staging tests depend on the type of gastrointestinal lymphoma and its location. In gastric MALT lymphoma, as already mentioned, once the diagnosis or suspicion of this pathology has been made, a second esophagogastroduodenoscopy with numerous biopsies (generally 20–30) must be performed according to an adequate protocol. This is because gastric MALT lymphoma is often multifocal and can also transform into DLBCL [31]. In addition, 25% of gastric MALT lymphomas present with multi-organ involvement. They need an extensive staging including colonoscopy with biopsies and magnetic resonance imaging (MRI) of the salivary and lacrimal glands [36]. In stomach tumors, locoregional staging is also performed with ultrasound endoscopy.

20.5 Gastric Lymphomas

The most commonly involved site of the gastrointestinal tract is the stomach (60–75% of cases) followed by small bowel, ileocecal region, and rectum. Gastric lymphoma alone accounts for 3–5% of all malignant tumors of the stomach. Gastric lymphomas can be classified histologically as marginal zone B-cell lymphomas of the mucosa-associated lymphoid tissue (MALT) type, diffuse large B-cell lymphomas (DLBCL), follicular lymphomas, mantle cell lymphomas, Burkitt's lymphomas, T-cell lymphomas, and plasmacytomas. MALT lymphoma and DLBCL make up nearly 90% of all gastric lymphomas. The marginal zone B-cell lymphoma of MALT type occurs in 38% of the cases, while diffuse large B-cell lymphoma (DLBCL) occurs in 59%. Other types such as mantel cell lymphoma, follicular lymphoma, and peripheral T-cell lymphoma occur rarely. Males are two to three times more likely to develop gastric lymphoma than females [37].

H. pylori plays a role in the development of most MALT lymphomas by inducing a state of chronic inflammation, which leads to an increased risk of malignant transformation through B-cell proliferation, mediated by tumor-infiltrating T cells [38]. *H. pylori* may play a similar role in the development of DLBCL, and few studies have shown complete remission after eradication therapy alone [6, 38].

In MALT gastric lymphomas, the most significant histological finding is the presence of lymphoepithelial lesions characterized by invasion and partial destruction of the mucous glands by tumor cells.

20.5.1 Clinical Presentation

The age of most gastric lymphoma patients is over 50 with a relative predilection in males. Clinical symptoms of gastric lymphoma are nonspecific and indistinguishable from other benign and malignant conditions. Consequently, the diagnosis can often be delayed. The most common complaints of patients with gastric lymphoma are epigastric pain, weight loss, nausea, and vomiting. Constitutional symptoms (fever, night sweat, and weight loss) are not common. Occasionally, an abdominal mass is palpable. Lymphadenopathy is rare, and patients often have no physical signs. Perforation, bleeding, or obstruction are uncommon, but when present, surgical intervention may be necessary.

It is widely known that perforation occasionally occurs in patients receiving chemotherapy. Some Eastern studies reported that perforation of gastric lymphoma in patients receiving chemotherapy occurs in about 0.9–1.1% of cases. On the other hand, spontaneous perforation of malignant gastric lymphoma is rare compared with perforation of gastric lymphoma in patients receiving chemotherapy, and its risk seems to be related with the size of the tumor [39].

The causes of perforation of gastric lymphoma under chemotherapy are different from those in patients who are not under chemotherapy. Ono et al. reported that in the former, weakening of the gastric tissue associated with rapid tumor necrosis, tumor lysis, and exuberant granulation due to chemotherapy play a role [40]. Shiomi et al. described two different patterns of spontaneous perforation. First, the spontaneous perforation resulting from an ulcer and tumor necrosis that has reached the subserosa; second, the perforation resulting from an ulcer in the absence of tumor [41].

Patients can have gastrointestinal bleeding ranging from occult bleeding leading to iron deficiency anemia to acute blood loss presenting as hematemesis, hematochezia, or melena (about 20–30% of patients with gastric DLBCL report gastrointestinal bleeding) [37]. Although ulcers are the most common cause of upper gastrointestinal bleeding (59%), compared to malignant tumors (2–4%), gastric MALT lymphoma has been reported to present as upper gastrointestinal bleeding at the time of diagnosis only in the 15.6% of cases [42].

20.5.2 Investigations

Endoscopy without biopsies cannot distinguish gastric lymphoma from gastric cancer. In gastric lymphomas, endoscopy identifies three main nonspecific patterns: ulceration, diffuse infiltration, and polypoid mass [43]. Although the morphological patterns are not specific, endoscopy is the fundamental examination in gastric lymphoma as it may allow the initial diagnosis on deep biopsy samples and is fundamental in the follow-up of patients. EUS can assess the extent of the lesion, which is usually hypoechoic, and its invasion. The growth of infiltrative carcinomas tends to be vertical in the gastric wall, while lymphomas tend to grow horizontally with greater involvement of the perigastric lymph nodes [44]. EUS shows the depth of

20.5.4 Immediate Treatment

Patients with gastric lymphoma can be treated in emergency in different ways, depending on the complication at presentation. Invasion into surrounding organs such as the hepatobiliary system and pancreas, although rare, can lead to numerous complications, including biliary obstruction, infection, and pancreatitis. In those cases, the surgeon must act accordingly. Among the most common complications, a massive upper gastrointestinal bleeding is a life-threatening emergency condition that requires intervention as soon as possible. A gastrosplenic fistula might be the underlying cause of bleeding in those patients. Fluid resuscitation and intensive care support are paramount to restore the hemodynamic stability. Urgent endoscopy (<6 h), especially in high-risk patients, has recently been described as an independent predictor of lower mortality rates; current guidelines also state that for acute overt nonvariceal upper GI bleeding in high-risk patients such as those who are hemodynamically unstable, very early endoscopy (<12 h) is recommended [53]. In patients presenting with bleeding, an adjunct of endoscopy can be an angioembolization. Surgery remains the treatment of choice when noninvasive hemostatic treatments are unsuccessful. With regard to perforation, it is widely known that this complication, albeit rare, occurs in patients receiving chemotherapy. Jointly with fluid resuscitation and intensive care support, surgery plays a critical role once the diagnosis of perforation is made with clinical examination, blood tests, and imaging techniques. Patients with large and voluminous transmural gastric lymphomas are those at greatest risk of treatment-related complications. To reduce the risk of perforation or other complications in these patients, a dose reduction is recommended for the first course of chemotherapy [51]. Differently, gastric outlet obstruction is more common compared to bleeding and perforation. In such cases, patients are treated conservatively with nasogastric tube drainage and total parenteral nutrition. In case of complete or near-complete obstruction, after placing the nasogastric tube to drain the stomach, some authors suggest administering steroids at high doses (dexamethasone, 10 mg intravenously every 6 h), with a rapid response [54]. Thereafter, radiotherapy and/or chemotherapy may be given. When conservative treatment fails, surgical intervention is necessary in order to resolve the obstruction and restore the gastrointestinal tract continuity. In minor obstructive cases, patients can be further evaluated with noninvasive tests and then decide whether to continue with medical or surgical therapy.

20.5.5 Surgical Treatment

As seen, surgical resection is no longer the primary treatment of choice for gastric lymphoma. Radiotherapy and chemotherapy, alone or in combination, achieve good relative outcomes without the morbidity and mortality associated with surgery [55]. With the same oncological results, there is an improvement in the quality of life of patients treated conservatively [51]. Furthermore, avoiding surgery means avoiding any delay in the initiation of systemic therapy. The surgical approach should be reserved for tumor-related complications such as perforation, obstruction, and major hemorrhage or in the case of persistent disease confined to the stomach after primary conservative therapy [6, 51, 54, 55]. The position and extension of the gastric tumor, as well as obtaining adequate safety margins, determine the extent of the resection: total versus partial gastrectomy. Based on the higher level of digestive and food-related problems after total gastrectomy, stomach-preserving surgery (subtotal gastrectomy, with accurate lymphadenectomy) should be preferred whenever possible.

It should be remembered that according to some authors, incomplete resection of the disease does not affect overall and disease-free survival if the patient receives adjuvant chemotherapy [56, 57]. However, gastrectomy should be considered if a giant ulcer and necrotic matter on the ulcer floor are present at upper gastrointestinal endoscopy because of the possibility of gastric perforation [58]. In addition to subtotal and total gastrectomy, the emergency surgeon may consider some alternative procedures that could fall within the definition of damage control surgery [59]. If the gastric perforation is smaller than 2 cm, a direct suture can be performed, associated or not with an omental patch. This surgery can be performed laparoscopically, favoring a faster postoperative recovery. In addition to the suture, the edges of the perforation must be removed and sent for histologic examination. In addition, the patient will then undergo a control gastroscopy 6 weeks after he or she recovers from the surgical procedure [60]. In patients with gastric obstruction due to lymphoma, of advanced age, or in poor clinical conditions, palliative interventions such as jejunostomy or gastrojejunostomy bypass can be considered [61].

20.6 Small Bowel Lymphomas

Lymphomas represent about 15–20% of all tumors of the small intestine and about 20% of primary gastrointestinal lymphomas [62, 63]. The most frequent site of localization of lymphomas of the small intestine is the ileum (60–65%), followed by the jejunum (20–25%) and the duodenum (6–8%) [6]. Small bowel lymphomas can affect any age group, becoming more common in the elderly, but some subtypes are more common in young people. The median age of onset in the United States is 66, and men account for 60% of patients [63]. As previously mentioned, some risk factors for the development of primary small bowel lymphomas have been identified. These include *H. pylori* infection, *C. jejuni* infection, EBV infection, chronic inflammatory bowel disease, celiac disease, and immunosuppression. Organ-transplant patients have an increased risk of developing lymphomas. Posttransplant lymphomas are often linked to Epstein-Barr virus infections. B-cell lymphomas account for approximately 90% of posttransplant lymphoproliferative disorders (PTLDs) [64]. The histological subtypes of the small bowel lymphomas are very heterogeneous and are of both B-cell and T-cell type. Most small bowel lymphomas are B-cell derived, and the most frequent histological type of small bowel lymphomas is diffuse large B-cell lymphoma (DLBCL), accounting for approximately 40% of all small bowel lymphomas, followed by low-grade follicular B-cell lymphomas

[65, 66]. Other histological subtypes are low-grade marginal zone B-cell MALT lymphoma, Burkitt's lymphoma, mantle cell lymphoma (MCL), immunoproliferative small intestinal disease (IPSID), and enteropathy-associated T-cell lymphoma (EATL). Burkitt's lymphomas frequently affect the terminal part of the ileum and often appear as an abdominal mass. Its onset is associated with EBV and HIV infection, it mainly affects children, and, as mentioned, there are three variants [67, 68]. MCL usually presents in advanced forms of the disease and mainly affects individuals over the age of 50. The gastrointestinal tract is involved in only 20% of MCLs, and the sites involved are generally the ileum and the jejunum. It presents with numerous small polyps of the mucosa, also called multiple lymphomatous polyposis (MLP) [69, 70]. IPSID, also known as alpha-chain disease, is a variant of MALT lymphoma that occurs in the small intestine. It mainly affects children and young adults and localizes in the proximal portion of the small intestine [71]. This type of GI lymphoma is associated with *C. jejuni* infection and is histologically characterized by the presence of centrocyte-like lymphocytes with IgA heavy chains. T-cell lymphomas account for only 10–20% of all small bowel lymphomas, with T-cell lymphoma-associated enteropathy being the most common [72]. Patients with celiac disease are at greater risk of developing this type of gastrointestinal lymphoma; in fact, in the general population, gastrointestinal T-cell lymphomas are about 7%, while in patients with celiac disease, the frequency is 40% [73]. The EATL is an intestinal intraepithelial T-cell lymphoma, which is most frequently localized in the jejunum and ileum. It is more frequent in northern Europe where celiac disease is more frequent [11].

20.6.1 Clinical Presentation

Small bowel lymphomas usually have nonspecific symptoms such as abdominal pain and positive fecal occult blood. A palpable mass is more frequent in small bowel lymphomas than in adenocarcinomas. Patients generally report symptoms lasting weeks to months [74]. In many patients, the clinical presentation is related to occlusive episodes, which may be characterized by nausea, vomiting, constipation, or mechanical obstruction possibly due to intussusception [75, 76]. Small bowel lymphomas may present to the surgeon's attention in emergency with bleeding in 10% of cases or with intestinal perforation in 5–10% of cases [74]. In one-third of patients, involuntary weight loss occurs. B-symptoms (fever, fatigue, and night sweats) are present in 15–50% of patients and are usually associated with high-grade or advanced lymphomas [74, 77]. In celiac patients who develop malabsorption despite adopting a gluten-free diet, lymphoma should be suspected. As mentioned, one of the manifestations of a small intestine lymphoma is intussusception and more than 50% of the primary malignant neoplasms of the small intestine that cause intussusception are lymphomas. All symptomatic intussusceptions of the adult must be resected due to the 70% risk of a growing lesion, of which about half are malignant [78].

20.6.2 Investigations

The diagnosis of small bowel lymphoma is difficult due to nonspecific presentation. A history of fever and night sweats (B-symptoms) can increase the suspicion of lymphoma. Clinical examination rarely helps, as abdominal lymphadenopathy, hepatosplenomegaly, or a palpable mass in the abdomen is rarely identified. Chronic anemia, or positive fecal occult blood, can lead to an endoscopic examination to look for the source of bleeding. However, most small bowel lymphomas are located in areas that cannot be reached with a standard endoscopic examination. The limitations of standard endoscopy have been partially overcome by capsule endoscopy (CE) and double-balloon push-and-pull enteroscopy. The CE can be useful in reaching the terminal ileum, but its use is limited by the lack of availability, the inability to perform biopsies, and the possible complication of capsule retention [79]. The double-balloon push-and-pull enteroscopy technique has the advantage of being able to perform biopsies and polypectomies [6] but is associated with complications such as intestinal perforation [80]. Radiological findings are often not specific in the diagnosis of small intestine lymphoma. Gastrointestinal contrast studies can identify stenosis, compression, or dilation of the involved bowel. CT findings are various and nonspecific (Fig. 20.2). CT may show an enlarging mass with thickening of the wall of the small intestine or flattening of the folds of the mucosa, but also polypoid forms with multiple nodules, infiltrative lesions, fistulizing forms, and invasive mesenteric forms with extraluminal masses. In Burkitt's lymphoma, a single bulky mass in the lower right quadrant is common; IPSID generally involves the proximal portion of the small intestine with disseminated nodules and thickening and irregularities of the mucosa. EATL can present with nodules, ulcers, and

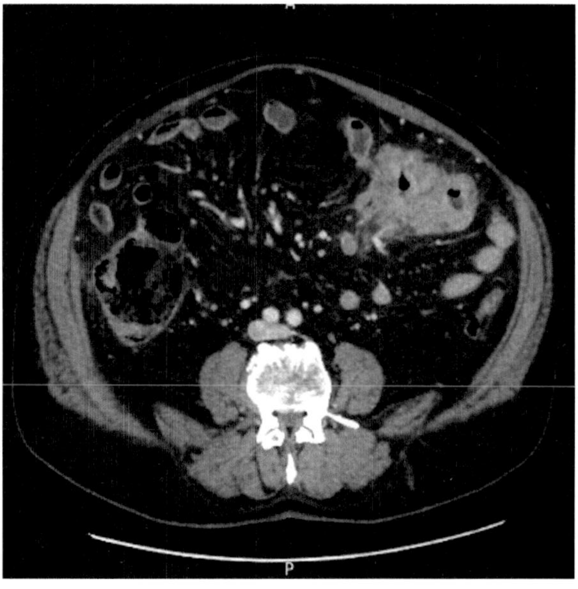

Fig. 20.2 CT scan of perforated small bowel lymphoma

strictures [81]. Follicular lymphomas, MCL, and MALT lymphoma rarely present with polypoid lesions [82]. CT is essential in patients presenting as emergencies with acute abdomen, if they are in stable general clinical conditions, and can be essential for the triage of those patients.

20.6.3 Surgical Treatment

The treatment of patients presenting as an emergency with small bowel lymphoma depends on various factors including his or her clinical conditions, the need for a histological diagnosis, the histologic type of lymphoma, and the stage of the disease. In patients presenting with acute mechanical obstruction, including intussusception, or perforation or massive bleeding, the main treatment is surgery [83]. In 30–50% of cases, patients with lymphoma of the small intestine present as an abdominal emergency [5, 84]. Often, in emergency, it is impossible to have a precise diagnosis before the emergency laparotomy and a suspect of lymphoma can arise only at laparotomy or on the histologic examination of the surgical specimen of a removed perforated (or obstructing) mass of the small bowel. In this group of patients, the aim of the intervention is to remove the segment of small intestine that causes the symptoms, obtaining an adequate tissue for histological diagnosis. Therefore, it must be kept in mind that the cause of the occlusion or perforation may be the lymphomatous tissue. In fact, intestinal perforations occur in 10% of patients with small bowel lymphoma, and in half of the cases, this is the presenting symptom [64]. The frequency of perforation in the first month of chemotherapy is high. Aggressive high-grade B-cell lymphomas and PTLDs appear to have the greatest risk of perforation, and prophylactic resection has been proposed in these groups, but at present, there are no robust data to support this advice [64, 66]. Another indication for surgery is the need to obtain a histological diagnosis. In fact, the therapeutic strategy may differ according to the histological type of lymphoma. Whenever a minimally invasive biopsy cannot be obtained for diagnosis (such as with an endoscopy), surgery has both a diagnostic and therapeutic value. In this case, it is advisable to perform a clear-margin segmental bowel resection with primary anastomosis. If possible, the associated mesentery should be included in the resection to facilitate the staging with the analysis of the proximal lymph nodes. In the meta-analysis by Lightner et al., the authors indicate that, unlike gastric lymphomas, surgery plays an important role in the elective treatment of small bowel lymphomas, with the exception of follicular lymphomas [85]. In the study by Lu et al., the authors report better survival in patients with primary nonmetastatic small bowel lymphoma who underwent primary site surgical resection and chemotherapy compared to patients who underwent surgery alone [86]. MALT lymphomas of the small intestine are treated according to their severity and the conditions of the patient. Local forms can be treated with surgical or endoscopic resection, while some cases are treated by eradicating the *H. pylori* infection. In the advanced and multifocal forms, the therapy of choice is multi-agent chemotherapy. In cases of follicular lymphoma (FL), which often involve the duodenum, in the initial stages, some authors suggest a watch-and-wait strategy, while in the symptomatic and advanced forms, the treatment is based on surgery and CHOP chemotherapy (cyclophosphamide, doxorubicin, vincristine, and prednisone) [87, 88]. The early stages of IPSID respond to antibiotic therapy (tetracyclines or ampicillin and metronidazole), while advanced forms are generally treated with anthracycline-based chemotherapy and antibiotics. This type of lymphoma can rarely be treated with surgery because it often presents in a diffuse form [6]. In the paper by Koniaris et al. [83], patients with Burkitt's lymphoma are divided into two groups: those at low risk and those at high risk. Low-risk patients with localized and resectable disease with negative resection margins should first undergo surgery and then chemotherapy. Patients at high risk, with diffuse, unresectable disease, elevated LDH levels, and involvement of bone marrow or cerebral spinal fluid, should undergo intensive chemotherapy. Complications of Burkitt's lymphoma, related to the growth of the neoplastic mass, in addition to intestinal perforation, gastrointestinal bleeding, and mechanical obstruction, include jaundice and pancreatitis due to ductal compression, and retroperitoneal invasion. The latter can lead to compression of the vena cava, lymphedema, and obstruction of the urinary tract. Surgery in many of these cases must aim to resolve the acute event in order to start chemotherapy as soon as possible.

20.7 Colorectal Lymphomas

Colorectal lymphomas account for approximately 6–12% of all gastrointestinal lymphomas [6]. Primary colorectal lymphomas are rare, and most of them are secondary forms of diffuse lymphomas. Primary lymphomas represent approximately 0.2–0.6% of malignant neoplasms of the large bowel; in fact, compared to the stomach and small intestine, the colon and rectum are uncommon sites of lymphoma [89]. The colonic segments most affected by primitive lymphomas are the cecum, the ascending colon, and the rectum, probably because the lymphoid tissue is more represented in these regions [90]. Various studies have shown a prevalence in male sex with twice the involvement of men compared to women [6, 89]. Patients are generally affected in the fifth to seventh decades of life. Risk factors associated with the onset of primary colonic lymphomas include two conditions: immunosuppression (linked to HIV infection, immunosuppression in transplants, and prolonged use of corticosteroids) and inflammatory bowel diseases (IBD) [85, 89]. Plasmablastic lymphoma (PBL), an aggressive variant of DLBCL, typical of the oral cavity can also be found in the anal canal in HIV+ patients [91]. Also in the large bowel, most primary lymphomas are B-cell derived. The most frequent type is diffuse large B-cell lymphoma (DLBCL), but intestinal lymphomas of the large intestine also include low-grade B-cell lymphomas such as MALT, MCL, and T-cell-derived lymphomas. MALT lymphomas of the colon are extremely rare, and unlike MALT gastric lymphoma, the role of *H. pylori* in their pathogenesis is not well defined [92]. Mantle cell lymphomas (MCLs) affect the colon usually within systemic forms [93]. Peripheral T-cell lymphomas represent more aggressive forms, with a poor prognosis and a higher frequency of perforation. These are rare lymphomas in

Western countries and more frequent in Asian ones with an increasing frequency [94].

20.7.1 Clinical Presentation

Colorectal lymphoma patients generally have nonspecific symptoms. The most frequent symptoms are abdominal pain, anorexia and weight loss, palpable abdominal mass, and blood in the stool [89]. More rarely, patients with colon lymphoma present urgently to the surgeon for perforation, rectal bleeding, or mechanical obstruction. Abbott et al. reported that colic perforations in lymphomas are less frequent than those in the small intestine and are more frequent in T-cell lymphomas than in B-cell lymphomas (23% vs. 3%) [95]. The same authors in their review report that gastrointestinal bleeding is the presenting feature in 2.2–22% of large bowel lymphomas. Rarely, colonic lymphomas can present in emergency as emphysematous colitis [96].

20.7.2 Investigations

The diagnosis of colonic lymphoma depends on the care setting, whether in emergency or as elective case. In fact, in an emergency due to gastrointestinal bleeding, obstruction, or perforation, the diagnosis is made by CT. Non-emergency patients usually complain of change in bowel habit, anorexia, weight loss, positive fecal occult blood, and a palpable mass (without signs of obstruction). The diagnosis is made by endoscopic examination and biopsy, which is the gold standard [97]. Endoscopically, the most frequent appearance is that of a single large ulcerated mass, although polypoid lesions may be present and, very rarely, annular lesions [98]. The radiological appearance of colon lymphomas on CT and double-contrast barium enema are highly variable and include focal and diffuse lesions [6]. The focal lesions can be polypoid, infiltrative, mucosal nodularity, or mucosal fold thickening [81]. Diffuse forms can be both nodular and ulcerative. Colon lymphoma lesions are generally larger and involve a longer segment than adenocarcinomas and are more frequently located near the ileocecal valve with direct extension into the terminal ileum [99]. Peripheral T-cell lymphomas may have ulcerative features similar to granulomatous diseases such as tuberculosis or Crohn's disease [100].

20.7.3 Surgical Techniques

There are few studies regarding the treatment of colorectal lymphomas due to the rarity of this disease, and most of them are small, retrospective, and observational. The treatment of colorectal lymphomas is based on surgery and chemotherapy. In fact, historically for these pathologies, the purpose of surgery is to remove a lesion that can cause problems of obstruction, perforation, and bleeding, while chemotherapy increases survival. The main treatment is a combination of surgery and chemotherapy [101]. Early-stage colorectal lymphomas are treated with surgery followed by polychemotherapy, while advanced-stage lymphomas are treated with multidrug chemotherapy [102, 103]. In the review by Beaton et al., the authors conclude by indicating how the choice between chemotherapy and surgery in colorectal lymphomas depends on the type of presentation, with patients with acute abdomen going more likely towards the surgical approach [79]. Furthermore, surgical treatment, in addition to preventing complications and providing a possible cure (with or without adjuvant therapy), provides important prognostic information, including histology, extent, and stage of the tumor [104]. Adjuvant chemotherapy has led to improved outcomes [89, 102, 103]. Chemotherapy regimens, alone or as adjuvant therapy, for colorectal lymphoma are usually the multi-agent type using the CHOP scheme (cyclophosphamide, doxorubicin, vincristine, and prednisone). With the introduction of the chemotherapy protocols for new active monoclonal drugs such as rituximab [105], the role of surgery is questionable. However, patients with fistulae, perforation, obstruction, and bleeding should be treated surgically as first choice. In fact, in the article by Cai et al., out of 43 patients [106], 56% required emergency operations. Similarly, Zhai et al. report that out of 46 patients [107], 13 required emergency surgery. Emergency treatment of colorectal lymphomas depends on the complication being treated. In the event of perforation, the resection of the affected area with or without anastomosis is performed by laparoscopy or open surgery. Similarly, an obstructing colon lymphoma can be treated with resection, whether or not associated with a stoma, or with an endoscopic stent. If the patient is in stable clinical conditions, a conservative chemoradiotherapy approach can also be attempted. Patients presenting with acute gastrointestinal hemorrhage from lymphoma of the large intestine, in addition to being treated with supportive therapy, can be managed endoscopically or with CT angiography and embolization.

References

1. Bonadonna G, Robustelli Della Cuna G, Valagusa P. Medicina Oncologica. 8th ed. Elsevier Masson: Milano; 2007.
2. Bowzyk Al-Naeeb A, Ajithkumar T, Behan S, Hodson DJ. Non-Hodgkin lymphoma. BMJ. 2018;362:k3204.
3. de Leval L, Jaffe ES. Lymphoma classification. Cancer J. 2020;26(3):176–85.
4. Swerdlow SH, Campo E, Harris NL, et al. WHO classification of tumours of haematopoietic and lymphoid tissues. Lyon, France: International Agency for Research on Cancer; 2017.
5. Freeman C, Berg JW, Cutler SJ. Occurrence and prognosis of extranodal lymphomas. Cancer. 1972;29:252–60.
6. Ghimire P, Wu GY, Zhu L. Primary gastrointestinal lymphoma. World J Gastroenterol. 2011;17(6):697–707.
7. Ghai S, Pattison J, Ghai S, O'Malley ME, Khalili K, Stephens M. Primary gastrointestinal lymphoma: Spectrum of imaging findings with pathologic correlation. Vol. 27, Radiographics. 2007. p. 1371–1388.

8. Gurney KA, Cartwright RA, Gilman EA. Descriptive epidemiology of gastrointestinal non-Hodgkin's lymphoma in a population-based registry. Br J Cancer. 1999;79(11–12):1929–34.
9. Lo Re G, Federica V, Midiri F, et al. Radiological features of gastrointestinal lymphoma. Gastroenterol Res Pract. 2016;2016:2498143.
10. Dawson IM, Cornes JS, Morson BC. Primary malignant lymphoid tumours of the intestinal tract. Report of 37 cases with a study of factors influencing prognosis. Br J Surg. 1961;49:80–9.
11. Bautista-Quach MA, Ake CD, Chen M, Wang J. Gastrointestinal lymphomas: morphology, immunophenotype and molecular features. J Gastrointest Oncol. 2012;3:209–25.
12. Pizzi M, Sabattini E, Parente P, Bellan A, Doglioni C, Lazzi S. Gastrointestinal lymphoproliferative lesions: a practical diagnostic approach. Pathologica. 2020;112(3):227–47.
13. Olszewska-Szopa M, Wróbel T. Gastrointestinal non-Hodgkin lymphomas. Adv Clin Exp Med. 2019;28(8):1119–24.
14. Rizvi MA, Evens AM, Tallman MS, Nelson BP, Rosen ST. T-cell non-Hodgkin lymphoma. Blood. 2006;107:1255–64.
15. Elenitoba-Johnson KSJ, Lim MS. New insights into lymphoma pathogenesis. Annu Rev Pathol. 2018;13:193–217.
16. Psyrri A, Papageorgiou S, Economopoulos T. Primary extranodal lymphomas of stomach: clinical presentation, diagnostic pitfalls and management. Ann Oncol. 2008;19:1992–9.
17. Ferreri AJ, Montalbán C. Primary diffuse large B-cell lymphoma of the stomach. Crit Rev Oncol Hematol. 2007;63:65–71.
18. Swerdlow SH, Campo E, Harris NL, et al. Extranodal marginal zone lymphoma of mucosa-associated lymphoid tissue (MALT lymphoma). In: Swerdlow SH, Campo E, Harris NL, et al., editors. World Health Organization classification of tumours of haematopoietic and lymphoid tissues (4th edition). Lyon: IARC Press; 2008. p. 214–7.
19. Lecuit M, Abachin E, Martin A, et al. Immunoproliferative small intestinal disease associated with campylobacter jejuni. N Engl J Med. 2004;350:239–48.
20. Matasar MJ, Zelenetz AD. Overview of lymphoma diagnosis and management. Radiol Clin N Am. 2008;46(2):175–98. vii
21. Azab MB, Henry-Amar M, Rougier P. Prognostic factors in primary gastrointestinal non-Hodgkin's lymphoma. A multivariate analysis, report of 106 cases, and review of the literature. Cancer. 1989;64:1208–17.
22. Rohatiner A, D'Amore F, Coiffier B, et al. Report on a workshop convened to discuss the pathological and staging classifications of gastrointestinal tract lymphoma. Ann Oncol. 1994;5:397–400.
23. May A, Nachbar L, Pohl J, et al. Endoscopic interventions in the small bowel using double balloon enteroscopy: feasibility and limitations. Am J Gastroenterol. 2007;102:527–35.
24. Kobayashi K, Katsumata T, Saigenji K. Clinical usefulness of single-balloon enteroscopy in the diagnosis and treatment of small-intestinal diseases. In: Niwa H, editor. New challenges in gastrointestinal endoscopy. Springer; 2008. p. 243–50.
25. Flieger D, Keller J, May A, et al. Capsule endoscopy in gastrointestinal lymphomas. Endoscopy. 2000;37:1174–80.
26. Boot H. In: Thesis, editor. Gastric MALT-lymphoma. Studies on diagnosis, pathogenesis and treatment. Amsterdam: Thesis Publishers; 1997.
27. Fischbach W, Dragosics B, Kolve-Goebeler M-E, et al. Primary gastric B-cell lymphoma: results of a prospective multicenter study. Gastroenterology. 2000;119:1191–202.
28. Boot H, de Jong D. Diagnosis, treatment decisions, and follow-up in primary gastric lymphoma. Gut. 2002;51:621–2.
29. Fischbach W. Gastric mucosa-associated lymphoid tissue lymphoma: a challenge for endoscopy. Gastrointest Endosc. 2008;68:632–4.
30. Liu H, Ye H, Ruskone-Fourmestraux A, et al. T(11;18) is a marker for all stage gastric MALT lymphomas that will not respond to H. pylori eradication. Gastroenterology. 2002;122:1286–94.

31. Boot H. Diagnosis and staging in gastrointestinal lymphoma. Best Pract Res Clin Gastroenterol. 2010;24(1):3–12.
32. Boveri E, Arcaini L, Merli M, et al. Bone marrow histology in marginal zone B-cell lymphomas: correlation with clinical parameters and flow cytometry in 120 patients. Ann Oncol. 2009;20:129–36.
33. Raderer M, Vorbeck F, Formanek M, et al. Importance of extensive staging in patients with mucosa-associated lymphoid tissue (MALT-type)-lymphoma. Br J Cancer. 2000;83:454–7.
34. Jerusalem G, Beguin Y, Fassotte MF, et al. Whole-body positron emission tomography using 18F-fluorodeoxyglucose for posttreatment evaluation in Hodgkin's disease and non-Hodgkin lymphoma has higher diagnostic and prognostic value than classical computed tomography scan imaging. Blood. 1999;94:429–33.
35. Isai CR, Lu P, Blaufox MD. A meta-analysis of 18F-2-deoxy-2-fluoro-D-glucose positron emission tomography in the staging and restaging of patients with lymphoma. Cancer. 2005;104:1066–74.
36. Raderer M, Wöhrer S, Streubel B, et al. Assessment of disease dissemination in gastric compared with extragastric mucosa-associated lymphoid tissue lymphoma using extensive staging: a single-center experience. J Clin Oncol. 2006;24:3136–41.
37. Juárez-Salcedo LM, Sokol L, Chavez JC, Dalia S. Primary gastric lymphoma, epidemiology, clinical diagnosis, and treatment. Cancer Control. 2018;25(1):1073274818778256.
38. Hussell T, Isaacson PG, Crabtree JE, Spencer J. Helicobacter pylori-specific tumour-infiltrating T cells provide contact dependent help for the growth of malignant B cells in low-grade gastric lymphoma of mucosa-associated lymphoid tissue. J Pathol. 1996;178:122–7.
39. Ohkura Y, Lee S, Kaji D, Ota Y, Haruta S, Takeji Y, Shinohara H, Ueno M, Udagawa H. Spontaneous perforation of primary gastric malignant lymphoma: a case report and review of the literature. World J Surg Oncol. 2015;13:35. https://doi.org/10.1186/s12957-015-0458-0.
40. Ono K, Matsumura S, Sakamoto K, Kobayashi S, Kamano T, Iwasaki R. A case of gastric malignant lymphoma with perforation during chemotherapy. Gan To Kagaku Ryoho. 1997;24(1):105–8.
41. Shiomi H, Watanabe E, Umeda T. A case report of perforated gastric malignant lymphoma. Jpn J Cancer Clin. 1997;43:25–8.
42. Bestari MB, Palungkun IG, Hernowo BS, Abdurachman SA, Nugraha ES. Low-stage gastric MALT lymphoma causing life-threatening upper gastrointestinal bleeding. Case Rep Gastroenterol. 2019;13(3):376–84.
43. Taal BG, Burgers JM. Primary non-Hodgkin's lymphoma of the stomach: endoscopic diagnosis and the role of surgery. Scand J Gastroenterol Suppl. 1991;188:33–7.
44. Püspök A, Raderer M, Chott A, Dragosics B, Gangl A, Schöfl R. Endoscopic ultrasound in the follow up and response assessment of patients with primary gastric lymphoma. Gut. 2002;51:691–4.
45. Al-Akwaa AM, Siddiqui N, Al-Mofleh IA. Primary gastric lymphoma. World J Gastroenterol. 2004;10:5–11.
46. Lupescu IG, Grasu M, Goldis G, Popa G, Gheorghe C, Vasilescu C, Moicean A, Herlea V, Georgescu SA. Computer tomographic evaluation of digestive tract non-Hodgkin lymphomas. J Gastrointestin Liver Dis. 2007;16:315–9.
47. Radan L, Fischer D, Bar-Shalom R, Dann EJ, Epelbaum R, Haim N, Gaitini D, Israel O. FDG avidity and PET/CT patterns in primary gastric lymphoma. Eur J Nucl Med Mol Imaging. 2008;35:1424–30.
48. Stathis A, Chini C, Bertoni F, Proserpio I, Capella C, Mazzucchelli L, Pedrinis E, Cavalli F, Pinotti G, Zucca E. Long-term outcome following helicobacter pylori eradication in a retrospective study of 105 patients with localized gastric marginal zone B-cell lymphoma of MALT type. Ann Oncol. 2009;20:1086–93.
49. Greiner A, Knörr C, Qin Y, Sebald W, et al. Low-grade B cell lymphomas of mucosa-associated lymphoid tissue (MALT-type) require CD40-mediated signaling and Th2-type cytokines for in vitro growth and differentiation. Am J Pathol. 1997;150(5):1583–93.

50. Raderer M, Wöhrer S, Kiesewetter B, et al. Antibiotic treatment as sole management of helicobacter pylori-negative gastric MALT lymphoma: a single center experience with prolonged follow-up. Ann Hematol. 2015;94(6):969–73.
51. Egger ME, Ikoma N, Badgwell BD. Primary gastric malignancies. In: The MD Anderson surgical oncology handbook. 6th ed. Wolters Kluwer Health Adis (ESP); 2018. p. 417–9.
52. Ferrucci PF, Zucca E. Primary gastric lymphoma pathogenesis and treatment: what has changed over the past 10 years? Br J Haematol. 2007;136:521–38.
53. Gralnek IM, Dumonceau JM, Kuipers EJ, et al. Diagnosis and management of nonvariceal upper gastrointestinal hemorrhage: European Society of Gastrointestinal Endoscopy (ESGE) guideline. Endoscopy. 2015;47(10):a1–46.
54. Yoon SS, Coit DG, Portlock CS, Karpeh MS. The diminishing role of surgery in the treatment of gastric lymphoma. Ann Surg. 2004;240(1):28–37.
55. Stabile BE, Smith BR. Cancer of the stomach: surgical management. In: Principles and practice of surgical oncology. Multidisciplinary approach to difficult problems. Lippincott Williams & Wilkins, a Wolters Kluwer Business; 2010. p. 685–7.
56. Speranza V, Lomanto D. Primary gastric lymphoma. In: Holzheimer RG, Mannick JA, editors. Surgical treatment: evidence-based and problem-oriented. Munich: Zuckschwerdt; 2001. https://www.ncbi.nlm.nih.gov/books/NBK6966/.
57. Salles G, Herbrecht R, Tilly H, et al. Aggressive primary gastrointestinal lymphomas: review of 91 patients treated with the LNH-84 regimen. A study of the groupe d'etude des lymphomes agressifs. Am J Med. 1991;90:77–84.
58. Ohkura Y, Lee S, Kaji D, et al. Spontaneous perforation of primary gastric malignant lymphoma: a case report and review of the literature. World J Surg Oncol. 2015;13:35.
59. Chen G, Zhang MM, Zhu JM, Mao J, Li YM. Damage control surgery saves patient with gastric lymphoma from radical gastrectomy. J Coll Physicians Surg Pak. 2021;31(8):978–81.
60. Søreide K, Thorsen K, Harrison EM, et al. Perforated peptic ulcer. Lancet. 2015;386(10000):1288–98.
61. Cao YJ, Duan J, Liu LF, Wei X, Ren L, Zhang LN, Zhang W. Individualized treatment and palliative Care for a 90-year-old patient with primary gastric diffuse large-B cell lymphoma: 4 year follow-up and inspiration. Chin Med Sci J. 2021;36(1):72–7.
62. Schottenfeld D, Beebe-Dimmer JL, Vigneau FD. The epidemiology and pathogenesis of neoplasia in the small intestine. Ann Epidemiol. 2009;19:58–69.
63. Bilimoria KY, Bentrem DJ, Wayne JD, Ko CY, Bennett CL, Talamonti MS. Small bowel cancer in the United States: changes in epidemiology, treatment, and survival over the last 20 years. Ann Surg. 2009;249(1):63–71.
64. Opelz G, Daniel V, Naujokat C, Dohler B. Epidemiology of pretransplant EBV and CMV serostatus in relation to posttransplant non-Hodgkin lymphoma. Transplantation. 2009;88(8):962–7.
65. Howell JM, Auer-Grzesiak I, Zhang J, Andrews CN, Stewart D, Urbanski SJ. Increasing incidence rates, distribution and histological characteristics of primary gastrointestinal non-Hodgkin lymphoma in a north American population. Can J Gastroenterol. 2012;26(7):452–6.
66. Scott KS, James RH. Tumors of the small bowel in Morita Ys. In: Balch CM, editor. Textbook of complex general surgical oncology. McGraw-Hill Companies; 2018. p. 1637–42.
67. Biko DM, Anupindi SA, Hernandez A, Kersun L, Bellah R. Childhood Burkitt lymphoma: abdominal and pelvic imaging findings. AJR Am J Roentgenol. 2009;192:1304–15.
68. Choi SY, Kim SJ, Kim WS, et al. Aggressive B cell lymphomas of the gastrointestinal tract: clinicopathologic and genetic analysis. Virchows Arch. 2011;459:495–502.
69. Nguyen V, Nguyen B, Petris GD, et al. Education and imaging. Gastrointestinal: gastrointestinal involvement of mantle cell lymphoma. J Gastroenterol Hepatol. 2012;27:617.
70. Hirata N, Tominaga K, Ohta K, et al. A case of mucosa-associated lymphoid tissue lymphoma forming multiple lymphomatous polyposis in the small intestine. World J Gastroenterol. 2007;13:1453–7.
71. Al-Saleem T, Al-Mondhiry H. Immunoproliferative small intestinal disease (IPSID): a model for mature B-cell neoplasms. Blood. 2005;105:2274–80.

72. Garrido A, Luque A, Vázquez A, et al. Primary small bowel neoplasms as a complication of celiac disease. Gastroenterol Hepatol. 2009;32:618–21.
73. Ludvigsson JF, Lebwohl B, Rubio-Tapia A, et al. Does celiac disease influence survival in lymphoproliferative malignancy? Eur J Epidemiol. 2013;28(6):475–83.
74. Koch P, del Valle F, Berdel WE, et al. Primary gastrointestinal non-Hodgkin's lymphoma: I. anatomic and histologic distribution, clinical features, and survival data of 371 patients registered in the German multicenter study GIT NHL 01/92. J Clin Oncol. 2001;19(18):3861–73.
75. Ibrahim EM, Ezzat AA, El-Weshi AN, et al. Primary intestinal diffuse large B-cell non-Hodgkin's lymphoma: clinical features, management, and prognosis of 66 patients. Ann Oncol. 2001;12(1):53–8.
76. Zinzani PL, Magagnoli M, Pagliani G, et al. Primary intestinal lymphoma: clinical and therapeutic features of 32 patients. Haematologica. 1997;82(3):305–8.
77. Donohue JH, Schnelldorfer T. Small bowel tumors. In: Silberman H, Silberman AW, editors. Principles and practice of surgical oncology multidisciplinary approach to difficult problems. Lippincott Williams & Wilkins, a Wolters Kluwer business; 2010. p. 814–6.
78. Onkendi EO, Grotz TE, Murray JA, Donohue JH. Adult intussusception in the last 25 years of modern imaging: is surgery still indicated? J Gastrointest Surg. 2011;15(10):1699–705.
79. Beaton C, Davies M, Beynon J. The management of primary small bowel and colon lymphoma—a review. Int J Color Dis. 2012;27(5):555–63.
80. Mitsui K, Tanaka S, Yamamoto H, et al. Role of double-balloon endoscopy in the diagnosis of small-bowel tumors; the first Japanese multicenter study. Gastrointest Endosc. 2009;70(3):498–504.
81. Gollub MJ. Imaging of gastrointestinal lymphoma. Radiol Clin N Am. 2008;46:287–312, ix.
82. Chung HH, Kim YH, Kim JH, Cha SH, Kim BH, Kim TK, Kim AR, Cho SJ. Imaging findings of mantle cell lymphoma involving gastrointestinal tract. Yonsei Med J. 2003;44:49–57.
83. Koniaris LG, Drugas G, Katzman PJ, Salloum R. Management of gastrointestinal lymphoma. J Am Coll Surg. 2003;197(1):127–41.
84. Fleming ID, Turk PS, Murphy SB, et al. Surgical implications of primary gastrointestinal lymphoma of childhood. Arch Surg. 1990;125:252–6.
85. Lightner AL, Shannon E, Gibbons MM, Russell MM. Primary gastrointestinal non-Hodgkin's lymphoma of the small and large intestines: a systematic review. J Gastrointest Surg. 2016;20(4):827–39.
86. Lu PW, Fields AC, Yoo J, Irani J, Goldberg JE, Bleday R, Melnitchouk N. Surgical management of small bowel lymphoma. J Gastrointest Surg. 2021;25(3):757–65.
87. Dickson BC, Serra S, Chetty R. Primary gastrointestinal tract lymphoma: diagnosis and management of common neoplasms. Expert Rev Anticancer Ther. 2006;6:1609–28.
88. Yamamoto S, Nakase H, Yamashita K, et al. Gastrointestinal follicular lymphoma: review of the literature. J Gastroenterol. 2010;45:370–88.
89. Dionigi G, Annoni M, Rovera F, Boni L, Villa F, Castano P, Bianchi V, Dionigi R. Primary colorectal lymphomas: review of the literature. Surg Oncol. 2007;16(Suppl 1):S169–71.
90. Fan CW, Changchien CR, Wang JY. Primary colorectal lymphoma. Dis Colon Rectum. 2000;43:1277–82.
91. Foukas PG, de Leval L. Recent advances in intestinal lymphomas. Histopathology. 2015;66(1):112–36.
92. Niino D, Yamamoto K, Tsuruta O, et al. Regression of rectal mucosa-associated lymphoid tissue (MALT) lymphoma after antibiotic treatments. Pathol Int. 2010;60:438–44.
93. Hollie N, Asakrah S. MALT lymphoma of the colon: a clinicopathological review. J Clin Pathol. 2020;73(7):378–83.
94. Said J, Pinter-Brown L. Clinical and pathological diagnosis of peripheral T-cell lymphoma and emerging treatment options: a case-based discussion. Clin Adv Hematol Oncol. 2009;7:S1, S4–13; quiz S15.
95. Abbott S, Nikolousis E, Badger I. Intestinal lymphoma—a review of the management of emergency presentations to the general surgeon. Int J Color Dis. 2015;30(2):151–7.

96. Chou YH, Hsu HL, Lee JC, Lin BR, Liu KL. Emphysematous colitis of ascending colon with portal venous air caused by diffuse large B-cell lymphoma. J Clin Oncol. 2010;28:e496–7.
97. Stanojevic GZ, Nestorovic MD, Brankovic BR, Stojanovic MP, Jovanovic MM, Radojkovic MD. Primary colorectal lymphoma: an overview. World J Gastrointest Oncol. 2011;3:14–8.
98. Vetro C, Romano A, Amico I, et al. Endoscopic features of gastro-intestinal lymphomas: from diagnosis to follow-up. World J Gastroenterol. 2014;20(36):12993–3005.
99. Levine MS, Rubesin SE, Pantongrag-Brown L, et al. Non-Hodgkin's lymphoma of the gastrointestinal tract: radiographic findings. Am J Roentgenol. 1997;168:167–72.
100. Lee HJ, Han JK, Kim TK, et al. Primary colorectal lymphoma: spectrum of imaging findings with pathologic correlation. Eur Radiol. 2002;12:2242–9.
101. Tondini C, Giardini R, Bozzetti F, Valagussa P, Santoro A, Bertulli R, et al. Combined modality treatment for primary gastrointestinal non-Hodgkin's lymphoma: the Milan cancer institute experience. Ann Oncol. 1993;4:831–7.
102. She WH, Day W, Lau PY, et al. Primary colorectal lymphoma: case series and literature review. Asian J Surg. 2011;34(3):111–4.
103. Pandey M, Swain J, Iyer HM, Shukla M. Primary lymphoma of the colon: report of two cases and review of literature. World J Surg Oncol. 2019;17(1):18.
104. Zighelboim J, Larson MV. Primary colonic lymphoma. J Clin Gastroenterol. 1994;19:135–8.
105. Salar A, Domingo-Domenech E, Estany C, et al. Combination therapy with rituximab and intravenous or oral fludarabine in the first-line, systemic treatment of patients with extranodal marginal zone B-cell lymphoma of the mucosa-associated lymphoid tissue type. Cancer. 2009;115:5210–7.
106. Cai S, Cannizzo F Jr, Bullard Dunn KM, Gibbs JF, CzuczmanM RA. The role of surgical intervention in non-Hodgkin's lymphoma of the colon and rectum. Am J Surg. 2007;193:409–12; discussion 412.
107. Zhai L, Zhao Y, Lin L, Tian Y, Chen X, Huang H, Lin T. Non-Hodgkin's lymphoma involving the ileocecal region: a single-institution analysis of 46 cases in a Chinese population. J Clin Gastroenterol. 2012;46(6):5091.

Miscellaneous Rare Malignancies: GIST 21

Massimo Sartelli and Sara Liverotti

21.1 Introduction

Stromal tumors were referred to as smooth muscle neoplasms of gastrointestinal tract [1]. Mazur et al. [2] named these tumors gastrointestinal stromal tumors (GISTs) to collectively refer to a group of mesenchymal tumors of neurogenic or myogenic differentiation, which lacked the immunohistochemical features of Schwann cells and did not have the ultrastructural characteristics of smooth muscle cells. GISTs are the most common mesenchymal tumors of the gastrointestinal tract, accounting for 1–3% of all gastrointestinal malignancies. Throughout the whole length of the gastrointestinal tract, GISTs arise most commonly from the stomach followed by small bowel. Less frequently, they can occur in the colon, rectum, appendix, esophagus, mesentery, omentum, or retroperitoneum.

The clinical presentations of GISTs are highly variable according to their site and size [3].

The clinical presentation depends on the primary localization of the neoplasm and tumor size; however, in 18%, it is asymptomatic [4].

Prognosis varies greatly depending on the malignant potential of the tumor, defined by tumor size, tumor location, mitotic rate, and presence of tumor rupture during surgery [5].

Most GISTs are primarily treated with surgery; however, the tyrosine kinase inhibitor (TKI) imatinib has proven to be effective in prolonging the survival of patients with a high risk of recurrence after surgery and cases with locally advanced, unresectable, and/or metastatic disease [6].

Sensitivity to imatinib therapy depends on the type of initial KIT/PDGFRA mutation [7].

GISTs can occur in emergency for two main reasons: bleeding and obstruction [8, 9].

M. Sartelli (✉) · S. Liverotti
Department of Surgery, Macerata Hospital, Macerata, Italy

A. Tarasconi et al. (eds.), *Oncologic Surgical Emergencies*, Hot Topics in Acute Care Surgery and Trauma, https://doi.org/10.1007/978-3-031-36860-8_21

21.2 Emergency Surgery in GISTs

Clinically, about 70% of patients with GIST are symptomatic, and gastrointestinal bleeding is the most common clinical symptom (in 30–40% of cases) [10]. Many patients seek medical treatment due to gastrointestinal bleeding. There are also many cases of patients that suffer an uncontrollably massive hemorrhage of the gastrointestinal tract and require emergency surgery.

Bleeding occurring into the peritoneal cavity due to a ruptured GIST leads to acute abdominal pain presenting as a surgical emergency. Bleeding into the gastrointestinal tract lumen, causing hematemesis, melena, or anemia, is usually more chronic on presentation.

The National Comprehensive Cancer Network (NCCN) treatment guidelines and the National Institutes of Health (NIH) risk stratification classify tumor rupture as a risk factor for recurrence. However, there are only few studies of the influence of GIST-induced gastrointestinal bleeding on prognosis [11].

A retrospective analysis of prognosis of GIST was used to assess the prognostic effects of hemorrhage of digestive tract induced by mucosal invasion of primary gastrointestinal stromal tumors and related mechanisms. The conclusion of the study was that GISTs with gastrointestinal hemorrhage are more likely to recur, which indicates poor prognosis. Therefore, gastrointestinal hemorrhage may be used as a significant indicator to assess the prognosis of patients [11].

A CT scan or angiography plays a role in the diagnosis of acute bleeding, in elucidating a cause and detecting active hemorrhage.

CT scan is the most commonly used modality in patients with abdominal emergency [12]. CT can point to a specific organ as the source of the bleeding, detect active hemorrhage, and provide information on how long ago the hemorrhagic episode took place.

The presence of a bleeding mass of uncertain nature may result in a challenging situation for the surgeon, who is forced to perform an emergency surgical procedure without knowing the exact nature of the tumor and hence the extent of resection required [13].

Obstruction can be the result of several different characteristics including

- The continued growth of the lesion with direct occlusion of the bowel
- The intussusception with the tumor acting as the lead point resulting in obstruction
- A volvulus-like torsion of the bowel around the tumor, if its growth pattern is extraluminal, resulting in obstruction [9]

In cases of small bowel obstruction where there is no obvious cause, a CT scan is recommended, and when a solid lesion of the small bowel is identified, the possibility of a GIST tumor should be considered.

21.3 Treatment

The surgical technique depends on the size and location of the tumor. Small asymptomatic gastric GISTs (less than 2 cm) with no high-risk EUS features can be managed conservatively with endoscopic surveillance at 6–12-month intervals.

At present, surgical resection remains the mainstay approach in treating the patients with localized, nonmetastatic GISTs.

Multivisceral and radical surgery should be avoided where possible. Segmental or wedge resection with an aim to obtain histologically negative margins is sufficient.

Studies comparing laparoscopic versus open resection of GISTs typically involve small comparative groups and often do not control for tumor size or stage of disease. However, recent findings support the use of laparoscopy as a viable and potentially more effective approach to GIST resection [14].

Laparoscopy has been recommended for selected GISTs present in favorable anatomic locations like the anterior wall of the stomach, jejunum, and ileum. The same surgical principles as in open surgery are applicable in laparoscopic surgery for GIST, also in the emergency setting.

The safety and appropriate use of laparoscopy in surgical resection of GIST tumors have been well documented; however, in an acute setting, the experience of the surgeon is important in successfully completing an oncologically safe procedure [15, 16].

21.4 Conclusion

GISTs can develop anywhere along the gastrointestinal tract from the esophagus to the rectum; however, stomach and small intestine are the most common locations for GIST.

Bleeding occurring into the peritoneal cavity due to a ruptured GIST can lead to acute abdominal pain presenting as a surgical emergency. Bleeding into the gastrointestinal tract lumen, causing hematemesis, melena, or anemia, is usually more chronic on presentation. Obstruction can be the result of several different characteristics including the continued growth of the lesion with direct occlusion of the bowel; the intussusception with the tumor acting as the lead point results in obstruction or a volvulus-like torsion of the bowel around the tumor.

At present, surgical resection remains the mainstay approach in treating the patients with localized, nonmetastatic GISTs.

References

1. Joensuu H. Gastrointestinal stromal tumor (GIST). Ann Oncol. 2006;17(Suppl 10):x280–6.
2. Mazur MT, Clark HB. Gastric stromal tumors. Reappraisal of histogenesis. Am J Surg Pathol. 1983;7:507–19.

3. Sorour MA, Kassem MI, Ael-H G, El-Riwini MT, Abu NA. Gastrointestinal stromal tumors (GIST) related emergencies. Int J Surg. 2014;12(4):269–80.
4. Giordano A, Moroni F, Di Filippo G, Cammelli F, Baraghini M, Giudicissi R, Vellei S, Feroci F, Cantafio S. Emergency duodenal resection for giant GIST with acute gastrointestinal bleeding a case report. Ann Ital Chir. 2021;10:S2239253X21036707.
5. Demetri GD, von Mehren M, Blanke CD, Van den Abbeele AD, Eisenberg B, Roberts PJ, et al. Efficacy and safety of imatinib mesylate in advanced gastrointestinal stromal tumors. N Engl J Med. 2002;347(7):472–80.
6. Dematteo RP, Gold JS, Saran L, Gonen M, Liau KH, Maki RG, et al. Tumor mitotic rate, size, and location independently predict recurrence after resection of primary gastrointestinal stromal tumor (GIST). Cancer. 2008;112(3):608–15.
7. Debiec-Rychter M, Sciot R, Le Cesne A, Schlemmer M, Hohenberger P, van Oosterom AT, et al. KIT mutations and dose selection for imatinib in patients with advanced gastrointestinal stromal tumours. Eur J Cancer. 2006;42(8):1093–103.
8. Khuri S, Gilshtein H, Darawshy A, Bahouth H, Kluger Y. Primary small bowel GIST presenting as a life-threatening emergency: a report of two cases. Case Rep Surg. 2017;2017:5.
9. Morrison JE, Hodgdon IA. Laparoscopic management of obstructing small bowel GIST tumor. JSLS. 2013;17(4):645–50.
10. Nilsson B, Bümming P, Meis-Kindblom JM. Gastrointestinal stromal tumors: the incidence, prevalence, clinical course, and prognostication in the preimatinib mesylate era—a population-based study in western Sweden. Cancer. 2005;103(4):821–9.
11. Liu Q, Li Y, Dong M, Kong F, Dong Q. Gastrointestinal bleeding is an independent risk factor for poor prognosis in GIST patients. Biomed Res Int. 2017;2017:7152406.
12. Razik A, Madhusudhan KS, Aggarwal A, Panwar R, Srivastava DN. Gastrointestinal stromal tumor of the jejunum with active bleeding demonstrated on dual-energy MDCT angiography: a case report. Curr Probl Diagn Radiol. 2017;S0363–0188(17):30271–2.
13. Rajendra R, Pollack SM, Jones RL. Management of gastrointestinal stromal tumors. Future Oncol. 2013;9:193–206.
14. Inaba CS, Dosch A, Koh CY, Sujatha-Bhaskar S, Pejcinovska M, Smith BR, Nguyen NT. Laparoscopic versus open resection of gastrointestinal stromal tumors: survival outcomes from the NCDB. Surg Endosc. 2019;33(3):923–32.
15. Nguyen SQ, Divino CM, Wang JL, Dikman SH. Laparoscopic management of gastrointestinal stromal tumors. Surg Endosc. 2006;20(5):713–6.
16. Alam I, Kheradmand F, Alam S, Jamil A, Wilson I, Hurley M. Laparoscopic management of acutely presenting gastrointestinal stromal tumors: a study of 9 cases and review of literature. J Laparoendosc Adv Surg Tech A. 2007;17(5):626–33.

22 Miscellaneous Rare Malignancies: Desmoplastic

Nicola de'Angelis and Francesco Marchegiani

22.1 Introduction

Desmoid tumors are rare neoplasms classified as low-grade soft tissue sarcomas [1, 2], also identified with the terms "aggressive fibromatosis," "deep fibromatosis," "musculoaponeurotic fibromatosis," or "desmoid fibrosis."

Firstly described by MacFarlane in 1833 [3], these tumors arise from fibrocyte-like cells affecting muscle connective tissue, fasciae, and aponeuroses.

They account for less than 3% of the sarcomas and less than 0.03% of all neoplasms [4]. Desmoid tumors develop between 15 and 60 years, with a peak age of 30–40 years, and they are more common in females [5, 6].

Despite the controversial etiology, the origin of these tumors is multifactorial with several risk factors identified: genetic factors, endocrine factors, antecedent trauma, and surgery itself [7].

Desmoid tumors can be sporadic but are often associated with adenomatous familial polyposis (AFP) and Gardner's syndrome. For AFP, a model of development was suggested resembling the adenoma-carcinoma sequence where the accumulation of genetic abnormalities brings to a malignant phenotype. The main stimulus driving the progression of mesenteric fibrosis is surgery itself, but it is not rare to find a desmoid tumor at index surgery in AFP patients [7, 8].

Desmoids account for 10–14% of deaths of Gardner's syndrome patients due to intestinal obstruction or perforation, making it the second leading cause of death after colorectal carcinoma [9].

Possible localizations of these tumors are the arms, the limbs, and the trunk both intra- and extraperitoneal. The desmoids can be classified into abdominal and

N. de'Angelis (✉) · F. Marchegiani
Unit of Colorectal and Digestive Surgery, DIGEST Department, University of Paris Cité, Beaujon University Hospital (AP-HP), Clichy, France

A. Tarasconi et al. (eds.), *Oncologic Surgical Emergencies*, Hot Topics in Acute Care Surgery and Trauma, https://doi.org/10.1007/978-3-031-36860-8_22

extra-abdominal. Abdominal desmoids are the most common, and they can be subclassified into abdominal wall tumors, when the tumor develops within the muscles of the abdominal wall, and into intra-abdominal tumors, when the tumor develops within the abdominal cavity [10].

Desmoid tumors do not show a metastatic potential as other sarcomas, but their local aggressive growth and the high local recurrence rate can be considered as devasting as other intra-abdominal malignancies.

Standard treatments stand on nonsteroidal anti-inflammatory drugs, hormone therapy, chemotherapy, surgery, and radiation therapy [2]. The natural history of the disease is poorly understood, and long periods of stabilization or spontaneous regression were observed resulting in a new "watch-and-wait" policy based on observation [6].

During the evolution of abdominal desmoid tumors, the local disease progression can lead to perforation or invasion of surrounding organs, which inevitably leads to an emergency treatment.

In this context, many reports are available in literature showing the involvement of the majority of intra-abdominal organs. The emergent presentation of desmoid tumors is defined as rare and unique by each author, mainly because of the low incidence of the disease. If all the reports are taken into account, common clinical features can be noted and subsequently clinical advices can be drawn.

Unfortunately, the level of evidence is very low given the nature of the available literature.

The aim of this chapter is to define the treatment of desmoid tumors in an emergency setting.

22.2 Diagnosis in Emergency Setting

Emergent clinical presentation drives the diagnostic, and no instrumental exams should be performed if there is a risk of delaying the treatment of a life-threatening condition.

The complete medical history could suggest the presence of a hereditary syndrome associated with desmoid tumors. Physical signs for Gardner's syndrome could be searched rapidly.

Blood analysis including routine tests and inflammatory markers can be useful to rule out the diagnosis.

Multimodality imaging including ultrasound (US), computerized tomography (CT), and magnetic resonance (MR) is useful, but the most reported modality in emergency is the CT scan with contrast enhancement.

The common US feature is the echogenicity of the mass, which varies depending on the amount of collagen, fibrosis, and cellular components of the lesion. In an emergency setting, the presence of pneumoperitoneum and a mass with suspect characteristics are enough to perform a CT scan with contrast injection.

The main elements to search in a CT scan performed with the suspicion of a complicated desmoid tumor are generic and useful to define the risky features: the presence of a mass which can have different appearances (in case of abscess, rupture, or perforation), the presence of free intra-abdominal air, the presence of liquid related to a perforation, the presence of liquid related to a hemorrhage, the presence of hydro-aerial levels, and the presence of infiltration of vessels and vital organs.

If an MRI can be performed, it could help to better define the nature of the mass and the involvement of surrounding structures. In fact, the relationship of the desmoid tumor to vessels and vital organs could play a role in the preoperative planning in order to drive the feasibility of the surgical approach.

The MRI features are important as for all the soft tissue tumors, but no clear descriptions are available concerning the imaging in emergency setting. The dense cellularity of desmoids typically generates T1 and T2 low signal intensity but various patterns of enhancement after injection of gadolinium. As for CT scan, when a lesion is complicated by abscess, rupture, or perforation, the overmentioned characteristics can change [11].

Multimodality imaging is useful even for the treatment response evaluation and for the surveillance of these tumors [5].

Differential diagnosis should be posed between a wide range of neoplasia: gastrointestinal stromal tumors (GIST), carcinomas, lymphomas, solitary fibrous tumors, inflammatory myofibroblastic tumors, sclerosing mesenteritis, and retroperitoneal fibrosis [12].

Only a biopsy with histopathology could define the exact diagnosis of the mass, but typically this will not be available in an emergency setting.

22.3 Clinical Presentations in Emergency Setting

Two mechanisms determine the diversity of clinical presentations: the compression on surrounding anatomical structures and the invasion of surrounding organs. This explains why desmoid tumors bear no specific symptoms but can determine a range of clinical scenarios ranging from hydronephrosis, intestinal obstruction, and vascular or neural compression to hollow organ perforation, fistulation, and bleeding.

In a cohort of 62 patients in follow-up for a diagnosis of desmoid tumors, Ophir et al. [13] described a complication rate of 63%. Twelve patients underwent an emergency surgery due to perforation ($n = 6$), obstruction ($n = 5$), and bleeding ($n = 1$). The described postoperative outcomes are not always acceptable with two patients requiring total parenteral nutrition and a recurrence rate of 25%.

Several literature reports are available, and the main clinical presentations in an emergency scenario are reported.

22.3.1 Perforation

Perforation of hollow organs generates fluid and gas leakage from the digestive tube. Several authors described the presence of a suspect hollow-viscus perforation, which revealed a desmoid tumor at the final histopathology.

Shah et al. [14] reported the case of a patient presenting at the emergency department with fever and abdominal pain, showing intra-abdominal free air at the CT scan performed. The patient underwent an emergency laparotomy showing a 9 cm tumor of the transverse colon. The surgeon performed a colonic resection. The resection was radical; no other lesions were described in the abdomen; and 1 year after the operation, the patient did not show any recurrence.

Yalav et al. [15] reported the case of a patient presenting with acute abdomen and free abdominal air detected at X-ray. No CT scan was performed before the intervention, and an emergency laparotomy revealed a gastric perforation due to a 14 cm mass, which was removed with a distal gastrectomy. The authors described a local recurrence after 7 years.

Intestinal perforation can happen even during a chemotherapeutic treatment for desmoid tumors. Li et al. [16] reported two cases of patients affected by Gardner's syndrome who were treated by chemotherapy (doxorubicin-dacarbazine-meloxicam) and experienced intestinal perforation. The mechanism is explained by the sensitivity of desmoid tumors to chemotherapy, which leads to necrosis, tumor shrinkage, and consequently perforation with peritonitis. The reported cases were successfully treated with intestinal resection and direct anastomosis in emergency setting even if one of the two patients received a covering stoma. The postoperative course was uneventful, and the patients underwent resumption of the chemotherapy.

22.3.2 Abscess Formation

A small perforation or a covered perforation can lead to an abscess formation. Small abscesses are usually asymptomatic and tend to resolve spontaneously or aided by antibiotic therapy. Unfortunately, when the abscess is related to the tumoral invasion, the evolution is unfavorable. The explanation for this clinical presentation stands on different possible mechanisms, and it is still debated. The most accredited hypothesis is that the invasion of the tumor into the bowel wall could lead to parietal ischemia, intestinal bacteria translocation, and subsequent abscess formation with or without the presence of a fistula [17].

In 2006, Cholongitas et al. [18] performed a left colectomy for a refractory abscess, which revealed a sporadic desmoid tumor.

A similar case was reported by Jain et al. [19] concerning a transverse colon perforation with pericolic collection, which revealed the presence of a desmoid tumor at that level. The authors were able to avoid an emergent resection with a defunctioning ileostomy and a postponed colon resection after 4 weeks.

In 2012, Haddad et al. [20] reported the case of a 9 cm abscess of the mesentery with air-fluid levels which brought to an emergency laparotomy revealing a mass, which at histopathology was a desmoid tumor.

Similarly, Bellamy et al. [21] reported on a bowel resection and direct anastomosis for a mesenteric mass with abscess, which resulted in a desmoid tumor.

More recently, Omori et al. [22] presented the case of a suspected ascending colon perforated diverticulitis, supported by consistent radiological findings.

However, the abscess detected was refractory to conservative treatments and, when clinical signs worsened, the authors performed a laparotomy showing a scarring tissue attached to the abscess and to the lateral wall of the ascending colon, spreading to retroperitoneum. A right colectomy was performed together with the abscess resection. The histopathology revealed a desmoid tumor with negative surgical margins.

22.3.3 Obstruction

The invasion or the compression of the digestive tract results in stenosis of the lumen. Therefore, the occlusion can represent a possible clinical presentation of desmoid tumors regardless of tumor dimensions.

Several series were published concerning patients affected by AFP who received a previous surgery and had a diagnosis of desmoid tumors. The rates of bowel occlusion are very high, ranging from 27 to 58% [23–25].

Yalav et al. [15] recently published a case series of desmoid tumors operated on during 9 years. One patient presented with a bowel obstruction due to a 27 cm mass and required an extensive bowel resection. No recurrence was visible at a follow-up of 62 months confirming the efficacy of the up-front surgery in emergency setting. Unfortunately, no definitions of the resection's extension nor the quality of life after the resection were reported arising questions on the eventual short bowel syndrome that a young patient could bear after an aggressive surgery.

The obstruction can even be related to an extra-abdominal desmoid involving the bowel. Chen et al. [26] reported the case of a patient which presented with colonic obstruction due to a suspected colon cancer. The patient underwent an emergent laparotomy, which demonstrated a mass of around 5 cm involving the splenic flexure of the colon, invading the spleen and the left 11th and 12th ribs. The authors performed a left hemicolectomy with diversion ileostomy together with a wide excision of the left lateral chest wall tumor and removal of the left 11th and 12th ribs. The final histopathology showed a desmoid tumor arising from intercostal muscles. The surgical margins were not free from disease, and the authors concluded that the adopted emergent surgical resection was suboptimal.

22.3.4 Hemoperitoneum

The direct involvement of vessels, despite the small dimension of the tumors, can lead to an erosion and a massive bleeding. Georgiades et al. [27] reported in 2012 the case of a young patient presenting with hemorrhagic shock, which led to an emergent laparotomy revealing a small tumor (1.5 cm by 0.5 cm) strangulating the splenic artery. The authors performed a resection of the tumor en bloc with splenic artery. The pathology revealed the presence of a desmoid tumor entrapping part of the pancreas and the vessels.

22.3.5 Ascites

Both the perforation of hollow viscera and the rupture of a mesenteric desmoid can produce abundant ascites. The nature of the ascites can be hardly defined by the CT scan, mainly adopting the Hounsfield values.

Tan et al. [28] reported the emergent case of a patient presenting with acute abdomen, a mass involving the mesentery at CT scan and diffuse ascites. The emergency laparotomy revealed the perforation of the mass with abundant purulent ascites. The authors performed an extensive resection of the mass together with the bowel devascularized by the interruption of the mesentery.

22.3.6 Combined Presentations

In rare cases, the combination of different mechanisms leads to a clinical presentation, which can be confused with a different pathological condition. That was the case of an abdominal mass mimicking an acute appendicitis, which led to hemoperitoneum and peritonitis, described by Asenov et al. [12] in 2019. The mass consisted of cystic and solid areas, and it involved the jejunum and its mesentery and was adherent to ileocecal junction. The authors performed a toilette of the peritoneal cavity and a small bowel resection with negative margins. The final histopathology revealed a sporadic desmoid tumor.

As a result of multiple mechanisms, the presence of more than one complicated desmoid can generate a mixed presentation. Abdalla et al. [29] described the case of a patient who presented with acute abdomen, and a CT scanner revealed a double mass, one occluding the lumen and the other surrounded by free fluid. At exploratory laparotomy, one tumor was perforated while the other had completely invaded a small bowel segment. The histopathology performed on the double resection revealed the presence of two concomitant desmoid tumors.

22.4 Surgery

Desmoid tumor management is multidisciplinary including watch and wait, surgery, radiation, and chemotherapy [5]. Up-front surgery has been the first-line treatment for desmoid tumors until 2000. Many studies were published concerning the outcomes of surgery, and they showed a high rate of recurrence. Factors correlated to the recurrence were analyzed, and a prognostic nomogram was realized [30]. Thanks to these observations, the overall management of this disease changed, and the functional preservation became the predominant aim. The current surgical treatment is individualized, and it is aimed to reduce the local failure without losing an acceptable morbidity rate and without impairing the quality of life.

Furthermore, the observation that a high percentage of desmoid tumors can have a spontaneous regression further reduced the up-front surgery adoption while a watch-and-wait policy emerged [31].

The intimate relationship of desmoid tumors to the mesenteric vessels, their infiltration, and the potential subsequent hemorrhage have led towards a reluctance to surgical excision and the reliance on medical treatments. However, desmoid tumors can bear complications requiring emergency surgery: abscess formation, perforation, peritonitis, hemoperitoneum, and obstruction.

No indications exist regarding the extension of the resection to perform, and even if several papers assessed the imperative importance of a free microscopic margin while performing a desmoid tumor resection [32], no high-quality evidence is present in literature to determine the efficacy of a free margin in preventing a local recurrence. In a multivariate analysis performed on 495 elective cases, Crago et al. [30] found that age, tumor size, and tumor site were independent predictors of recurrence but margin status (R1 vs. R0) was not associated with worse outcomes. However, in the cohort of small tumors (diameter <5 cm), R0 resection was associated with longer local recurrence-free survival. The same association was not found for larger lesions.

Furthermore, there is no evidence regarding the extension of the free margin adopted and the risk of local control failure.

It is difficult to translate in an emergency setting the principles of elective surgery, but a stepwise approach is recommended taking into account both the life-threatening complication and the oncological evolution of the disease. The adoption of a damage control concept could be useful and could offer time to perform a definitive treatment. Firstly, the management of acute abdomen is imperative in order to control the life-threatening condition (mainly bleeding and contamination). When the underlying possible cause is identified in a desmoid tumor, a resection with negative gross margin should be performed. It is of primary importance to avoid the R2 surgical resections especially in a palliative context because the surgical injury itself results in further tumor progression. However, no extended resections are recommended due to the high recurrence rate of these tumors and the low quality of life resulting from massive resections (Table 22.1).

The absence of histopathology in emergency setting further complicates the clinical decision because of the wide spectrum of abdominal malignancies with common macroscopical features and clinical presentations, highlighting the need for a nonoperative management aimed to control the systemic condition and to postpone surgery with a preoperative planning, a histopathological diagnosis, and an adequate patient preparation.

Table 22.1 Principles of emergency surgery

Control the life-threatening condition
Perform a resection with negative gross margin but avoid extensive mutilating surgery
Reduce palliative resection (no R2)
Postpone the definitive surgery if extensive treatments are required
Adopt integrated approaches (interventional radiology, endoscopy)

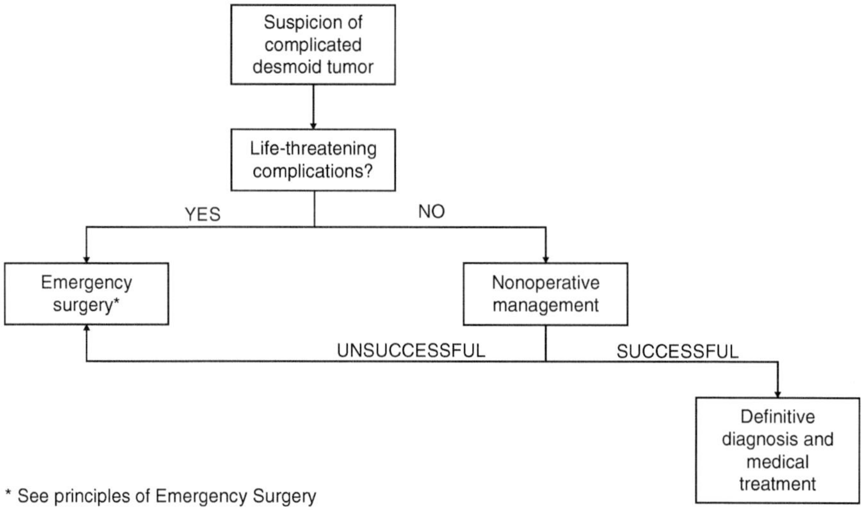

Fig. 22.1 Decisional flowchart

The nonoperative management does not exclude the surgical treatment, and it is part of the described stepwise approach. The level of attention should be high when a nonoperative management is adopted due to the high risk of clinical deterioration as described by Ong et al. [33] who reported the case of a patient with an acute abdomen and sepsis, approached with a nonoperative management. The authors started the diagnostic workup, which revealed a mass related to the jejunum. A biopsy was planned due to the initial clinical and biological improvement, but after 4 days of hospitalization, the patient worsened and an emergent laparotomy was required. A mass adherent to the jejunum together with an abscess cavity and free purulent fluid was found. The patient underwent a segmental intestinal resection, which revealed a desmoid tumor at histopathology. Unlike previous reports, no fistulas were found between the abscess and the bowel (Fig. 22.1).

22.5 Nonoperative Management

In an emergency context, patients often present with malnutrition, pain, sepsis, and hemorrhage, bearing a high surgical risk and a potential low survival rate.

The clinical scenario drives the nonoperative management, and life-threatening complications do not leave the opportunity to rule out differential diagnosis with imaging and histopathology.

However, not every acute clinical presentation of desmoid tumors should be treated with emergency surgery (Table 22.2).

Table 22.2 Principles of nonoperative management

Patient resuscitation
Patient surveillance (intensive care unit if necessary)
Antibiotic therapy
Pain control
Blood transfusion if necessary
Evaluation of the nutritional status and parenteral nutrition
Radiological drains if needed
Definitive diagnosis and proper medical/surgical management

Asare et al. [34] showed that no systematic approach nor guidelines exist for patients presenting in an emergency setting with soft tissue sarcoma-related complications. In a small cohort of 16 patients admitted from 1998 to 2018 at MD Anderson Cancer Center, the authors adopted a protocol made of antibiotic therapy, parenteral nutrition, and drain placement with the aim to avoid an emergent, nononcological resection. The results were encouraging with 75% of patients with ruptured or fistulized tumors, which were able to receive a preoperative chemotherapy or radiotherapy without facing an up-front emergency laparotomy.

Similarly, Alemanno et al. [35] discussed the current guidelines on desmoid tumors highlighting the absence of a well-defined indication in case of complications. Given the available evidence, a possible sequence in emergency setting could be the adoption of a nonoperative approach followed by surgery in case of complications (Fig. 22.1).

In a recent report, Tawada et al. [36] were in favor of nonoperative management even in case of a giant perforated desmoid tumor with acute peritonitis.

In case of abscesses and collections, percutaneous drainage is a feasible option when a desmoid tumor is suspected or when the desmoid tumor is in the differential diagnosis list. One of the first experiences of nonoperative treatment was reported in 1995 by Maldjian et al. [17] who demonstrated that in patients affected by Gardner's syndrome, percutaneous drainage, associated with antibiotic therapy, results in clinical improvement. In two out of three patients, the authors were able to visualize the presence of a fistula between the small bowel and the desmoid mass, thus helping the preoperative planning.

Furthermore, the skepticism associated with the drainage of desmoid tumor abscesses, collections, or purulent ascites due to the fear of cancer seeding does not find a place in literature [34].

As stated before, the failure of nonoperative management can determine the need for an emergent surgery. Huang et al. [37] reported the case of a patient diagnosed with a desmoid tumor of the mesentery, which received multiple drainage placement due to the presence of an intratumoral abscess and, after the multiple failure to control the sepsis, was operated on.

References

1. World Health Organization. Soft tissue and bone tumours. 5th ed. Geneva: OMS; 2020.
2. National Comprehensive Cancer Network. Soft tissue sarcoma. 2021. https://www.nccn.org/professionals/physician_gls/pdf/sarcoma.pdf.
3. MacFarlane J. Clinical reports of the surgical practice of the Glasgow Royal Infirmary. Med Chir Rev. 1833;18:126–35.
4. Bertani E, Testori A, Chiappa A, et al. Recurrence and prognostic factors in patients with aggressive fibromatosis. The role of radical surgery and its limitations. World J Surg Onc. 2012;10:184.
5. Ganeshan D, Amini B, Nikolaidis P, Assing M, Vikram R. Current update on Desmoid fibromatosis. J Comput Assist Tomogr. 2019;43:29–38.
6. Alman B, Attia S, Baumgarten C, et al. The management of desmoid tumours: a joint global consensus-based guideline approach for adult and paediatric patients. Eur J Cancer. 2020;127:96–107.
7. Sanchez-Mete L, Ferraresi V, Caterino M, Martayan A, Terrenato I, Mannisi E, Stigliano V. Desmoid tumors characteristics, clinical management, active surveillance, and description of our FAP case series. JCMM. 2020;9:4012.
8. Clark SK, Smith TG, Katz DE, Reznek RH, Phillips RK. Identification and progression of a desmoid precursor lesion in patients with familial adenomatous polyposis. Br J Surg. 1998;85:970–3.
9. Turina M, Pavlik CM, Heinimann K, Behrensmeier F, Simmen H-P. Recurrent desmoids determine outcome in patients with Gardner syndrome: a cohort study of three generations of an APC mutation-positive family across 30 years. Int J Color Dis. 2013;28:865–72.
10. Sakorafas GH, Nissotakis C, Peros G. Abdominal desmoid tumors. Surg Oncol. 2007;16:131–42.
11. Azizi L, Balu M, Belkacem A, Lewin M, Tubiana J-M, Arrivé L. MRI features of mesenteric desmoid tumors in familial adenomatous polyposis. Am J Roentgenol. 2005;184:1128–35.
12. Asenov Y, Genadiev S, Timev A, Panaiotova J, Hadjiiska V, Veselin T, Sedloev T. Ruptured desmoid tumor imitating acute appendicitis—a rare reason for an emergency surgery. BMC Surg. 2019;19:194.
13. Ophir G, Sivan S, Hana S, et al. Abdominal desmoid: course, severe outcomes, and unique genetic background in a large local series. Cancer. 2021;13:3673.
14. Shah IA, Toor SA, Gerogiannis I. A rare case of desmoid fibromatosis of the transverse colon mimicking a perforated malignancy. Oxf Med Case Reports. 2021;2021:omab031.
15. Yalav O, Erdogan O, Teke Z, Doran F. Primary mesenteric fibromatosis: a single center experience. Ann Ital Chir. 2020;91:283–90.
16. Li W, Zhou Y, Li Q, Tong H, Lu W. Intestinal perforation during chemotherapeutic treatment of intra-abdominal desmoid tumor in patients with Gardner's syndrome: report of two cases. World J Surg Onc. 2016;14:178.
17. Maldjian C, Mitty H, Garten A, Forman W. Abscess formation in desmoid tumors of Gardner's syndrome and percutaneous drainage: a report of three cases. Cardiovasc Intervent Radiol. 1995;18:168. https://doi.org/10.1007/BF00204144.
18. Cholongitas E, Koulenti D, Panetsos G, Kafiri G, Tzirakis E, Thalasinou P, Papatheodoridis GV. Desmoid tumor presenting as intra-abdominal abscess. Dig Dis Sci. 2006;51:68–9.
19. Jain P, Shah P, Bhansali M. Unusual presentation of an uncommon abdominal pathology. Ann R Coll Surg Engl. 2010;92:e19–21.
20. Haddad J, Alam H, Keriakos K, Azzi M. Reporting an unusual case of mesenteric desmoid tumor. J Med Liban. 2012;60:176–81.
21. Bellamy F, Gunawardene A, Osipov V, Aljanabi I. Intra-abdominal desmoid tumour presenting as an acute abdomen. ANZ J Surg. 2019;89:1654–5.
22. Omori S, Ito S, Kimura K, et al. Intra-abdominal Desmoid-type fibromatosis mimicking diverticulitis with abscess: a case report. In Vivo. 2021;35:1151–5.

23. Clark SK, Neale KF, Landgrebe JC, Phillips RK. Desmoid tumours complicating familial adenomatous polyposis. Br J Surg. 1999;86:1185–9.
24. Soravia C, Berk T, McLeod RS, Cohen Z. Desmoid disease in patients with familial adenomatous polyposis. Dis Colon Rectum. 2000;43:363–9.
25. Xhaja X, Church J. Small bowel obstruction in patients with familial adenomatous polyposis related desmoid disease. Color Dis. 2013;15:1489–92.
26. Chen C-I, Sun C-K. Desmoid fibromatosis of intercostal muscle causing colonic obstruction: a case report and literature review. Int J Color Dis. 2016;31:1047–8.
27. Georgiades C, Vallianou N, Argyrakos T, Aristodimou A, Kolovelonis G, Sioula E. An unusual case of desmoid tumour presenting as haemorrhagic shock. Ann R Coll Surg Engl. 2012;94:e81–2.
28. Tan KK, Yan Z, Liau KH. Emergency surgery for a ruptured intra-abdominal desmoid tumour. Ann Acad Med Singap. 2010;39:497–8.
29. Abdalla S, Wilkinson M, Wilsher M, Uzkalnis A. An atypical presentation of small bowel obstruction and perforation secondary to sporadic synchronous intra-abdominal desmoid tumours. Int J Surg Case Rep. 2016;20:147–50.
30. Crago AM, Denton B, Salas S, Dufresne A, Mezhir JJ, Hameed M, Gonen M, Singer S, Brennan MF. A prognostic nomogram for prediction of recurrence in Desmoid fibromatosis. Ann Surg. 2013;258:347–53.
31. Kasper B, Baumgarten C, Garcia J, et al. An update on the management of sporadic desmoid-type fibromatosis: a European consensus initiative between sarcoma PAtients EuroNet (SPAEN) and European Organization for Research and Treatment of cancer (EORTC)/soft tissue and bone sarcoma group (STBSG). Ann Oncol. 2017;28:2399–408.
32. Harati K, Jaenisch A, Behr B, Goertz O, Harati A, Hirsch T, Stricker I, Lehnhardt M, Daigeler A. Effect of surgical margins on prognosis in aggressive fibromatosis: a single-institutional analysis of 90 patients. Oncol Lett. 2017;14:5129. https://doi.org/10.3892/ol.2017.6864.
33. Ong F, Aziz F, Fedorine S. Rare case of mesenteric fibromatosis (desmoid tumour) associated with an acute abdomen and sepsis. ANZ J Surg. 2021;91:1298–300.
34. Asare EA, Davis CH, Chiang Y, Sabir S, Rajkot NF, Phillips PR, Roland CL, Torres KE, Hunt KK, Feig BW. Management and outcomes of ruptured, perforated or fistulized tumors of mesenchymal origin. J Surg Oncol. 2020;121:474–9.
35. Alemanno G, Zambonin D, Sturiale A, Cavalli T, Bellucci F, Pesi B, Di Martino C, Giudici F, Tonelli F. A multidisciplinary approach to desmoid tumors. When intra-abdominal fibromatosis degenerates into an abscess, which is the right treatment? Int J Surg Case Rep. 2013;4:757–60.
36. Tawada M, Misao Y, Sugimoto T, Tanaka H. Ruptured mesenteric desmoid-type fibromatosis without emergency surgery: a rare case report. Int J Surg Case Rep. 2021;85:106208.
37. Huang K, Stuart H, Lyapichev K, Rosenberg AE, Livingstone AS. Mesenteric desmoid tumour presenting with recurrent abdominal abscess and duodenal fistula: a case report and review of literature. Int J Surg Case Rep. 2017;37:119–23.

23 Surgical Emergencies in Cancer Surgeries: Sarcoma

Tyler J. Mouw and Robert D. Winfield

23.1 Introduction

Soft tissue sarcoma (STS) is a broad term which is commonly used to describe a family of neoplastic processes encompassing upwards of 60 distinct histologies, which can have varied clinical courses in terms of aggressiveness, local control, and metastatic potential. In general, these are rare clinical entities which comprise fewer than 1% of all cancers [1]. The histologies most likely to be encountered are liposarcoma, leiomyosarcoma, and pleomorphic sarcoma, and these span the continuum with respect to behavior and patterns of spread. While tumor histology can be associated with specific distributions or body locations, it is possible for these to arise in any area of the body. For surgeons, it is most useful to organize sarcomas into two broad groups consisting of extremity or trunk (specifically the abdominal wall) sarcomas and retroperitoneal (RP) or intra-abdominal sarcomas, as these categorizations can have implications in oncologic management and treatment sequencing that may impact presentations or decision-making in an emergent setting. For the purposes of this chapter, soft tissue sarcomas will be discussed using these broad categorizations. In general, surgical emergencies caused by sarcomas are rare. When they do occur, they tend to follow the same pattern of presentations involving hemorrhage, obstruction, infection, or perforation that may prompt any surgeon to operate emergently. We will discuss issues arising from the primary tumor and those arising from treatment complications/morbidity separately in this chapter.

T. J. Mouw
Department of Surgery, Texas Tech University Health Sciences Center, Lubbock, TX, USA
e-mail: tyler.mouw@ttuhsc.edu

R. D. Winfield (✉)
Department of Surgery, University of Kansas Medical Center, Kansas City, KS, USA
e-mail: rwinfield@kumc.edu

A. Tarasconi et al. (eds.), *Oncologic Surgical Emergencies*, Hot Topics in Acute Care Surgery and Trauma, https://doi.org/10.1007/978-3-031-36860-8_23

23.2 Extremity Sarcoma

STS most commonly arises in the extremities, comprising as much as 60% of sarcoma cases [2]. Given the similarities to bony sarcomas, surgical management of extremity STS across the United States is most often shared between subspecialties of general surgery and orthopedic surgery. The oncologic management of extremity sarcoma has evolved over time. Where radical resections and amputations were once mainstay approaches, limb salvage has become the standard of care when possible [3]. Histologies commonly encountered in the extremities include liposarcoma and what are referred to as the "SCARE" sarcomas (synovial sarcoma, clear cell sarcoma, angiosarcoma, rhabdomyosarcoma, and epithelioid sarcoma). The "SCARE" sarcomas are notable primarily because of an increased propensity for lymphatic patterns of metastases, which may warrant surgical staging or therapeutic dissection of nodal basins [4]; however, the exact role of sentinel node biopsy and nodal dissection in these cancers is still a topic of investigation. The primary prognostic factor in extremity sarcoma is tumor grade. Low-grade tumors are primarily well-differentiated liposarcomas which have little to no metastatic potential, while higher grade sarcomas, including dedifferentiated liposarcomas and other histologies, should be worked up for metastatic disease prior to invasive testing or intervention. The mainstay of treatment is surgical resection to negative margins. Local control can be augmented with radiation therapy (XRT). In general, preoperative RT is preferred as targeting the tumor margins directly results in a more focal treatment area as opposed to irradiating a post-resection bed. This can be particularly useful with tumors near joints, as the joints can be particularly sensitive to radiation toxicity. While the variability in histologies and locations makes it difficult to succinctly describe the likelihood of surgical emergencies associated with extremity STS, these tumors tend to be space occupying rather than infiltrative and rarely present as the causative factor in a patient requiring emergent surgical intervention. Many emergent and urgent presentations have been described in limited case series only.

23.2.1 Extremity Sarcoma: Tumor-Related Emergencies

Extremity STS will typically arise from tissues of fat, muscle, nerve sheath, or vascular origin. The tissue of origin may have specific implications for the presentation and may alter the likelihood of emergent presentations. However, these tumors are most frequently diagnosed due to the presence of a painless mass in the extremity.

23.2.1.1 Hemorrhage

Although rare, extremity STS may initially present with hemorrhage. Whereas most extremity STS will present as a painless mass, hemorrhage may be associated with pain and more abrupt swelling as opposed to classic presentations [5, 6]. In most cases, hemorrhage is self-limiting as the tumor capsule and extremity compartments will contain the bleed [7]. One concern worth mentioning is that hemorrhagic sarcomas can be misdiagnosed as simple hematomas, which may delay definitive diagnosis by several months [5–7]. Follow-up imaging is important, especially for patients who present with spontaneous bleeds who otherwise have few hemorrhagic risk factors.

For cutaneous sarcomas or any tumor which has been neglected and allowed to erode through the skin, ongoing or uncontrolled hemorrhage may be encountered. If the situation allows, stabilization of the patient and transfer to a center with subspecialty expertise are always advised. If surgery due to continued bleeding is warranted, MRI is a useful tool to delineate tumor margins to allow for a complete resection. The decision to operate should consider the morbidity of the resection based on tumor size and location. This should be weighed against standard wound management techniques based on the volume of hemorrhage.

23.2.1.2 Obstruction

Tumor growth or lymphatic metastasis may impinge venous or lymphatic outflow resulting in obstruction. Although rare, cases of extremity compartment syndrome and so-called "pseudocompartment syndrome" due to sarcoma have been reported [8, 9]. While prompt decompression may be undertaken, in cases of presumed compartment syndrome with an atypical presentation (absence of trauma or vascular insufficiency) or intraoperative findings (abnormal appearance of the musculature on fascial decompression), sarcoma may be considered in the differential diagnosis. Problematic lymphedema may also develop; however, this tends to be insidious and chronic in nature.

23.2.2 Extremity Sarcoma: Treatment-Related Emergencies

For high-grade tumors, and those near to sensitive structures such as nerves or joints, preoperative radiotherapy is preferred. The efficacy of systemic therapies is somewhat limited for most sarcomas and therefore surgical resection is the mainstay of treatment, with radiotherapy used primarily to augment local control. Emergencies arising from the management of sarcomas include issues that arise during the diagnostic workup as well as anticipated complications associated with resection.

23.2.2.1 Hemorrhagic

Significant bleeds are a concern following STS resection, as tumors can commonly involve major neurovascular structures. Significant bleeds requiring transfusion were noted in as many as 16% of extremity STS cases in a large National Surgical Quality Improvement Program (NSQIP) study [10].

Bleeding associated with the workup of soft tissue masses may lead to scenarios where emergent intervention is warranted. Surgical dogma has suggested that histologies such as angiosarcoma should not be biopsied out of concern for causing hemorrhage. Case reports of this complication specific to extremity sarcoma are rare. The current sarcoma guidelines do support biopsy irrespective of histology subtype. Consideration can be made to perform fine needle aspiration rather than core biopsy if a concern for bleeding exists; however, this technique may underestimate tumor grade [3].

23.2.2.2 Infectious

On rare occasion, treatment effect may result in a large burden of necrotic tumor, which could become infected and present with sepsis. In such cases, management is not dictated by the presence of tumor and the standard approaches of resuscitation and source control should be followed. This may include debridement of dead tumor, and this should be performed just as with debridement of other necrotic tissue (e.g., until viable tissue is encountered).

23.3 Retroperitoneal Sarcoma

Retroperitoneal (RP) sarcoma as a term usually describes any sarcoma deep to the abdominal fascia—as distinct from superficial trunk sarcomas, which are typically managed with a similar strategy to extremity sarcoma. These tumors include a number of different histologies but are most commonly well-differentiated or dedifferentiated liposarcoma and leiomyosarcoma. Because of the relatively few anatomical boundaries in the retroperitoneum, these tumors can often silently grow massive prior to becoming clinically evident. In the elective setting, the mainstay of management is to achieve an R0 (microscopic negative) resection, which is not always feasible given tumor size and adjacency to vital structures. Liposarcomas can progress along a continuum from well differentiated to dedifferentiated. Well-differentiated liposarcoma will typically appear on axial imaging to have the same density or signal as abdominal fat. Multiple septations or areas with a more solid component raise concerns for a dedifferentiated component to the tumor. Positive resection margins in large well-differentiated liposarcomas are common and frequently unavoidable even with an aggressive resection strategy. Well-differentiated liposarcomas have no metastatic potential but do tend to recur locally. Only poorly differentiated sarcomas, including other histologies along with dedifferentiated liposarcoma, have the potential to metastasize. For this reason, it is the practice at many centers to reserve aggressive en bloc resection of adjacent organs only for areas with concern for dedifferentiation. If there is any concern for dedifferentiation or the presence of a poorly differentiated sarcoma, staging imaging should be obtained if possible as this may inform the goals of an emergent operation. Intraoperative frozen section has limited utility, and this can vary with different histologies. It is not helpful in well-differentiated frozen section as the freezing process disrupts tissue to a problematic degree. With solid tumors, frozen section may not clearly differentiate between tumor and stromal or desmoplastic responses with atypia. For this reason, aggressive en bloc resection is typically pursued when feasible.

23.3.1 RP Sarcoma: Tumor-Related Emergencies

Because of the typical slow-growing behavior of well-differentiated liposarcoma and the lack of a confined space in the retroperitoneum, it is uncommon for RP sarcomas to present emergently. When they do, obstruction is the most likely presentation. This is more likely when the tumor is centered within the bowel mesentery as tumors arising posterior to the peritoneal compartment will typically push organs away as they grow. Management of complete obstruction should follow the tenets detailed above. In the acute setting and for well-differentiated tumors, an aggressive approach with en bloc resection of adjacent organs may result in undue morbidity without significantly changing the likelihood of durable local control. Therefore, a mitigating approach with diversion or limited resection may be appropriate based on the level of obstruction. En bloc resection of organs involved with poorly differentiated tumors is appropriate.

Non-bowel obstructive symptoms may be more commonly encountered by general surgeons. Ureteral obstruction has also been described [11]. In these cases, ureteral stenting or diversion with percutaneous nephrostomy tube placement should be prioritized to manage the acute issue and allow for elective surgical management of the tumor. Vascular obstruction can also occur with retroperitoneal sarcomas. This is particularly true for leiomyosarcomas, which can arise from the muscular layers of large central vessels [12–14]. In general, venous occlusive disease does not require emergent operative intervention as the venous system has time to compensate with collateralization around the growing mass.

On rare occasion, sarcomas have been reported as the primary cause of intestinal perforation [15]. Management in these patients should adhere to the general principles of supportive care, adequate resuscitation, and source control that one would employ in other causes of perforation. It should be understood that it may not be possible to safely remove the offending tumor at the initial intervention, and so securing enteral access for nutritional support is a priority.

23.3.2 RP Sarcoma: Treatment-Related Emergencies

Sarcomatosis is the wide distribution of sarcoma tumors throughout the abdominal cavity. Surgical violation or spontaneous rupture of the tumor is named a risk factor for this presentation, and as such, it is important to avoid fracturing the tumor capsule, which may result in peritoneal seeding. The primary downstream sequela of this complication which may present emergently is obstruction. The definitive management of this entity in highly selected patients is complete cytoreduction [16]. For the general surgeon who encounters such a patient presenting with obstruction, the initial management should be conservative with bowel rest and resuscitation. If operative intervention is required due to failure to improve or signs of clinical deterioration, we recommend simple bowel excisions or bypass procedures to minimize morbidity while addressing the acute issue. Cytoreduction in the setting of an acutely ill patient is only reasonable with minimal disease that would otherwise be removed with the necessary bowel resections.

Treatment-related emergencies for RP sarcomas are primarily due to the use of XRT. The recent publication of the "Surgery With or Without Radiation Therapy in Untreated Nonmetastatic Retroperitoneal Sarcoma" (STRASS) trial [17] is expected to change the treatment landscape of retroperitoneal sarcoma. This trial randomized patients to surgery with or without preoperative XRT. Their results showed no difference in survival with a trend toward worsened perioperative morbidity and the possibility of preoperative morbidity in the radiotherapy group. As such, routine use of neoadjuvant radiotherapy is no longer recommended for RP sarcoma. Even in selective use, abdominal radiotherapy predisposes patients to visceral fistula formation, stenosis, and abdominal abscesses. Review of the radiation fields or discussion with a radiation oncologist may be warranted before approaching these issues to gain an appreciation of the scope of the effected tissues. Radiation-related complications are unlikely to require heroic measures to obtain adequate source control or to relieve obstruction, so temporizing measures are reasonable if there is any uncertainty about the extent of radiation-exposed tissues. As with other abdominal complications, the placement of feeding access should be strongly considered if any operative intervention is undertaken.

23.4 Summary

Surgical emergencies due to acute presentations of sarcomas or issues resulting from prior therapy are relatively rare in nature. At times, a high index of suspicion will be required to identify sarcoma as the underlying cause of the disease state seen, and general surgeons should be aware of specific management considerations in these cases to include the roles of intraoperative biopsy, en bloc resections, and tumor debulking. Most often, standard principles of surgical management will suffice in the acute management of these patients, while subsequent multidisciplinary oncologic care can be initiated following stabilization.

References

1. Mastrangelo G, Coindre JM, Ducimetiere F, Dei Tos AP, Fadda E, Blay JY, Buja A, Fedeli U, Cegolon L, Frasson A, Ranchere-Vince D, Montesco C, Ray-Coquard I, Rossi CR. Incidence of soft tissue sarcoma and beyond: a population-based prospective study in 3 European regions. Cancer. 2012;118(21):5339–48. https://doi.org/10.1002/cncr.27555.
2. Puri A, Gulia A. Management of extremity soft tissue sarcomas. Indian J Orthop. 2011;45(4):301–6. https://doi.org/10.4103/0019-5413.82332.
3. Network NCC. Soft tissue sarcoma. National Comprehensive Cancer Network. 2021. https://www.nccn.org/professionals/physician_gls/pdf/sarcoma.pdf. Accessed 28 Jan.
4. Maduekwe UN, Herb JN, Esther RJ, Kim HJ, Spanheimer PM. Pathologic nodal staging for clinically node negative soft tissue sarcoma of the extremities. J Surg Oncol. 2021;123(8):1792–800. https://doi.org/10.1002/jso.26465.

5. Mann HA, Hilton A, Goddard NJ, Smith MA, Holloway B, Lee CA. Synovial sarcoma mimicking haemophilic pseudotumour. Sarcoma. 2006;2006:27212. https://doi.org/10.1155/SRCM/2006/27212.
6. Naito N, Ozaki T, Kunisada T, Kawai A, Dan'ura T, Morimoto Y, Inoue H. Synovial sarcoma with a large hematoma in the inguinal region. Arch Orthop Trauma Surg. 2000;120(9):533–4. https://doi.org/10.1007/s004029900109.
7. Ward WG Sr, Rougraff B, Quinn R, Damron T, O'Connor MI, Turcotte RE, Cline M. Tumors masquerading as hematomas. Clin Orthop Relat Res. 2007;465:232–40. https://doi.org/10.1097/BLO.0b013e31815953a7.
8. Marlborough F, V. R. Lower extremity sarcoma mimicking acute compartment syndrome. JPRAS Open. 2015;3:29–34. https://doi.org/10.1016/j.jpra.2015.02.003.
9. Scheipl S, Leithner A, Radl R, Beham-Schmid C, Ranner G, Linkesch W, Windhager R. Myeloid sarcoma presenting in muscle-tissue of the lower limb: unusual origin of a compartment-syndrome. Am J Clin Oncol. 2007;30(6):658–9. https://doi.org/10.1097/01.coc.0000189704.33839.f9.
10. Gallaway KE, Ahn J, Callan AK. Thirty-day outcomes after surgery for primary sarcomas of the extremities: an analysis of the NSQIP database. J Oncol. 2020;2020:7282846. https://doi.org/10.1155/2020/7282846.
11. Squires MH, Ethun CG, Donahue EE, Benbow JH, Anderson CJ, Jagosky MH, Salo JC, Hill JS, Ahrens W, Prabhu RS, Livingston MB, Gower NL, Needham M, Trufan SJ, Fields RC, Krasnick BA, Bedi M, Abbott DE, Schwartz P, Votanopoulos K, Chouliaras K, Grignol V, Roggin KK, Tseng J, Poultsides G, Tran TB, Cardona K, Howard JH. A multi-institutional validation study of prognostic nomograms for retroperitoneal sarcoma. J Surg Oncol. 2021;124(5):829–37. https://doi.org/10.1002/jso.26586.
12. Chiu WHK, Lo AW, Lee JK. Leiomyosarcoma of the portal vein: a case report and review of the literature. BJR Case Rep. 2017;3(2):20160125. https://doi.org/10.1259/bjrcr.20160125.
13. Kieffer E, Alaoui M, Piette JC, Cacoub P, Chiche L. Leiomyosarcoma of the inferior vena cava: experience in 22 cases. Ann Surg. 2006;244(2):289–95. https://doi.org/10.1097/01.sla.0000229964.71743.db.
14. Oliveira N, Dias E, Lima R, Oliveira F, Cassio I. Primary iliac venous leiomyosarcoma: a rare cause of deep vein thrombosis in a young patient. Case Rep Med. 2011;2011:123041. https://doi.org/10.1155/2011/123041.
15. Kopplin L, Kim J. Retroperitoneal sarcoma: a rare cause of intestinal perforation in two cases. J Surg Case Rep. 2011;2011(5):3. https://doi.org/10.1093/jscr/2011.5.3.
16. Bonvalot S, Cavalcanti A, Le Pechoux C, Terrier P, Vanel D, Blay JY, Le Cesne A, Elias D. Randomized trial of cytoreduction followed by intraperitoneal chemotherapy versus cytoreduction alone in patients with peritoneal sarcomatosis. Eur J Surg Oncol. 2005;31(8):917–23. https://doi.org/10.1016/j.ejso.2005.04.010.
17. Bonvalot S, Gronchi A, Le Pechoux C, Swallow CJ, Strauss D, Meeus P, van Coevorden F, Stoldt S, Stoeckle E, Rutkowski P, Rastrelli M, Raut CP, Hompes D, De Paoli A, Sangalli C, Honore C, Chung P, Miah A, Blay JY, Fiore M, Stelmes JJ, Dei Tos AP, Baldini EH, Litiere S, Marreaud S, Gelderblom H, Haas RL. Preoperative radiotherapy plus surgery versus surgery alone for patients with primary retroperitoneal sarcoma (EORTC-62092: STRASS): a multicentre, open-label, randomised, phase 3 trial. Lancet Oncol. 2020;21(10):1366–77. https://doi.org/10.1016/S1470-2045(20)30446-0.

Miscellaneous Rare Malignancies: Pseudomyxoma Peritonei

24

Jingjing Yu, Brittany G. Sullivan, Lourdes Swentek, and Maheswari Senthil

24.1 Introduction

Pseudomyxoma peritonei (PMP) is commonly used to describe mucinous ascites and peritoneal implants, often from a ruptured appendiceal mucinous tumor [1]. Although the term PMP represents a clinical syndrome, it is nonspecific as it fails to distinguish between peritoneal dissemination from a mucinous adenocarcinoma or from that of a mucinous neoplasm. Since management and prognosis of mucinous peritoneal dissemination vary widely based on the nature of the primary tumor and type of peritoneal dissemination, it is crucially important to avoid describing this condition as merely PMP. Mucinous peritoneal dissemination commonly arises from ruptured appendiceal mucinous neoplasms (AMNs) and occasionally from mucinous neoplasms of ovary, colon, urachus, and pancreas [2]. In this chapter, we provide a detailed description of the current nomenclature of AMNs and PMP, common clinical presentations, and management.

24.2 Epidemiology

AMNs are rare and make up <1% of gastrointestinal cancers in the United States [3] with roughly 1500 cases diagnosed annually [3]. Incidence of these tumors is 0.12 cases per one million persons per year [4]. Furthermore, AMN is diagnosed

J. Yu · B. G. Sullivan · M. Senthil (✉)
Division of Surgical Oncology, Department of Surgery, University of California Irvine Medical Center, Orange, CA, USA
e-mail: jingjiy7@hs.uci.edu; bgsulliv@hs.uci.edu; maheswas@hs.uci.edu

L. Swentek
Division of Trauma and Critical Care Surgery, Department of Surgery, University of California Irvine Medical Center, Orange, CA, USA
e-mail: lyrobles@hs.uci.edu

A. Tarasconi et al. (eds.), *Oncologic Surgical Emergencies*, Hot Topics in Acute Care Surgery and Trauma, https://doi.org/10.1007/978-3-031-36860-8_24

incidentally in 0.2–0.3% of all appendectomy specimens [5]. In a Surveillance, Epidemiology, and End Results (SEER) program study, women accounted for 55% of the appendiceal tumor population and the majority were Caucasian patients (75%) [4]. Over the last four decades, the overall incidence of AMNs has increased along with a decrease in age at diagnosis [4]. Although the majority of AMNs are diagnosed after peritoneal dissemination, they generally have better prognosis than colorectal peritoneal carcinomatosis [4].

24.3 Classification of Appendiceal Mucinous Neoplasms

AMNs represent a heterogenous group of neoplasms with various malignant potential. Until recently, the terminology and classification of AMNs had been widely inconsistent, resulting in significant confusion in reporting and management. Since histologic differentiation significantly influences the prognosis, a classification system that allows for clear delineation of biologic behavior is essential to guide management.

In 2016, the Peritoneal Surface Oncology Group International (PSOGI) published a new consensus for the classification of AMN using a modified Delphi process [2] (Table 24.1). Within this classification system, mucinous appendiceal tumors without evidence of infiltrative invasion are classified as either low-grade or high-grade appendiceal mucinous neoplasm (LAMN or HAMN) based on the absence or presence of high-grade cellular atypia. Mucinous tumors of the appendix that show infiltrative invasion are categorized as mucinous adenocarcinomas of the appendix and can be further grouped as well, moderately, or poorly differentiated.

Table 24.1 Classification of mucinous neoplasms of the appendix adapted from PSOGI Consensus

Terminology	Histologic features
Low-grade appendiceal mucinous neoplasm (LAMN)	Mucinous neoplasm with low-grade cytology: – Loss of muscularis mucosa – Fibrosis of submucosa – Pushing invasion or expansile, diverticulum-like growth – Dissection of acellular mucin in wall – Mucin and/or cells outside of appendix
High-grade appendiceal mucinous neoplasm (HAMN)	Mucinous neoplasm with architectural features of LAMN with high-grade cytology but no infiltrative invasion
Mucinous adenocarcinoma: – Well differentiated – Moderately differentiated – Poorly differentiated	Mucinous neoplasm with infiltrative invasion: – Tumor budding – Small, irregular glands – Activated fibroblasts/myofibroblasts with vesicular nuclei
Poorly differentiated mucinous adenocarcinoma with signet ring cells	Mucinous neoplasm with <50% signet ring cells
Mucinous signet ring cell carcinoma	Mucinous neoplasm with >50% signet ring cells

Of note, signet ring cells seen on histology automatically confer a poor prognosis and are considered poorly differentiated [2]. Acknowledging the negative impact of the signet ring component on prognosis, the categorization of mucinous adenocarcinoma of the appendix is further divided into mucinous adenocarcinoma with signet ring cells if the tumor is composed of <50% signet ring cells and mucinous signet ring cell carcinoma if the tumor is composed of >50% signet ring cells.

24.4 Pathophysiology of PMP

When mucinous appendiceal tumors rupture, mucin and epithelial tumor cells are released into the intraperitoneal space and float freely in the peritoneal fluid. Peritoneal mucinous disease spreads as a result of physiologic flow of intraperitoneal fluid and gravity, also known as the redistribution phenomenon [6, 7]. Gravity causes the fluid to collect in the pelvis, allowing tumor cells to accumulate in the rectovesical pouch or the pouch of Douglas. Negative pressure created by respiration causes fluid to move along the right paracolic gutter toward the right hemidiaphragm and be absorbed by the lymphoid lacunae and lymphoid aggregates. As a result of this distribution and absorption, the pelvis, paracolic gutters, diaphragm, and greater and lesser omentum become the most common sites of peritoneal disease. Parts of the bowel that are anchored to the retroperitoneum (rectosigmoid colon, ileocecal valve, and pylorus) are also more heavily involved compared to areas of the small bowel and its mesentery, which are more mobile [6]. It is important for surgeons to understand the commonly affected sites to ensure visualization of these areas during exploration.

24.5 Classification of PMP

Histologic classification of PMP is prognostically significant. The current classification of PMP was also developed via a modified Delphi process sponsored by PSOGI and includes four groups (Table 24.2) [2]. LAMN- and HAMN-associated

Table 24.2 Classification of PMP adapted from PSOGI Consensus

Terminology	Histological features
Acellular mucin	Mucin in peritoneal cavity without neoplastic cells
Low-grade mucinous carcinoma peritonei OR disseminated peritoneal adenomucinosis (DPAM)	Low cellularity, minimal cytological atypia, no infiltrative growth
High-grade mucinous carcinoma peritonei OR peritoneal mucinous carcinomatosis (PMCA)	High cellularity, high-grade cytological atypia, with infiltrative growth
High-grade mucinous carcinoma peritonei with signet ring cells OR peritoneal mucinous carcinomatosis with signet ring cells (PMCA-S)	Any lesion with signet ring cells

peritoneal disseminations are typically either acellular mucin or diffuse peritoneal adenomucinosis (DPAM). Although the term low-grade mucinous carcinoma peritonei is interchangeably used with DPAM, the word carcinoma is misleading as these are not invasive cancers. Peritoneal mucinous carcinomatosis (PMCA) is a result of dissemination from mucinous adenocarcinoma. Tumors with signet ring cells are classified separately from other high-grade lesions because of their worse prognosis [2, 8].

24.6 Clinical Presentation

AMNs can present with varied signs and symptoms based on the extent of disease. Since the mucinous lesion in the appendix usually grows slowly, patients commonly remain asymptomatic and present often after rupture of the tumor with peritoneal dissemination. When the tumor ruptures, patients usually do not recall associated abdominal pain. As disease progresses and mucin accumulates, patients may develop vague abdominal symptoms and bloating. Eventually, in advanced cases, patients can experience abdominal pain, palpable masses, bowel obstruction, and weight loss [1].

Given the lack of specific symptoms and signs, most patients are diagnosed incidentally by cross-sectional imaging or at the time of laparoscopy/laparotomy for other medical conditions [1]. In a few rare occasions, AMNs are diagnosed prior to rupture (Fig. 24.1). In a retrospective study by Shariff et al., that evaluated the mode of presentation of 1070 patients with perforated epithelial appendiceal tumors and PMP, 30.3% of patients presented with abnormality on cross-sectional imaging and 16.8% of patients were diagnosed incidentally at the time of surgery [9]. Other modes of presentation included acute appendicitis (19%), ovarian mass (19.2% of women), and new onset of a hernia (9.9%).

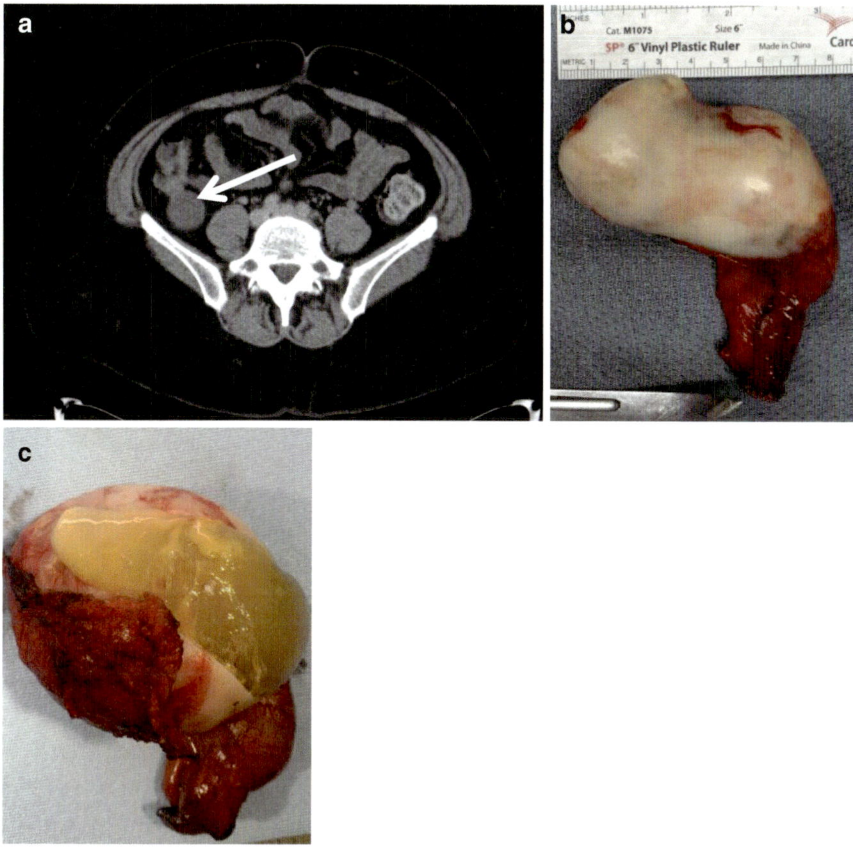

Fig. 24.1 Unruptured appendiceal mass. (**a**) Cross-sectional CT imaging of unruptured appendiceal mass (white arrow). (**b**, **c**) Gross specimen of unruptured LAMN with intraluminal mucin found once the appendix was dissected open

24.7 Evaluation and Management

24.7.1 Localized AMNs

Since AMNs can present as appendicitis, general surgeons may encounter them during surgical exploration for appendectomy. Evaluation of the appendix for signs of serosal perforation and evidence of extra-appendiceal mucin should be performed and documented. Extreme care should be taken to avoid rupture of the tumor during surgical manipulation [1]. Unruptured LAMNs and HAMNs can be managed with simple appendectomy when feasible as they are not associated with lymph node metastasis (Fig. 24.1). Additional colon resection may be necessary if the proximal margin is positive for mucin. If postoperative pathology shows evidence of adenocarcinoma, a right hemicolectomy is indicated for appropriate lymph node staging

[10]. In a large retrospective study of stage I–III mucinous appendiceal cancers, lymph node metastasis was detected in 21.1% of patients; higher grade (moderately differentiated: OR 2.16, $p < 0.0001$; poorly or undifferentiated: OR 3.07, $p < 0.0001$) and lymphovascular invasion (OR 7.28, $p < 0.0001$) were independent predictors of lymph node metastasis [11]. In general, as per the American Society of Colorectal Surgeons (ASCRS) guidelines, right hemicolectomy is recommended for most appendiceal adenocarcinomas [12]. However, controversy exists around the need for right hemicolectomy in well-differentiated mucinous adenocarcinomas with peritoneal dissemination as the incidence of lymph node metastasis is low (6%) and right hemicolectomy may not offer survival benefit in the setting of cytoreductive surgery [13, 14].

24.7.2 AMNs with Peritoneal Dissemination

24.7.2.1 Initial Evaluation

AMNs with peritoneal dissemination can be detected on diagnostic imaging or during surgical exploration. When peritoneal dissemination is detected on diagnostic imaging, additional workup should be directed at identifying the site of the primary tumor and obtaining a histologic diagnosis. Lower and upper endoscopies are necessary to exclude malignancies of the stomach and colon as AMNs are usually diagnosed by exclusion [10]. Tumor markers including CEA, CA 19-9, and CA-125 should be obtained as they have been found to have prognostic value [15–17]. Percutaneous biopsy of peritoneal implants or omental mass is a reasonable choice [1]. Diagnostic laparoscopy is extremely helpful to confirm the diagnosis, assess the extent of peritoneal dissemination, and obtain tissue biopsies and should be entertained freely. During laparoscopy, specific documentation about the extent and nature of disease along with photographic documentation is valuable for subsequent management decisions [18]. Alternatively, since these patients should be referred to a peritoneal malignancy surgeon for definitive management, diagnostic laparoscopy can be deferred to the specialist surgeon.

It is possible that the general surgeon incidentally finds evidence of mucinous dissemination during laparoscopy/laparotomy for another disease, including presumed appendicitis or hernia. If mucinous deposits are incidentally discovered, biopsies of the peritoneal implants should be taken for histologic diagnosis. Preferably, the biopsies should include small representative samples of the disease from different locations obtained by sharp dissection. An appendectomy can be performed if there are signs of appendicitis or features suggestive of tumor. If the appendix looks normal, resection of the appendix is not necessary. When mucin is discovered in a hernia sac, the hernia sac should also be sent for histopathologic review [15]. Specimens should be removed from midline ports so they can be excised with later surgery if they become seeded with disease [15, 18]. Patients may also present with small bowel obstruction (SBO) if their disease is particularly advanced (Fig. 24.2) [1]. Treatment of PMP with SBO can vary from curative treatment to palliative gastrostomy tube depending on the grade, disease burden, and

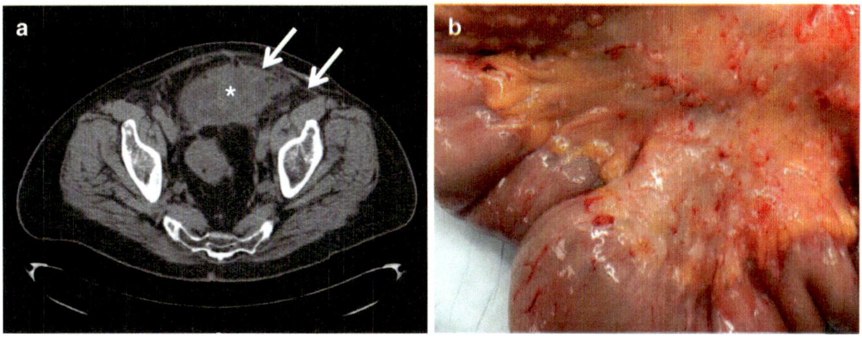

Fig. 24.2 Small bowel involvement from signet ring adenocarcinoma. (**a**) CT axial imaging showing thickened peritoneum (white arrows) and matted small bowel (asterisk). (**b**) Gross specimen of small bowel and mesentery with numerous implants

resectability of the disease. It is important to recognize that nontherapeutic explorations reduce the chance of successful cytoreduction in the future. Hence, it is vitally important to refer patients to a peritoneal malignancy center for subsequent care and long-term management.

24.7.2.2 Management

The main treatment of PMP is a combined approach of cytoreductive surgery (CRS) and hyperthermic intraperitoneal chemotherapy (HIPEC). The goal of CRS is to remove all macroscopic tumors through a combination of omentectomy, visceral resections, and peritonectomies. CRS is usually combined with HIPEC at the same setting to target microscopic disease [7]. Since survival of patients who undergo CRS/HIPEC for AMNs is excellent and decision about feasibility of CRS can only be determined by an experienced peritoneal malignancy surgeon, it is crucial to refer these patients to a peritoneal malignancy center. Once referred, the patient's disease burden and histopathology are carefully evaluated by a multidisciplinary team to decide if CRS/HIPEC is feasible and appropriate. CT imaging and laparoscopy are important to evaluate the burden of disease, while the subtype and grade of the AMN are assessed via histologic evaluation from pathology. Given the historically confusing and nuanced classification system of AMNs, a pathologist specialized in appendiceal neoplasms should be utilized for this assessment [19]. This is also why frozen sections on the initial operation are not recommended to help determine diagnosis and subsequent treatment.

The extent of peritoneal dissemination varies and can be localized to the right lower quadrant (Fig. 24.3), present with large ovarian mass (Fig. 24.4), or involve multiple organs throughout the abdomen (Fig. 24.5). For patients with LAMN or HAMN with acellular dissemination or DPAM, CRS/HIPEC is the treatment of choice (Fig. 24.6) and is associated with nearly 60–70% 10-year overall survival [1]. Systemic treatment is usually not indicated for LAMN and HAMN as these are not invasive cancers.

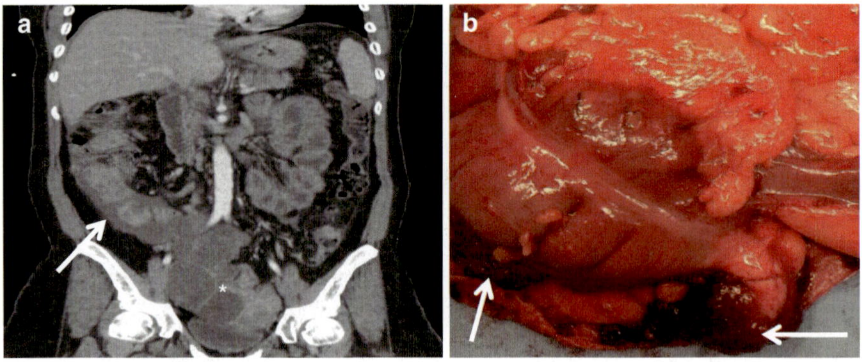

Fig. 24.3 Ruptured AMN with localized mucinous dissemination. (**a**) CT coronal image of large appendiceal mass with focal dissemination along the right paracolic gutter (white arrow) and pelvis (asterisk). (**b**) Gross specimen of ruptured AMN with mucin extravasation from the appendiceal tip and mucin along the right paracolic gutter (white arrows)

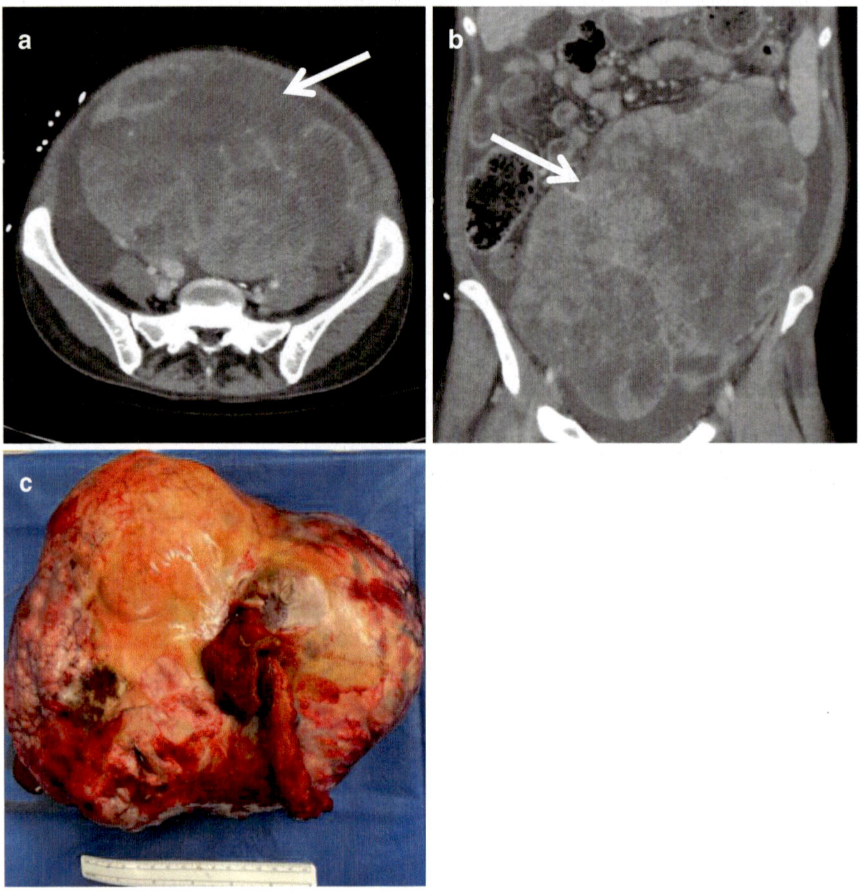

Fig. 24.4 Large ovarian tumor metastasis from mucinous adenocarcinoma. (**a**, **b**) CT axial and coronal images showing large ovarian mass (white arrows). (**c**) Gross specimen of large ovarian mass

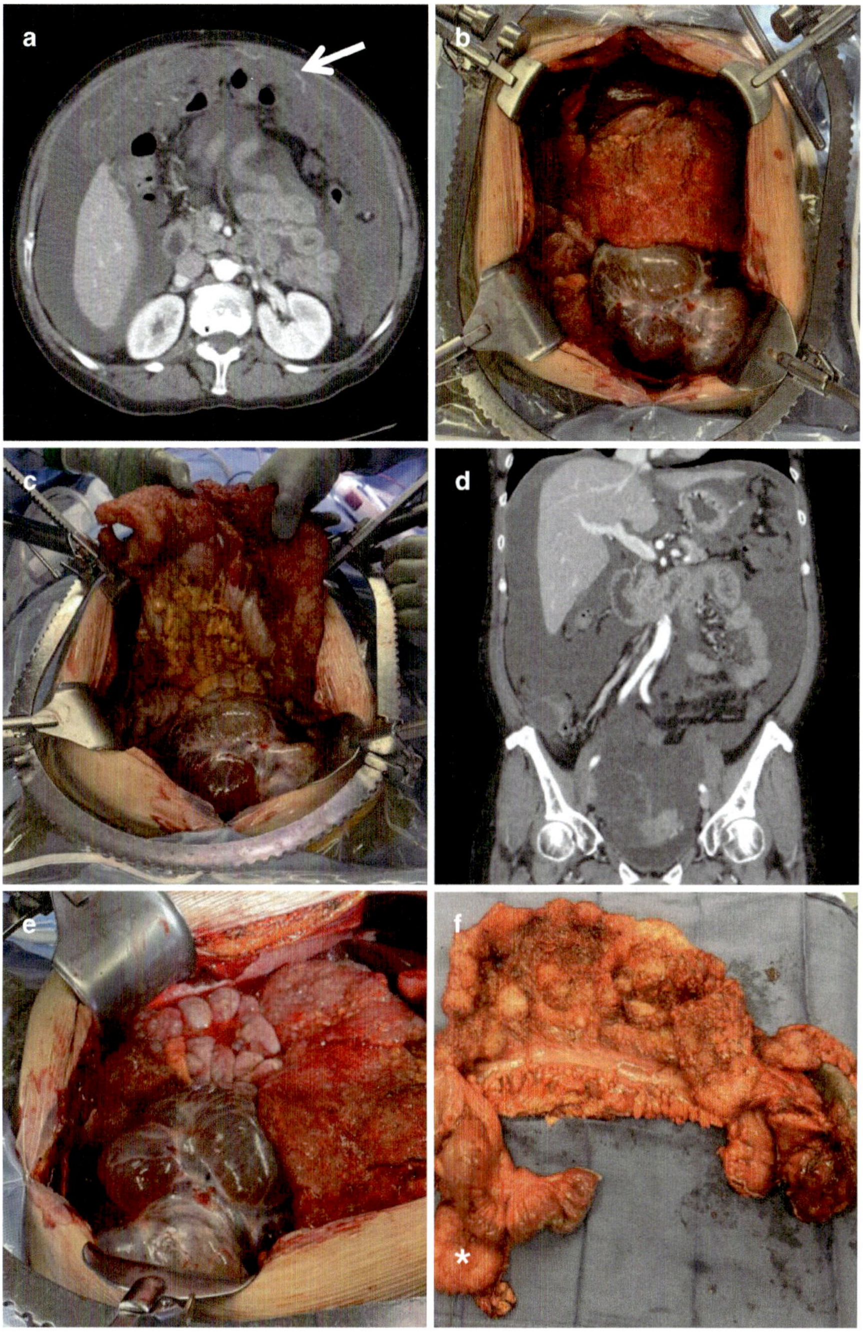

Fig. 24.5 Ruptured AMN with widely disseminated peritoneal mucinous disease. (**a** and **d**) CT axial and coronal sections highlighting large-volume ascites, pelvic mass, and omental caking (white arrow). (**b**, **c**, and **e**) Intraoperative photographs depicting large omental cake, large abdominal mass, and diffuse disseminated mucin. (**f**) Photograph of gross specimen including distal ileum, appendix (asterisk), subtotal colon, omental cake, distal pancreas, spleen, and gastric wedge resection

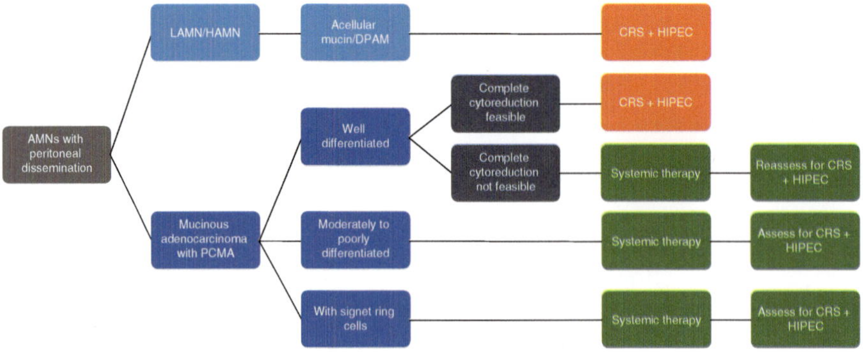

Fig. 24.6 Treatment algorithm for appendiceal mucinous neoplasms with peritoneal dissemination

The sequencing of treatment in mucinous appendiceal adenocarcinoma with peritoneal dissemination is influenced by the grade, peritoneal disease burden, and ability to achieve complete cytoreduction. The role of systemic chemotherapy, whether neoadjuvant or adjuvant, is not well defined and is often extrapolated from colon cancer despite the evidence that appendiceal cancers are genomically distinct entities from colon cancer [20, 21]. Nevertheless, due to the uncommon nature of appendiceal cancers and lack of specific treatment data, systemic treatment recommendations and regimen are often derived from current colon cancer treatment guidelines. Well-differentiated mucinous appendiceal adenocarcinoma is less likely to metastasize to distant organs and shows marginal responsiveness to systemic chemotherapy. Thus, in patients with well-differentiated appendiceal mucinous adenocarcinoma, with peritoneal metastases, CRS/HIPEC is the initial treatment of choice if complete cytoreduction is feasible. Systemic therapy is utilized mainly for patients in whom complete cytoreduction is not feasible. On the other hand, in patients with high-grade mucinous appendiceal adenocarcinoma or signet ring cell adenocarcinoma, systemic chemotherapy is routinely incorporated into the treatment regimen and is often administered perioperatively. CRS/HIPEC still remains an important treatment option, provided that complete cytoreduction is feasible and the patient is a candidate for CRS/HIPEC (Fig. 24.6) [10].

Although HIPEC is routinely combined with CRS in AMN with peritoneal metastases, there are no randomized controlled trials that have evaluated the benefits of HIPEC therapy in AMN. However, based on several large retrospective series and previous trial of patients with colorectal peritoneal carcinomatosis which also included appendiceal adenocarcinoma, expert consensus is to include HIPEC with mitomycin in the management of patients with AMN and peritoneal metastases [15]. There are significant controversies around the utility of HIPEC, duration, drug, and dose. Investigations utilizing 3-D tumor models are aiming to provide better guidance about intraperitoneal treatment regimens. Readers are referred to the chapter on peritoneal carcinomatosis elsewhere in this book for a more detailed description about the management of PMCA.

24.8 Complications and Outcomes

CRS/HIPEC for AMN with acellular mucin or DPAM is associated with a high, overall 5-year survival [22]. There are reports of peritoneal recurrences, for which repeat CRS/HIPEC can be considered. Outcomes for mucinous appendiceal adenocarcinoma after CRS/HIPEC depend on the grade and degree of differentiation of disease. Moderately differentiated mucinous adenocarcinoma treated with CRS/HIPEC has a 5-year survival rate of 30–60% with a high chance of peritoneal recurrence [22]. Poorly differentiated mucinous adenocarcinoma with signet ring cells has the worst prognosis after CRS/HIPEC with an overall 5-year survival of 10–40% [22].

Complications of CRS/HIPEC for AMN are similar to those of other major cancer resections and include thromboembolism, anastomotic leak, enteric fistula, abscess, and wound dehiscence [23]. Morbidity and mortality depend on the extent of peritoneal disease, patient comorbidities, and preoperative functional status. In a study by Chua et al. which included 2298 patients who underwent CRS for PMP from an AMN, major grade 3, 4, or 5 postoperative complications occurred in 24% of patients (grade 3 = requires interventional radiology or minimally invasive procedural treatment, grade 4 = requires return to the operating room, grade 5 = 30-day hospital stay or mortality). Independent factors associated with major operative complications were found to be at least two prior operations and peritoneal carcinomatosis index of more than 20 [24]. The overall survival rates were 80%, 74%, 63%, and 59% in 3, 5, 10, and 15 years, respectively [24].

24.9 Summary

PMP is a challenging disease entity as it has a wide range of presentations, biologic behavior, management options, and outcomes. Often, acute care surgeons are involved in the initial evaluation and diagnostic procedures; hence, knowledge of AMNs and PMP is extremely valuable. As the majority of patients with PMP can achieve excellent long-term survival with cytoreduction and HIPEC, referral to a peritoneal malignancy surgeon early on for evaluation and definitive treatment is paramount.

References

1. Mittal R, Chandramohan A, Moran B. Pseudomyxoma peritonei: natural history and treatment. Int J Hyperth. 2017;33(5):511–9.
2. Carr NJ, Cecil TD, Mohamed F, Sobin LH, Sugarbaker PH, Gonzalez-Moreno S, et al. A consensus for classification and pathologic reporting of pseudomyxoma peritonei and associated appendiceal neoplasia. Am J Surg Pathol. 2016;40(1):14–26.
3. Shaib WL, Assi R, Shamseddine A, Alese OB, Staley C 3rd, Memis B, et al. Appendiceal mucinous neoplasms: diagnosis and management. Oncologist. 2017;22(9):1107–16.
4. Shaib WL, Goodman M, Chen Z, Kim S, Brutcher E, Bekaii-Saab T, et al. Incidence and survival of appendiceal mucinous neoplasms. Am J Clin Oncol. 2017;40(6):569–73.

5. Smeenk R, Van Velthuysen M, Verwaal V, Zoetmulder F. Appendiceal neoplasms and pseudomyxoma peritonei: a population based study. Eur J Surg Oncol. 2008;34(2):196–201.
6. Carr NJ. New insights in the pathology of peritoneal surface malignancy. J Gastrointest Oncol. 2021;12(Suppl 1):S216.
7. Mehta SS, Bhatt A, Glehen O. Cytoreductive surgery and Peritonectomy procedures. Indian J Surg Oncol. 2016;7(2):139–51.
8. Carr NJ, Bibeau F, Bradley RF, Dartigues P, Feakins RM, Geisinger KR, et al. The histopathological classification, diagnosis and differential diagnosis of mucinous appendiceal neoplasms, appendiceal adenocarcinomas and pseudomyxoma peritonei. Histopathology. 2017;71(6):847–58.
9. Shariff US, Chandrakumaran K, Dayal S, Mohamed F, Cecil TD, Moran BJ. Mode of presentation in 1070 patients with perforated epithelial appendiceal tumors, predominantly with pseudomyxoma peritonei. Dis Colon Rectum. 2020;63(9):1257–64.
10. The Chicago Consensus on peritoneal surface malignancies: management of appendiceal neoplasms. Cancer. 2020;126(11):2525–33.
11. Shannon AB, Goldberg D, Song Y, Paulson EC, Roses RE, Fraker DL, et al. Predictors of lymph node metastases in patients with mucinous appendiceal adenocarcinoma. J Surg Oncol. 2020;122(3):399–406.
12. Glasgow SC, Gaertner W, Stewart D, Davids J, Alavi K, Paquette IM, et al. The American Society of Colon and Rectal Surgeons, clinical practice guidelines for the management of appendiceal neoplasms. Dis Colon Rectum. 2019;62(12):1425–38.
13. Sugarbaker PH. When and when not to perform a right colon resection with mucinous Appendiceal neoplasms. Ann Surg Oncol. 2017;24(3):729–32.
14. Turaga KK, Pappas S, Gamblin TC. Right hemicolectomy for mucinous adenocarcinoma of the appendix: just right or too much? Ann Surg Oncol. 2013;20(4):1063–7.
15. Govaerts K, Lurvink R, De Hingh I, Van der Speeten K, Villeneuve L, Kusamura S, et al. Appendiceal tumours and pseudomyxoma peritonei: literature review with PSOGI/EURACAN clinical practice guidelines for diagnosis and treatment. Eur J Surg Oncol. 2021;47(1):11–35.
16. Taflampas P, Dayal S, Chandrakumaran K, Mohamed F, Cecil TD, Moran BJ. Pre-operative tumour marker status predicts recurrence and survival after complete cytoreduction and hyperthermic intraperitoneal chemotherapy for appendiceal Pseudomyxoma Peritonei: analysis of 519 patients. Eur J Surg Oncol. 2014;40(5):515–20.
17. Rizvi SA, Syed W, Shergill R. Approach to pseudomyxoma peritonei. World J Gastrointest Surg. 2018;10(5):49–56.
18. Soucisse ML, Lansom J, Alshahrani MS, Morris DL. Mucinous appendiceal neoplasms with or without pseudomyxoma peritonei: a review. ANZ J Surg. 2020;90(10):1888–94.
19. Darryl S, Alejandro P, Izquierdo FJ, Votanopoulos KI, Cusack JC Jr, Lana B, et al. The Chicago consensus on peritoneal surface malignancies: management of appendiceal neoplasms. Ann Surg Oncol. 2020;27(6):1753–60.
20. Jönsson JI, Boyce NW, Eichmann K. Immunoregulation through CD8 (Ly-2): state of aggregation with the alpha/beta/CD3 T cell receptor controls interleukin 2-dependent T cell growth. Eur J Immunol. 1989;19(2):253–60.
21. Tokunaga R, Xiu J, Johnston C, Goldberg RM, Philip PA, Seeber A, et al. Molecular profiling of Appendiceal adenocarcinoma and comparison with right-sided and left-sided colorectal cancer. Clin Cancer Res. 2019;25(10):3096–103.
22. Valasek MA, Pai RK. An update on the diagnosis, grading, and staging of appendiceal mucinous neoplasms. Adv Anat Pathol. 2018;25(1):38–60.
23. Simkens GA, van Oudheusden TR, Luyer MD, Nienhuijs SW, Nieuwenhuijzen GA, Rutten HJ, et al. Serious postoperative complications affect early recurrence after cytoreductive surgery and HIPEC for colorectal peritoneal carcinomatosis. Ann Surg Oncol. 2015;22(8):2656–62.
24. Chua TC, Moran BJ, Sugarbaker PH, Levine EA, Glehen O, Gilly FN, et al. Early-and long-term outcome data of patients with pseudomyxoma peritonei from appendiceal origin treated by a strategy of cytoreductive surgery and hyperthermic intraperitoneal chemotherapy. J Clin Oncol. 2012;30(20):2449–56.

Ethical Issues in Emergency Surgery

25

Giovanni D. Tebala, Roberto Cirocchi, Lucia Lazzereschi, Angus Livingstone, and Zoe Slack

25.1 Introduction

Ethics is a system of morality that is at the basis of the human code of conduct; medical ethics refers to the medical code of conduct. In other terms, medical ethics is a framework of natural and legal principles that governs our choices as doctors. Facing the growing effectiveness and complexity of elective and emergency surgical treatment along with the massive social changes we have been witnessing in the last few decades, in terms of increasing patients' expectations and multiculturality, the surgeon may feel overwhelmed and pressurised in his or her clinical choices. Nowadays, they cannot take into account only the clinical and pathophysiologic aspects of the treatment, but must also involve good use of resources while guaranteeing the best possible care for the single patient. Unfortunately, most surgeons are not prepared to face those ethical dilemmas and tend to base their choice only on their clinical judgement.

G. D. Tebala (✉)
Surgical Emergency Unit, Oxford University Hospitals NHS Foundation Trust, Oxford, UK

Digestive and Emergency Surgery Unit, Azienda Ospedaliera S. Maria, Terni, Italy
e-mail: g.tebala@aospterni.it

R. Cirocchi
Digestive and Emergency Surgery Unit, Azienda Ospedaliera S. Maria, Terni, Italy
e-mail: roberto.cirocchi@unipg.it

L. Lazzereschi · Z. Slack
Surgical Emergency Unit, Oxford University Hospitals NHS Foundation Trust, Oxford, UK
e-mail: lucia.lazzereschi1@nhs.net

A. Livingstone
Surgical Emergency Unit, Oxford University Hospitals NHS Foundation Trust, Oxford, UK

Stanford Law School, Stanford University, Stanford, CA, UK
e-mail: alivingstone@stanford.edu

A. Tarasconi et al. (eds.), *Oncologic Surgical Emergencies*, Hot Topics in Acute Care Surgery and Trauma, https://doi.org/10.1007/978-3-031-36860-8_25

The basic principles of medical ethics have been variably described [1], but the core values are the following:

1. **Autonomy.** Every adult and competent patient has the right to decide what happens to their bodies. This principle is crucial to informed consent.
2. **Fidelity and veracity.** The doctor-patient relation must be based on trust and truth, even when truth is not what the patient would expect.
3. **Beneficence and nonmaleficence.** Every decision on the care of a patient must be taken to his or her best interest, with the aim of doing good to that patient. However, beneficence must be extended to the wide community, beyond the single doctor-patient relationship, according to the utilitarian principle of "providing the greatest amount of good to the greatest amount of people". At the same time, the Hippocratic principle of "first do not harm" must guide our choices.
4. **Justice.** All medical decisions must be taken on the bases of fairness and equality. This principle is challenged every time that clinical choices are based on financial consideration. The concept of justice in medical practice is strictly related to the "political" meaning of justice, and it is quite a relative opinion, more than a universally accepted principle, and assumes different notations in government-managed vs. privately managed healthcare systems.

These principles will be discussed in their various applications.

The surgeon must acknowledge and recognise that every patient is somehow pulled out of his or her own environment and comfort zone and faces existential issues related to life and death, pain and body image. This may elicit anxiety, aggressive behaviour, fear and frustration, but the same feelings can be transferred to the doctor, in particular if he or she is not mentally prepared to face and control his or her feelings. Luckily, the old cliché of the cold, un-affective and emotionally detached surgeon has demonstrated its inconsistence, and surgeons are more and more able to set up an empathic relationship with their patients. The downside of this is the difficulty of acting objectively and to see the interest of the wider community, beyond the small bubble of the doctor-patient rapport. Good communication and reciprocal trust can help overcome the negative feelings and have a therapeutic added value.

The principles of medical ethics must guide each and every action of any doctor and find their specific application in several specific conditions in emergency and elective surgery.

25.2 Triage

The concept of "triage" was first introduced by Dominique Jean Larrey, Chief Surgeon of the Army of Napoleon Bonaparte, to sort ("trier" in French) the war casualties by priority and decide who should have been transferred first from the battlefield to the rearguard for immediate medical treatment. At that time, priority was given to the soldiers with less severe injuries who could be treated quickly and sent back to the frontline as soon as possible. Since then, the "triage" is being applied everyday, both in civil and military environments, to guide the prioritisation of multiple emergencies and decide the allocation of resources accordingly. Nowadays, the principles of triage are quite flexible and adapt to the circumstances; triaging emergency patients during a natural catastrophe or a war (multiple casualties) is different from our everyday hospital practice. The aim of "civil" triage is to provide the best treatment to the highest number of patients within the restraints of resources and time. Therefore, the prioritisation is based on clinical gravity, according to the multiple available definitions. In civil disaster triage, patients are grossly classified into (1) those who will probably die even if they are treated, (2) those who will survive even if left untreated (or treated at a later stage) and (3) those who will survive if treated but will probably die if not treated [2], and treated accordingly, giving priority to those of group 3. Somewhat differently, the aim of "military" triage has always been to provide the best care to soldiers who are expected to return quickly to the battlefield. In this last case, triage is based on military considerations—i.e. treat first those patients with mild injuries in order to maintain the manpower at the frontline. Strictly linked with the concept of "triage" is the definition of "multiple casualties" and "mass casualties". In the military jargon, the term of "multiple casualties" refers to the access of several trauma emergencies but within the capacity of the system, and by mass casualties they mean a condition when the system is overwhelmed and cannot cope [3]. This distinction is crucial in hostile environments (war, catastrophes) with limited resources. In case of multiple casualties in war environment, the "P" (= priority) system is used, where P1 identifies someone who needs immediate resuscitation with or without surgery or else they will not survive, P2 indicates someone who can tolerate a 30–60-min delay and P3 is for those who can wait and are not in immediate risk of death. On the contrary, the "T" (=triage) system is used in case of mass casualties when the system cannot guarantee treatment for everyone. It considers T1, needing immediate resuscitation and/or surgery but with an expectancy of good results (those with life-threatening injuries and poor prognosis are under the category T4); T2, patients who can tolerate a 30–60-min delay; T3, those who can tolerate a longer delay; and T4, those who have multiple severe life-threatening injuries not expected to survive and for whom any treatment in those overstretched circumstances will be futile. In the civilian environment, this system has been replaced by a colour code, where Red corresponds to patients who cannot wait due to life-threatening injuries, Yellow identifies patients who can tolerate a 2-h wait, Green are patients who must wait up to 4 h and Blue are patients who are dying or will die soon despite any treatment [3, 4].

The ATLS triage is inspired by the principle of "do the most good for the most patients using available resources" [4]. It classifies casualties according to the ABCDE scheme, where patients with airway problems ("A") must be treated first, followed by "B" (breathing), "C" (circulation and bleeding), "D" (neurologic disability) and "E" (minor injuries, not life threatening), because "in general, airway problems are more rapidly lethal than breathing problems, which are more rapidly lethal than circulation problems, which are more rapidly lethal than neurologic injuries" [4]. Clearly, these priorities may change in war conditions, when a triage sieve is applied, based on a simple algorithm where patients who are walking are considered T3 and can wait, those who cannot walk and do not breathe are considered dead and those with abnormal respiratory rate (>30 or <10) and those with normal respiratory rate but with long capillary refilling time (>2 s) are considered true immediate emergencies (T1). Those patients with normal respiratory rate and normal capillary refilling time, but not able to stand or walk, are considered T2 (urgent) [3].

The triage process is a clinical pathway but, probably much more than other procedures, has deep ethical implications. For instance, the decision not to treat a severe casualty who might be rescued in other less critical environmental conditions is hard for all the stakeholders. Nonetheless, the triage decisions must be based on clear, precise and agreed principles. The most frequently applied is the Bentham's utilitarian principle of providing "the greatest good to the greatest number" (which is also the basis of the ATLS methodology), but other considerations may replace this ethical principle. In particular, during critical situations and mass casualties, would the reverse be applicable? In other terms, would it be justified to treat first the patients with mild injuries so that we are sure we are using our limited resources effectively on those who have the highest chance of surviving? Or, on a battlefield, would it be more ethical if we treated first those fighters with limited injuries so that they can go back sooner to the frontline and possibly save civilian lives?

The ethical principles that should be applied are (1) fidelity, (2) veracity, (3) autonomy, (4) justice and (5) beneficence [5].

Fidelity is the trust relationship between the doctor and the patient. Sometimes, by law, it is seen as a contractual obligation. At a superficial reflection, fidelity might appear to be broken by the application of triage, when the care of a patient is delayed to make room for another sicker patient. However, the principle can be re-established on the basis of mutual trust when it is evident to both stakeholders (patient and doctor) that a choice has been made for the benefit of the larger community with a spirit of altruism [5].

Veracity is somehow a consequence and the basis of fidelity and represents the need of a truthful exchange of information between doctor and patient [5]. In the triage process, honesty and truth are paramount to make clear the principles at the basis of the triage. A patient whose care is delayed—but also a patient whose access to care is prioritised—has the right to be informed of the reasons why this happens. In most emergency departments, this information is clearly showed on posters and advertisements.

Respect for a patient autonomy is an ethical and legal obligation. Autonomy is about privacy, free choice and personal beliefs and has the necessary corollary of personal responsibility. However, autonomy of a patient is somehow subordinate to the clinical right to decide priorities for a wider and superior benefit. Patients cannot claim their right to autonomy if this impacts on someone else's life and well-being. The triaging doctor has the obligation to respect the autonomy of patients but also to educate them to understand the mechanism of triage. Sometimes, the principle of autonomy must be overruled in critical situations and also when specific patients are not able to understand and decide autonomously [5]. In these cases, the doctor must choose considering first the best interest of the community or large group and only subsequently the best interest of the single patient, on a spirit of justice.

While the three previous ethical principles were relative to the single patient, justice has a larger application and deals with the fairness that must be applied in the triage process. Fair—and equitable—triage does not mean that all patients have the same treatment [5], as this is contrary to the spirit of good allocation of resources. To be sure that the principle of justice is respected, it is important that policies and guidelines on triage are in place and followed by the individual triage officer. Even more important, the principle of justice in triage must be clearly explained to the general public. Repine et al. report the interesting example of an American soldier who may find unfair that an enemy prisoner who has just shot one of his fellows is treated before him or her because the Geneva Convention prescribes that casualties are triaged according to their clinical conditions and the available resources, irrespective of their status of ally or enemy and their nationality, and again highlight the importance of education and information on the "greater intent" of the Geneva Convention [5].

Beneficence is about acting in the best interest of a patient. While this is surely possible in non-emergency conditions, critical situations such as multiple casualties or mass casualties show that this principle is hugely relative, as triaging patients in austere environments with limited resources implies the choice to act in the best interest of prioritised patients, and not everyone, thus violating the beneficence principle [5]. The above-reported utilitarian principle of "providing the greatest good to the greatest number" must be the guide for the use of limited resources, even when it means positively deciding not to act in the best interest of someone to the advantage of someone else and, on a wider scale, of the larger community. Although it may appear morally unacceptable that a patient with serious injuries in a "mass casualties" situation is left aside to die without treatment, and definitely contrary to the beneficence principle, the thought that this choice is based on the duty of the doctor to save the largest number of people should reduce the moral burden. In an austere and hostile environment, the principle of effective use of limited resources for the best interest of the largest number of casualties may take priority with respect to the individual beneficence.

The application of the above-discussed ethical principles to the triage process, in particular in critical conditions, is a stressful and not-desirable job and is rarely straightforward. The application of rigid guidelines taking into account objective measures (heart rate, respiratory rate, saturation, trauma scores …) may help the triage officer to overcome the feeling of guilt and responsibility by objectifying what is, at the end, a personal judgement. On the other hand, the abuse of score systems based on general statistics [6], albeit advanced, does not seem fully justified on the basis that scores derived from regression analysis are for their very nature quite limited and usually apply only on the "average" patient, who does not exist in the real world. Deciding on the life or death of a patient only on the basis of a sterile calculation is not acceptable. As a consequence, the clinical prioritisation must be a human process that considers all the variables including personal experience, clinical acumen and patient's expectations. The triage officer, being him or her a doctor, a nurse or a paramedic, must be supported and debriefed as needed, and the triage choices must be periodically audited along with their outcomes using as standards not only the clinical results (mortality, morbidity, rescue rate …) but also, when possible, patients' satisfaction in relation to their expectations and beliefs.

25.3 Informed Consent

Consent, *noun*: "Voluntary agreement to or acquiescence in what another proposes or desires; compliance, concurrence, permission" [7].

Obtaining consent is a vital component of any medical intervention. It empowers the patient to make autonomous decisions regarding their care and simultaneously helps to protect doctors from accusations of assault and/or battery. This section begins by highlighting the requirements for consent to be valid, the principles upon which consent is founded, and how consent should be obtained. It goes on to describe common issues regarding consent that present themselves in surgical emergencies and how these might be addressed. Finally, a case will be explored that presents a working example of how to address these issues. Situations in paediatrics are outside the scope of this textbook and shall therefore be excluded. Due to the variation in legal policies in different countries, certain law-based options (for example, power of attorney, advance decisions) will also be excluded. In these cases, it is the duty of the doctor to know the law in their country of practice and act within its remits.

For consent to be valid, it must be informed, competent and voluntary [1]. By "informed", we mean the relevant information that a patient must have available to be able to adequately weigh up the pros and cons of the intervention in the context of their personal situation and feelings. In the case of emergency surgery, this will include (but may not be limited to) the nature of the operation—what it stands to achieve and the intended benefits, along with the associated risks; the benefits and risks of providing no intervention; and the benefits and risks of alternative interventions, should they exist. To be "competent", the patient must have the capacity to make the decision at hand. To have capacity, the patient must be able to [8]:

1. Understand the information relevant to the decision
2. Retain that information
3. Use or weigh that information as part of the decision-making process
4. Communicate that decision by any means

To be "voluntary", the patient must willingly make the decision without duress or undue influence. Examples of where these requirements may fail to be met are covered later in this section.

Consent is based on the principles of respect for autonomy and beneficence [9]. As per Kantian philosophy, an autonomous person is an end in themselves; they are not to be merely treated as a means to an end for others and are free to determine their own paths [10]. Thus, in a medical context, the accepted protocol is to follow the wishes of the patient, with the burden of moral proof on the physician attempting to circumvent said wishes. This extends the patient the right to choose treatment from a list of available options (including no treatment) but does not give the patient the right to demand a treatment if that treatment would not otherwise be offered under the circumstances. We can see that to do so would be against this Kantian principle; the doctor has a duty of care to the patient (see beneficence below) but cannot be used as a means to provide medical care that does not meet (nor actively go against) this duty. This ties in with beneficence, which is itself built on the following four sub-principles:

1. Do not cause harm.
2. Prevent harm.
3. Remove harm.
4. Do or promote good.

It is arguable whether the final principle here implies a duty or an ideal. It is also argued whether these principles should follow this particular hierarchy, following the centuries-old battle between deontological and utilitarian principles. Realistically, harm is often done to some extent in surgery; patients will experience pain, may have scarring and may lose the function of a particular structure or organ. For example, to remove a ruptured appendix would be to prioritise (3) over (1). As surgeons, the priorities between the above sub-principles, as well as the respect for autonomy, must be balanced to create an overall net positive of good over harm. In general, the ideals set out in the Nuremberg code can set an acceptable base standard (see below). While this would normally relate to principles of medical research, it provides a nice summary: "The degree of risk to be taken should never exceed that determined by the humanitarian importance of the problem to be solved" [9].

Who should obtain informed consent? Theoretically, this can be anyone who possesses the thorough understanding required to fully explain the procedure, intended benefits, risks and all other elements a patient needs to be able to make an informed decision. Practically, this would most likely mean the surgeon due to perform the procedure, or a more junior doctor that has received the training necessary to fulfil the above requirements. This could be in the form of official training, or on an ad hoc basis by witnessing the consenting process delivered by a competent individual enough times to be able to deliver the information themselves. Caution should be exercised in this latter case, and it would be advisable for the junior to be supervised in their earlier efforts to ensure that acceptable standards are met.

The first issues we consider relate to a series of scenarios in which a patient is unable to demonstrate capacity, thus resulting in a failure to meet the informed and/or competent criteria for valid consent. This may be due to learning disability, delirium, lack of consciousness or any other situation that results in a lack of capacity. The first option explored should be whether capacity can be restored. If interventions can be feasibly delayed until, for example, the cause of a delirium has been reversed, this provides an ideal platform for retaining autonomy. Of course, this in itself requires treatment decisions to be made on behalf of the patient; however, in instances where these treatments are more conservative in nature, with fewer or less severe risks, they can be considered the more appropriate option. In the absence of any pre-existing personal legal documentation or directives that may exist in the doctor's country or state of practice, the next option is to act in the "best interests" of the patient. Where possible, this should involve knowledge of the patient's prior wishes. Exploration of previously expressed wishes or knowledge of personal beliefs is vital, be it through the doctor's long-standing history with the patient, discussions with next of kin or carers or previously documented conversations with other healthcare workers. Insight into past wishes can provide guidance into patient-specific management ideals. Caution should be exercised at times; relatives and those close to the patient can have ulterior motives and may therefore portray sentiments that do not echo those of the patient. As a general rule, if interventions are likely to be successful with an acceptable post-intervention quality of life, and there is no definitive evidence that the patient's wishes would be otherwise, doctors should act to preserve life. Where it is not possible to ascertain the previous wishes of the patient, the patient's clinical condition, feasibility of surgery, likelihood of recovery and potential quality of life post-surgery should be considered and weighed up in the decision-making process.

Ulterior motives of next of kin link to duress, another potential issue that can arise in consent. As stated previously, consent must be given voluntarily. Fear or pressure from outside factors can lead to verbalisation of consent (or declining treatment) without its internal expression, thus rendering the consent non-voluntary. Instances like this are rare, but doctors must be vigilant and investigate any signs or suspicions that the consent or declining of treatment has been given non-voluntarily.

In summary, valid consent must be informed, competent and voluntary, and it is the duty of the doctor to ensure that these criteria are met. In certain cases, particularly pertinent to emergency surgery, barriers can arise that prevent any combination of these three requirements from being achieved. In these cases, if no personal legal orders have been established that provide clear insight into the patient's wishes, there must be an exploration of the "best interests" of the patient. This must factor in a number of criteria, including but not limited to likelihood of success, potential harms, post-intervention quality of life and any knowledge available about the patient's personal feelings, for example from family members. Where the latter is unclear or uncertain, doctors have a duty to act to preserve life. This section will now finish with a worked example that highlights some potential issues in clinical context.

Consider the following case:

Ms. Smith is a 54-year-old Jehovah's Witness who presents in need of emergency surgery. She demonstrates capacity and consents to surgery but declines blood transfusion under any circumstances. During the surgery, she suffers significant blood loss, which will be fatal if she does not undergo transfusion.

In this case, we have a clear example of a patient exercising their autonomy. Ms. Smith has the capacity and the right to refuse transfusion on any grounds, in this case religious. Doctors should seek to avoid paternalism wherever possible, and a disagreement in the reasoning behind a decision to forgo or choose a less effective treatment (provided that the patient has capacity) is not a reason to overrule an autonomous decision. Although Ms. Smith will likely die due to her refusal of transfusion, she should have been presented with this potential situation during the consenting process and therefore the choice ultimately lies with her. She has weighed and considered the harm of receiving a blood transfusion to be greater than the harm of death. Now, consider the following alteration:

Ms. Lee is a 54-year-old woman who presents unconscious in need of emergency surgery. It is believed that chances of a successful surgery are high and that she will suffer few long-term side effects. Her partner does not provide consent by proxy, stating that Ms. Lee would reject surgery on religious grounds.

Here, the conundrum becomes more nuanced. While the previous case provided us with a clear autonomous decision made by the patient, Ms. Lee, unable to consent on her own behalf, requires a decision be made in her best interests. Assuming that she will not regain capacity before surgery is required, and that there is insufficient time to consult the courts or follow any other legal protocol in the country in question, the decision must fall to the doctors, who must use whatever information is available to them. While her partner is able to provide some information, the situation puts at risk the life of a patient that would otherwise make a full recovery. Importantly, there is a lack of definitive proof of Ms. Lee's treatment preference; therefore, the following four options arise:

1. Treat the partner's information as false and proceed with surgery. The partner's information was incorrect, and the life of the patient has been rightly saved.
2. Treat the partner's information as false, and proceed with surgery. The partner's information was correct, and the patient has undergone a treatment that they would have fundamentally rejected on religious grounds if they had had the capacity.
3. Treat the partner's information as true, and do not proceed. The partner's information was false, and the patient dies unnecessarily.
4. Treat the partner's information as true, and do not proceed. The partner's information was true, and the patient did not receive treatment they would have otherwise declined.

This presents two decisions that were "correct", and two that were "incorrect", based on the validity of the partner's information. Although in this case consent by proxy is sought, the balance of harms must be weighed. Is it more harmful to allow a patient to die if they should otherwise have lived than to save a life that should otherwise have died? Again, this has the potential for paternalistic viewpoints; as mentioned above in Ms. Smith's case, a patient with capacity judged a particular life-saving treatment to be more harmful than death. Thus, harms alone cannot settle this issue. Ultimately, it is the *facts* that must be used to settle the case. All information provided regarding the patient's possible refusal of a surgery is hearsay. In the absence of clear evidence that this patient would indeed refuse surgery that would be considered to be in the best interests of the majority of patients in the same position, the surgery should be performed.

25.3.1 Jehovah's Witnesses and Blood Transfusions

The case of Jehovah's Witnesses represents a particular application of the informed consent process and raises several ethical and legal considerations that must be well known to emergency surgeons.

Jehovah's Witnesses (JWs) refuse transfusions of blood and its derivates on the basis of four paragraphs from the Bible:

1. *Every living and moving thing will be food for you; I give them all to you as before I gave you all green things. But flesh with the life-blood in it you may not take for food. (Gen 9:3,4)*
2. *If any man of Israel, or any other living among them, takes any sort of blood for food, my wrath will be turned against that man and he will be cut off from among his people. For the life of the flesh is in its blood; and I have given it to you on the altar to take away your sin: for it is the blood which makes free from sin because of the life in it. For this reason I have said to the children of Israel, No man among you, or any others living with you, may take blood as food. (Lev 17:10,12)*
3. *For it seemed good to the Holy Spirit and to us, to put on you nothing more than these necessary things; to keep from things offered to false gods, and from blood, and from things put to death in ways which are against the law, and from the evil desires of the body; if you keep yourselves from these, you will do well. May you be happy. (Act 15:28,29)*
4. *But as to the Gentiles who have the faith, we sent a letter, giving our decision that they were to keep themselves from offerings made to false gods, and from blood, and from the flesh of animals put to death in ways against the law, and from the evil desires of the body. (Act 21:25)*

As a general rule, JWs refuse blood transfusion and blood products, often even when it is their own blood (pre-deposit autologous blood donation), under the principle that the blood circulation should not be interrupted in any way. Therefore, most of them also refuse cell salvage unless there is direct reinfusion without blood storage. This is a very sensible matter for JWs as their acceptance of transfusions, even as a life-saving procedure, may lead to expulsion or exclusion from their own community. "Accepting a blood transfusion willingly and without regret is seen as a sin. The JW concerned would no longer be regarded as one of JWs" [11]. In 2000, the JW Church decided that they would no longer take action against a member who accepts a transfusion [11], but the influence of the community is very strong, and JWs often fear the ostracism of their community more than the possible negative consequences for their own health. On the other hand, receiving a transfusion against their will is not considered a sin and is not cause of exclusion. Usually, JWs carry with them a specific advance directive (the so-called "no-blood card") to inform the treating emergency doctor of their will to refuse any blood or blood product.

However, a minority of JWs may still accept transfusions or reinfusion of blood for themselves and their children in very special circumstances and may also accept infusion of blood products and use of cell saver. It is therefore crucial that the practitioner (i.e. the emergency physician or surgeon) takes into account the view of each individual JW with a direct, thorough and documented discussion when possible or takes into account advance directives or the opinion of those who have power of attorney. In the case of an incompetent patient (i.e. the one who is not able to understand, retain and use the information given by the doctor and is not able to communicate his or her decision), the opinion of family and friends should be taken into account, but it is not legally binding. On the contrary, the "no-blood card" is legally binding to the doctor but also releases him or her from any liability in case of a negative clinical outcome due to their decision. It is still unclear if a previously communicated decision of the patient—which is different from a formal advance directive—should be considered valid under any circumstances in the future, but previous decisions should not be taken for granted considering the patient's freedom to change their mind at any time. Similarly, the fact that a patient is a JW must not—under any circumstance—mean that he or she refuses blood and blood product unless this is not clearly stated by the patient himself or herself or by an advance directive. Administering blood or blood products—even as a life-saving decision—to a competent JW who has clearly stated his or her refusal may be considered an assault and could lead to criminal proceedings on the ground of violation of individual freedom [11]. On the contrary, in the case of a non-competent patient who needs a transfusion, in the absence of an advance directive or any other direct and clear statement, the decision stays with the treating doctor who may seek the opinion of family and friends. However, in most countries, this opinion is not binding. Knowing that a patient was a JW, but without an advance directive, does not bind the doctor to not transfuse. However, in such cases, if the transfusion is mandatory to save the patient's life, it would be advisable to seek a second opinion by a senior colleague or a court order. A strict and frank communication with the family is also mandatory to prevent legal issues.

Much more difficult is the case of children whose parents refuse transfusions for them on the bases of their parental authority. In these cases, the treating doctor has different options, but always bearing in mind that the best interest of a child is paramount in all decisions regarding them. In elective conditions, for example when offering and discussing a surgical operation where transfusions may likely be required (i.e. liver transplant or cardiac surgery), the doctor may agree with the parents not to use blood at all, despite posing a possible threat to the young patient, or they may agree to use blood only under special and critical circumstances or the doctor may decide to transfer the patient under another surgeon who may be willing to perform the operation without blood transfusion. In emergency, if no agreement can be found with the parents, it is advisable that the doctor seeks a court order authorising the transfusion. In the United Kingdom, this is regulated by the Children Act 1989. In some countries (in particular the United Kingdom, Australia, Canada and New Zealand), children over the age of 12 years who are mature enough to decide for themselves (so-called Gillick competent) may accept or refuse a medical treatment [12]. However, unlike adults, the decision of a child is not absolute and can be overruled by a court order.

Where appropriate and timely, it may be useful to contact the local JW Hospital Liaison Committee for a frank and overt discussion, but bearing in mind the principles hereby exposed.

25.4 Palliative Care

Palliative care is a branch of medical healthcare that aims to relieve symptomatic suffering in individuals that are nearing death or who are suffering from complex, debilitating illnesses. It does so by taking into consideration the patient's cultural, ethical and religious views to support a joint treatment plan to improve their quality of life. It is based on the four fundamental principles of bioethics: autonomy, beneficence, nonmaleficence and justice. Research in palliative care is more prevalent in medical settings and has been shown to be effective in improving symptomatic relief and providing treatment in alignment with patient preferences; very little has been researched within surgical settings [13]. Palliative surgery is regarded as such if the operation's primary aim is to provide symptomatic relief and improved quality of life caused by advancing disease or malignancy and not for curative intent [14]. Palliative surgery is also used to support and enable the delivery of non-surgical palliative treatment. There are many distinctive ethical issues, based around the four pillars of bioethics, that arise for surgeons when dealing with palliative surgery. These are discussed below and summarised in Table 25.1.

Physical and psychological vulnerability in palliative patients may impact the ability to gain informed consent, or for patients to weigh the options and make a decision. Informed consent in this patient group may require multiple discussions, and often breaks may need to be taken because of fatigue or confusion. Additionally, the patient may be under a range of influences, which may affect judgement such as pain, opiates, biochemical imbalances or pre-existing mental health issues [15]. A surgical procedure comes with potential morbidity and mortality and may exacerbate the patient's condition. Risks associated with carrying out an intervention and the impact they may have on the patient need to be carefully considered when discussing treatment options. This is less of an issue when palliative treatment is medical or pharmacological as the outcome does not affect morbidity in the same way that post-operative complications might [16]. Recovery from palliative surgery may

Table 25.1 Ethical issues encountered in palliative surgery. A list of the main issues encountered in palliative surgery by clinicians, divided based on the main principles of bioethics

Autonomy	Beneficence and nonmaleficence	Justice and medical fidelity
• Patients' vulnerability may affect the ability to understand and retain information • Patients' health can deteriorate rapidly • Patients' expectations of the surgical outcomes from the palliative operation may differ from reality • Patients may feel pressure from loved ones	• An intervention for symptomatic relief may lead to unintended harm in the form of post-operative complications • An intervention, even if successful, may lead to a lower baseline than the one pre-operation and lead to worsening outcomes and a longer recovery period	• It may be difficult to determine patient wishes on knowing about their disease progression and prognosis • It may be difficult to balance limited resources and palliative treatment that proves to be futile

lead to a loss of decision-making ability or capacity based on the procedure outcome, which makes informed consent more challenging.

An added challenge when offering palliative surgery in the context of patient autonomy involves determining how and up until which point the consent is valid if deterioration prior to surgery occurs. What should be done if the patient loses capacity and is no longer able to make the relevant decision? Who is supporting the patient at home, and will they make the right decisions for their loved one if burdened by grief? Advance care planning empowers patients to make decisions about management—this may well include decisions to refuse surgical intervention. Countries have different legal documents that fall within this category; in the United States they are called "advance directives", while in the United Kingdom they are classed as "advance decisions" (or "living will"). The crux is however the same: they are legally binding documents where individuals can record their refusal of treatment. The issue with these documents is that for them to be valid, specific treatment and interventions need to be recorded. However, the extent of what is and is not available may (a) change with time and with the clinical status of the patient and (b) the individual itself may change their mind as they reach the end of their life [17]. It is therefore pivotal to have a multidisciplinary team discussing this with palliative patients alongside with their next of kin and family members. It is imperative that the latter are involved by the clinician in the discussion, during the decision process or once the decision has been made based on what the patient prefers. This is to ensure that they are aware of what their loved one wants and to avoid patients feeling pressured by their families, which often occurs in the palliative care setting [18]. Families face numerous stressors including impending loss, grief, being available to offer support to their loved one and, if involved in their care, having the responsibility to make critical decisions that may impact their prognosis. They are often an incredible source of support for the patient but, due to the burden they carry, family disputes may arise [19]. Conflict needs to be carefully balanced by the clinician involved in the decision-making, as it could delay important treatment that can improve the patient's quality of life. Avoiding conflict altogether is unrealistic. Conversations focused on communicating the needs and concerns of all parties may mitigate the development of disputes and should focus on making sure that the patient retains their autonomy.

Lastly, patient's expectations of the surgical outcomes from palliative interventions may differ from reality. The relative success of a palliative intervention—whether it is to provide symptomatic relief or allow for further palliative treatment—may differ between the healthcare provider and the patient. If this disparity exists, why does the patient feel that their health needs have not been met? Has the operation minimised the burden of the disease the patient is suffering from [20]? Various external factors may lead to this situation: misinformation fuelled by hope from family members, poor communication between the professional and the patient on the possible surgical outcomes of the intervention and unrealistic expectations of how the intervention may affect their prognosis [21]. At the crux of this lies, once again, the importance of communicating and clearly explaining, when gaining consent, the expectations the surgeon has if the operation proves successful.

This will mitigate the risk of the patient expecting more or expecting the intervention to completely treat their illness and ensure that autonomy is maintained when a decision is made.

The main considerations when providing palliative surgery to patients should be focused on beneficence and nonmaleficence. The principle of beneficence focuses on relieving symptoms that impair the patient's quality of life. The patient's best interest is at the heart of decision-making, and this is even more critical when dealing with a palliative intervention that may lead to unintended post-operative complications that may cause significant morbidity. This ties in with the principle of nonmaleficence, which is the duty to cause no harm and, in palliative care, is focused on relieving symptoms that are causing harm to the patient. Conversely, careful consideration has to be held from an anaesthetic, physiotherapy and nutrition point of view if an operation aimed to relieve pain and other symptoms ends up leading to a lower baseline for the patient and therefore ends up causing further harm. Additionally, in contrast with the decline that chronic patients experience when receiving medical treatment for palliation, acutely ill palliative patients who may need interventional stenting or surgical treatment may acutely deteriorate [22]. When complications arise following these interventions in individuals who are already clinically compromised, the previous treatment plans and patient preferences may no longer be feasible. Crucially, palliative surgery needs to be discussed in the context of patients having prognostic understanding and that interventions may change or not be carried out if the best possible outcome is no longer consistent with the quality of life they were hoping for [22]. This can be difficult for surgeons as providing accurate information on outcomes and prognosis is often dependent on whether a palliative intervention can be carried out. In surgical relief of bowel obstruction, for example, medical management would be unable to completely relieve symptoms of nausea and vomiting, and long-term nasogastric aspiration may lead to discomfort that the patient may not want [15]. If intervention is possible, what are the burdens and the benefits of the operation and how do these apply specifically to the patient you are treating? The decision to carry out palliative surgery is patient centred—an individual's view of what would benefit their palliative condition might be completely different from another patient who is suffering with the same ailment but has different goals. This links back to the principle of autonomy and the need for advance care planning and establishing clear goals of care [23]. This is to assure not only autonomy but also that if a patient is unable to communicate their wishes in the future, no unnecessary harm and inappropriate treatment are provided.

Healthcare professionals have an obligation to advocate on behalf of their palliative patients to receive fair and appropriate treatment, in line with their wishes and beliefs. This can be difficult when patients request "futile care", a term used to determine medical or surgical interventions that clinically would result in very little or no benefit to the palliative patient. Some ethicists believe that futile care in palliation is ethically unjustifiable [14]. They believe that treatment that is not providing any measurable benefit should be discontinued especially as allocation of resources available needs to be considered to avoid healthcare inequity [24]. Ethicists that support futile care ultimately place autonomy above all other bioethical principles as their school of thought is underpinned by the overarching principle that it is the patient's right to determine what is appropriate, and never solely the surgeon's. If however futile care in palliative care is defined as treatment that is no longer benefiting the patient, who defines when such benefit ends? If the patient feels temporary relief or hope because of the intervention, is it not beneficial [25]? Clinicians need to have frank and open conversation with patients and explain the medical reasoning behind why interventions may not be medically appropriate or beneficial. Although a medical professional does not have to provide futile care that they believe to be immoral, they have an obligation for continued care, and involvement of other healthcare professionals and members of the multidisciplinary team may be needed in order for a decision to be made [14].

Justice goes hand in hand with the principle of medical fidelity, which mandates to approach patients with honesty and candour. It can often be difficult to determine how much patients wish to know when it comes to diagnosis and prognosis. Having effective patient-centred communication skills is essential to determine an individual's preference in order to then act accordingly. However, appropriate treatment prognosis can help the patient make autonomous decisions on their medical care, and a fine balance needs to be struck between sharing information that is medically necessary and withholding aspects of the disease in line with patient wishes.

In summary, when considering palliative surgery in patients, alongside applying principles of autonomy, beneficence, nonmaleficence, justice and medical fidelity lies the importance of open, frequent communication with the patient and their support system. By understanding our patient's cultural, religious and ethical views and understanding what is important to them, surgeons can provide ethical, high-quality end-of-life care.

25.5 Surgical Training

Patient-centred care, whereby patient choice and preferences are taken into consideration when discussing management options, is further integrating itself within healthcare systems around the world. Concerns are arising on the impact this could be having on surgical trainees, as patients may not feel comfortable being operated on by someone who is still learning [26]. This is especially prevalent in emergency surgery, where patients are clinically unwell and may require time-critical surgical intervention.

On the other hand, "you cannot learn to play the piano by going to concerts", and surgical trainees (and junior surgeons) must be allowed to perform operations by themselves under their own responsibility. The dilemma between the rights of the young surgeon to learn and the obligation to provide the best possible care to the patient can be resolved within an effective learning environment where both teaching and patient safety are paramount to the whole healthcare system. The crucial step is the one of "supervision" or "supervised self-education" where the trainee acquires his or her own competence and the supervisor guarantees safety and quality of the care provided [27].

A qualitative study carried out in Canada reported that surgical trainees, when consenting patients for surgery, were vague when discussing their specific role within the operating theatre [28]. Patient autonomy, a key component in the relationship between a surgeon and the patient, would be, in this case, compromised. The study reported that trainees felt that there was a lack of understanding from the general public on the training pathway. An increase in patient education on the training pathway may allow for better informed consent. Surgeons have legal and ethical obligations to disclose benefits, risks and alternative non-surgical treatments to patients. This should include information on trainee participation. However, patients were less likely to consent to a trainee assisting and operating, limiting their surgical exposure and having an impact on their training [28]. In order to avoid this, a clear discussion with the patient needs to be had by both the trainee and their senior. Independence provided to trainees by supervising surgeons is only done so once competencies have been demonstrated. This framework allows for trainees to progress to being safe surgeons and practitioners. Excluding surgeons in training comes with the risk of decreasing the ability and experience of trainees, which in turn could affect the quality of surgical care provided in the long term. Surgical training across the world largely involves increasing responsibility and independence as trainees progress and develop their clinical skills. The training pathway has to be respected, and trainees need to be given opportunities for continued development, but this has to be balanced with respect for the autonomy of the patient. Additionally, complete disclosure on the role of the trainee in surgery during the consent process may not always be possible as often the trainee's specific role is not established until the operation has begun. This has, in instances, led to "ghost" surgery, where the operation is carried out by an individual other than the one disclosed to the patient [29]. A handful of "ghost" surgery cases in the United States have led to malpractice suits. In countries where there is not a nationally funded healthcare system and patients are required to pay, such as in the United States, a patient's choice of surgeon is as important as the informed consent of the surgery [30]. In Perna v. Pirozzi (1983), for example, the patient had named only one surgeon while consenting. The operation had however been carried out by another professional, and the patient was given a cause of action for battery due to unconsented touching. The Supreme Court ruled that battery had occurred as the operation had been performed by another doctor other than the one that was agreed on with the patient [31]. This is less common in countries where the healthcare system is government funded, like in the United Kingdom and most European Countries, where patients only pay for surgery if they go private. Trainees in this case have no clinical rotations or blocks of training within private institutions, and the risk of "ghost" surgery is minimal. When consenting patients, a list of possible complications is provided, so that patients are aware of the issues that may occur after the operation. Although none of them might happen, it is good clinical practice to provide insight into the most common so that the informed consent is valid. The same approach should be applied when discussing who might be assisting in the operation. Usually, the information given to the patient contains a statement that warns them that it cannot be guaranteed that a specific surgeon would perform the procedure, even if he or she represents the patient's choice.

Informed consent within emergency surgery is more challenging: there is an element of time constraint due to possible deterioration, emotional stress and acute pain, which may lead to decreased comprehension of the information relayed to gain consent [32]. In these cases, surgeons must balance obtaining informed consent and the consequences of delayed treatment and associated risks. Involving trainees and discussing their involvement with patients may further delay treatment and would go against the *primum non nocere* credo, which the principles of nonmaleficence and beneficence originate from [33]. Where nonmaleficence aims to avoid the causation of harm, beneficence requires that every medical decision in a patient's treatment plan which may benefit the patient is balanced against all possible risks and costs. When training surgeons, this also applies to trainees carrying out parts of operations that are appropriate for their level of training. If all clinical assessments and surgical management in emergency surgery were carried out by seniors, the risk of causing harm would be mitigated, but medical education would be negatively impacted. Trainees would take longer to complete their training and delay achieving all their requirements, and there would be a shortage of qualified professionals. For training to be successful, alongside keeping patient safety at the forefront of decision-making, all parties involved need to balance the principles of patient choice, nonmaleficence and beneficence and the importance of continued education and trainee development. Trainees and their mentors need to recognise the limits of one's professional competence and surgical competence. Both are required in order to "do no harm" and can only be effectively learned and developed by doing [34]. While e-learning and simulation training in surgical settings are effective to develop team communication and clinical acumen and improve patient safety, it falls short when it comes to operating [35]. This is especially true in the context of emergency surgery. A simulation of a surgical procedure will take trainees through all the procedural steps allowing for safe, repeated practice. Although it closely mimics the clinical environment, ultimately trainees are aware that their actions will not harm the patient. This removes the opportunity for trainees to practise operating in time-sensitive situations such as emergency cases. The degree of inflammation and disease will vary based on the aetiology of the presentation and the patient's clinical status at the time of operation. Simulation training, although a safe learning experience that should supplement initial training and learning, removes elements in emergency surgery that trainees need to be exposed to in order to develop their operating ability in time-critical and acute situations [36].

Ultimately, individual trainees and supervising seniors need to make a clinical judgement on when, if, how and on who trainees can operate while taking into consideration patient autonomy and safety. This however cannot come at the expense of trainees; each patient has to be a case-by-case decision. Multiple factors will influence the decision: the clinical presentation, the degree of haemodynamic instability, the ability of the trainee, the type of operation, the extent of the disease and the number of seniors available. This will ensure that trainees can still develop their competencies and surgical ability within emergency surgery while maintaining patient care the number one priority.

25.6 Medicolegal Issues and Guidelines

Medical malpractice claims are increasing all over the world. As the relationship between practitioner and patient evolves, so does the management of the malpractice claim. Historically, the doctor–patient relationship was more personal than it is today. A family doctor in the past would know the patient, their past medical history and family history in much greater detail than any doctor can possibly hope to know today. This allowed doctors the time to provide treatment tailored to the patient, more individualised, and overall, care that was more holistic. However, with an increasing global population and subsequently increasing patient numbers, the doctor–patient relationship has become more disjointed and impersonal. With the advent of rigid guidelines, this relationship has become even more strict and contractual in nature with treatment less tailored to that of the individual patient and more focused on adhering to guidelines. This both suppresses personal relationships and supports the clinicians' ability to make decisions regarding that patient that are less holistic than they once would have been [37].

Since their introduction in the second half of the twentieth century, clinical guidelines have become the benchmark to which each clinician is expected to uphold their care. Although formal guidelines rationalising modern medicine were introduced in the twentieth century, even in ancient Egypt, practitioners were held accountable to the written rules. They were punished for not obeying these rules, sometimes, regardless of the outcome of the patient [38]. The Romans treated medical malpractice claims under the same jurisdiction as deliberate physical assault. Medical practice was most often carried out by the father of the household (*pater familias*) [39]. The Romans introduced the term "contract" with respect to medical treatment, but this was only possible between "free men", which was rare. After the Norman conquest of Britain in 1066, the English Common Law was established. Few sporadic cases were raised, but these had little effect on the overall practice of medicine [40]. As medicine evolved, it became more of a personal contract between the doctor and patient. Up until the eighteenth century, clinicians were largely protected from their malpractice mainly due to the lack of guidance and regulated standards [41].

Nowadays, in countries whose legal system derives from the Roman law (*Codex Justinianeus*), the legal action is managed by civil or criminal courts and is based on a fundamental set of rules, which are then applied to individual cases. Therefore, in those countries, medicolegal claims are benchmarked against established guidelines and regulations.

In the United Kingdom (and more generally in all the Commonwealth countries), a fundamental change came to the assessment of medical malpractice in 1957 after the "Bolam Case". During the Bolam vs. Friern Hospital Management Committee, a patient suffered physical injuries during electro-convulsant therapy after they failed to request sedatives or restraints. The patient argued that they had not been warned of the physical risk without sedatives and so had not requested them. The medical team counter-argued that it was not customary to warn patients of very small risks and sometimes the presence of sedatives and restraints caused greater risk than their absence did. A "reasonable body of evidence" which at the time was "a panel of average professionals of the same specialty" agreed with the medical team, but after this case, it was a requirement that "customary practice" also encompasses legal and acceptable standards [42]. In 1993, the assessment of medical malpractice evolved further after the "Bolitho vs. City and Hackney Health Authority case". This case added causation to the criteria. This means that the error must have affected the outcome. In the Bolitho vs. City and Hackney Health Authority, a paediatric registrar failed to attend a child with breathing difficulties because the batteries in their bleep were low. The child later died. The clinician successfully argued that had batteries been working and the alert received, they would have attended the child but would not have intubated them and so the error did not cause the adverse outcome in this case [42]. Both the Bolam and Bolitho tests are applied by a panel of average professionals of the same specialty, thus creating a strong framework where the medical profession defends itself by introducing a bias related to personal ideas and customary practice even when guidelines and evidence may have suggested differently [43]. Australia has rejected the Bolam test completely stating, "It is not the law that if all or most of the medical practitioners in Sydney habitually fail to take an available precaution to avoid foreseeable risk of injury to the patients that none can be found guilty of negligence" [44]. This viewpoint identifies and neatly summarises the inherent failings of the Bolam test in that it is fundamentally doctor centred. The Montgomery vs. Lanarkshire case in the United Kingdom also added that the quality of the information provided by the clinician should be judged by the patient and not the clinician [45]. The evolution of medical malpractice assessment in the United States has been similar to that of the United Kingdom. Initially derived from the UK system, and based upon "any act or omission by a physician during a treatment of a patient that deviates from accepted norms of practice in the medical community and causes an injury to the patient", similar cases have also added the criteria that "any expert opinion" must be based on scientific evidence that is "subjected to scientific peer review and published in scientific journals" [46]. Clearly, there is growing attention to the fact that the opinion of an "average professional" or a "panel of average professionals" may not be consistent with evidence and guidelines and can be biased towards customary practice.

It must be acknowledged, however, that guidelines may not always represent best practice and strongest evidence. Undoubtedly, they have multiple advantages and play a substantial role in modern healthcare, as they streamline health services, regulate treatments and improve equity across healthcare on the basis of "clinical evidence", but the process of creating formal guidelines may be long and subject to bias [47]. Therefore, they can be easily criticised, and professionals may choose to act on the basis of their own experience and beliefs more than guidelines. Detractors of guidelines state that, by their own nature, guidelines are not specific to any case and apply to the "average" patient. An adaptation to the single specific case is therefore necessary.

On the contrary, sometimes guidelines can be too "advanced" with respect to customary practice, and professionals may decide to continue with their customary practice without considering new evidence and guidance. This happens in particular when doctors are too defensive and risk-averse. An obvious consequence of this attitude is a possible conflict in the court between the opinion of the average professional or a panel of professionals (who may not follow the most recent guidelines) and a doctor who has followed the last evidence and guidance [42].

A specific example of where guidelines are different from common practice is in the surgical treatment of complicated acute diverticulitis when the medical treatment fails. Historically, this would have been treated with the one-century-old Hartmann's procedure. But an unacceptably high rate of these patients are never reversed and their long-term quality of life is severely affected, not to speak about the possible complications of the terminal stoma. The most up-to-date guidance advises that immediate anastomosis of the bowel does not carry increased risks and provides better outcomes for patients [48, 49]. Despite strong evidence and guideline, most surgeons will still carry out a Hartmann's procedure, either for customary practice or for defensive medicine. It is speculated that this is due to a surgeon's fear of an anastomotic leak, the like of which is heavily weighted, and although almost all surgeons will have a rate of anastomotic leaks, the such is still considered relatively unacceptable in the general surgical community and among surgical peers. Therefore, surgeons would avoid following the guidelines due to the perceived risk of an adverse outcome.

Same inconsistence can be seen in the treatment of acute cholecystitis, where recent guidelines [50] suggest immediate cholecystectomy—or anyway during the same index admission—while most surgeons would prefer a conservative medical treatment and a delayed operation, probably fearing—against evidence—that an emergency procedure would be more difficult and risky.

This leads to the fact that in both cases, a "panel of average professionals of the specialty" would not agree with the clinician if they had instead followed the guidelines.

It is therefore crucial to find a compromise between customary practice and guidelines.

The late Prof. Sackett proposed that clinicians should work by "… integrating individual clinical expertise with the best available external clinical evidence from systematic research …" [51]. This creates a potential grey area where clinicians are able to escape the guidance and avoid those practices that they fear. However, those who deviate from the guidance must be able to prove that they did so with experience and based on their best judgement. They must also be able to explain and demonstrate their reasoning and evidence for such a deviation as well as demonstrate causation by the Bolitho test.

Tebala et al. suggested that a more flexible approach be instated whereby the "experts" provide various acceptable options for the management of individual cases. These offerings may include examples that they do not agree with as individual clinicians but are supported by rigorous and reliable studies or common sense [42]. Clinical decisions should be made based upon evidence, supported by the doctor's experience and centred around the patient's beliefs and expectations.

As guidelines play a greater and greater role in medical practice, it is important that we address the interaction between clinician and guidelines, understand how they are interpreted and address how they are applied to each clinical case, because correct interpretation and appropriate application are likely to improve patient care.

25.7 Research

Experimentation on human subjects is a practice as old as medicine itself. From the Middle Ages, where corpses were exhumed and dissected publicly without the prior consent of the deceased nor their relatives [52], to more recent horrors such as the Tuskegee Study or the experiments led by Josef Mengele in Auschwitz and other concentration camps, medical research has a dark past. That said, medicine would not be where it is today without research, and thus ethical principles are required to govern the practice so that progress can be made without breaching human rights. This section will explore the principles that ethical research is built upon, using the infamous Tuskegee Experiment as an example of how accepted principles have been breached in the past.

25.7.1 Research in Comparison to Clinical Practice

The primary differences between clinical practice and research lie in the aims. In clinical practice, clinicians strive to deliver the treatment or intervention, which most closely matches the best interests of their individual patient at a particular time. Conflicts arise in determining these interests. In research, the participant may or may not benefit, or indeed may actively be harmed; the aim is to benefit all relevant patients going forward. Conflicts therefore arise in balancing the interests of the patients against those of medical science, and therefore gains in knowledge and the progression of evidence-based medicine must be weighed against risks imposed upon participants.

25.7.2 The Tuskegee Experiment and Belmont Report

Consider the following case study [53, 54]:

The *Tuskegee Study of Untreated Syphilis in the Negro Male*, commonly referred to as the *Tuskegee Experiment*, was conducted between 1932 and 1972 by the United States Public Health Service and the Centers for Disease Control and Prevention. Three-hundred ninety-nine African-American participants with latent syphilis were recruited for a 6-month epidemiological study to research the progression of the disease. The researchers reasoned that harm was not being done in that the participants were unlikely ever to receive treatment for syphilis. Participants were recruited with the incentive that they would receive free medical care. This was untrue. Subjects were never informed of their diagnosis by the researchers (some discovered it serendipitously) or the risks of transmission. The study ran long beyond the 6 months initially stated to the participants, and they were denied access to penicillin once it had been established as an effective treatment. By the end of the study in 1972, only 74 of the participants were alive. Twenty-eight had died of syphilis, 100 died of related complications, 40 of their wives had been infected and 19 of their children were born with congenital syphilis. President Bill Clinton formally apologised on behalf of the United States in 1997.

This experiment was in part responsible for the Belmont Report, issued in 1978 by the National Commission for the Protection of Human Subjects of Biomedical and Behavioral Research. It sets out three basic principles upon which medical research should be based [55]:

1. Respect for persons: Treating people as autonomous agents and protecting those with diminished autonomy
2. Beneficence: Adhering to the code "do not harm" and maximising possible benefits while minimising possible harms
3. Justice: Ensuring the fair and reasonable distribution of benefits and costs among participants without coercion or exploitation

It is clear that the Tuskegee Experiment would have failed all three of these criteria. Participants were denied the right to leave the study, harms were not minimised and participants were selected on an unjust basis and coerced with the false promise of certain benefits.

While the Belmont Report provides a brief outline of the ethical principles that should form the basis of medical research, more stringent criteria are required to further ensure that medical research occurs in as ethical a manner as possible. The remainder of this section explores these criteria, using the Tuskegee Experiment as a reference where appropriate.

25.7.3 The Nuremberg Code

The Nuremberg trials were a series of military tribunals conducted against high-ranking Nazi officials and industrialists at the end of World War II. The first of these was *United States* vs. *Karl Brandt* (Mengele himself had escaped to Argentina), otherwise known as the Doctor's Trial, in which medical doctors were accused of human experimentation and murder under the guise of euthanasia. Using unwilling participants selected from the concentration camps, subjects were exposed to such heinous experiments as intravenous injection of petroleum, ingestion of various poisons and infection with a range of viruses [9]. This led to the prescription of the Nuremberg Code, a set of research ethics and principles designed to govern the practice of human experimentation. This, together with the Belmont Report and Declaration of Helsinki, has formed the backbone of ethical regulation of clinical trials and research. The code can be found below [56]:

1. The voluntary consent of the human subject is absolutely essential.
2. The experiment should be such as to yield fruitful results for the good of society, unprocurable by other methods or means of study, and not random and unnecessary in nature.

3. The experiment should be so designed and based on the results of animal experimentation and a knowledge of the natural history of the disease or other problem under study that the anticipated results will justify the performance of the experiment.
4. The experiment should be so conducted as to avoid all unnecessary physical and mental suffering and injury.
5. No experiment should be conducted where there is an a priori reason to believe that death or disabling injury will occur, except, perhaps, in those experiments where the experimental physicians also serve as subjects.
6. The degree of risk to be taken should never exceed that determined by the humanitarian importance of the problem to be solved by the experiment.
7. Proper preparations should be made and adequate facilities provided to protect the experimental subject against even remote possibilities of injury, disability or death.
8. The experiment should be conducted only by scientifically qualified persons. The highest degree of skill and care should be required through all stages of the experiment of those who conduct or engage in the experiment.
9. During the course of the experiment, the human subject should be at liberty to bring the experiment to an end if he has reached the physical or mental state where continuation of the experiment seems to him to be impossible.
10. During the course of the experiment, the scientist in charge must be prepared to terminate the experiment at any stage, if he has probable cause to believe, in the exercise of good faith, superior skill and careful judgement required of him, that a continuation of the experiment is likely to result in injury, disability or death to the experimental subject.

It does not take much analysis to see that almost every one of the ten points set out in the Nuremberg Code was breached by the Tuskegee Experiment. (1) With a lack of insight into the nature or duration of the experiment, consent could not be informed and therefore was not valid. (2, 3) Though the information garnered may have yielded some benefit for society, the results could undoubtedly have been obtained through other means, and there was a clear lack of knowledge of the progression of the disease, hence the need for the experiment in the first place. (4–7, 10) These were clearly breached in a truly heinous manner, there was strong evidence at the time that syphilis could cause harm and further harm was caused through the denial of access to treatment. The risk to life of participants and those that had the potential to transmit the disease to far outweighed any justifiable gains in knowledge. (9) Clearly, this was violated, up to and beyond the prescription of the Nuremberg Code, as participants were denied access to penicillin up until the study's termination in 1972. (8) This was perhaps the only point of the code followed, depending on the interpretation of "skill and care". If this refers purely to the scientific method, and the need for it to be applied such that the experiment proceeds safely without the addition of unnecessary risk within the remit of the trial itself, then these criteria may be fulfilled; that is, though the trial itself constituted a humanitarian abomination in its unnecessary risk, additional risks were not compounded through the addition of people unqualified in their ability to run the experiment.

25.7.4 The Declaration of Helsinki

The Nuremberg Code provided a platform for ethical practice in research but did not address all necessary issues. For example, by demanding "voluntary consent" as an imperative, certain groups, collectively unable to demonstrate the capacity required to provide consent (children, patients with certain psychiatric conditions), would see a lack of progression in treatment. Thus, certain changes were required. The Declaration of Helsinki, first prescribed in 1964 and most recently updated in 2013, addressed some of these shortcomings. Due to its length, an abridged version, highlighting the major changes from the Nuremberg Code, is included below [57]:

25.7.4.1 General Principles

"*The health of my patient will be my first consideration*", "*A physician shall act in the patient's best interest when providing medical care*" and "*While the primary purpose of medical research is to generate new knowledge, this goal can never take precedence over the rights and interests of individual research subjects*". This idea is not explicitly stated in the Nuremberg Code; the welfare of the patient is paramount, and a gain in knowledge should not be at their expense. As discussed earlier in this chapter, this essentially references the Kantian principle that an autonomous person is not a means to an end, but an end in themselves.

> *"No national or international ethical, legal or regulatory requirement should reduce or eliminate any of the protections for research subjects set forth in this Declaration".*
>
> *"Groups that are underrepresented in medical research should be provided appropriate access to participation in research".*
>
> *"Appropriate compensation and treatment for subjects who are harmed as a result of participating in research must be ensured".*

25.7.4.2 Risks, Burdens and Benefits

"*In medical practice and in medical research, most interventions involve risks and burdens. Medical research involving human subjects may only be conducted if the importance of the objective outweighs the risks and burdens to the research subjects*". This more explicitly states that not only must the benefits outweigh the risks, but it must also outweigh the risks and burdens imposed upon the participants, and therefore a large risk to a small number of people is not outweighed by a small benefit to an entire population.

25.7.4.3 Vulnerable Groups and Individuals

> *"Some groups and individuals are particularly vulnerable and may have an increased likelihood of being wronged or of incurring additional harm. All vulnerable groups and individuals should receive specifically considered protection".*

> *"Medical research with a vulnerable group is only justified if the research is responsive to the health needs or priorities of this group and the research cannot be carried out in a non-vulnerable group. In addition, this group should stand to benefit from the knowledge, practices or interventions that result from the research".*

25.7.4.4 Scientific Requirements and Research Protocols

"The design and performance of each research study involving human subjects must be clearly described and justified in a research protocol". This includes a statement of the ethical considerations and the manner in which the principles in the Declaration of Helsinki have been addressed. It also requires information such as funding, affiliations, conflicts of interest, and incentives and compensation provided to subjects.

25.7.4.5 Research Ethics Committees

"The research protocol must be submitted for consideration, comment, guidance and approval to the concerned research ethics committee before the study begins". This committee must be independent and transparent in its functioning. They maintain the right to monitor the study throughout its course and must be made aware of any changes in protocol.

25.7.4.6 Privacy and Confidentiality

> *"Every precaution must be taken to protect the privacy of research subjects and the confidentiality of their personal information".*

25.7.4.7 Informed Consent

"Participation by individuals capable of giving informed consent as subjects in medical research must be voluntary". Note the addition of the word *"capable"*, allowing as discussed for research to take place for the benefit of those that could not give consent. This research must not breach any of the other principles of the Declaration.

> *"For a potential research subject who is incapable of giving informed consent, the physician must seek informed consent from the legally authorised representative. These individuals must not be included in a research study that has no likelihood of benefit for them unless it is intended to promote the health of the group represented by the potential subject, the research cannot instead be performed with persons capable of providing informed consent, and the research entails only minimal risk and minimal burden".*

"Research involving subjects who are physically or mentally incapable of giving consent, for example, unconscious patients, may be done only if the physical or mental condition that prevents giving informed consent is a necessary characteristic of the research group. In such circumstances the physician must seek informed consent from the legally authorised representative. If no such representative is available and if the research cannot be delayed, the study may proceed without informed consent provided that the specific reasons for involving subjects with a condition that renders them unable to give informed consent have been stated in the

research protocol and the study has been approved by a research ethics committee. Consent to remain in the research must be obtained as soon as possible from the subject or a legally authorised representative". This latter point may be of particular relevance to emergency surgery, where patients may be incapacitated as a result of their clinical condition.

"For medical research using identifiable human material or data, such as research on material or data contained in biobanks or similar repositories, physicians must seek informed consent for its collection, storage and/or reuse. There may be exceptional situations where consent would be impossible or impracticable to obtain for such research. In such situations the research may be done only after consideration and approval of a research ethics committee". Again, this may hold particular relevance in emergency surgery, where specimens may be taken for research purposes. The most famous case of a breach of this principle is that of Henrietta Lacks, from whom a sample of cervical cancer was taken without her consent that would go on to become HeLa, the world's first immortal cell line, which has been the subject of significant debate regarding consent, privacy and ownership of tissue [58].

25.7.4.8 Use of Placebo

"The benefits, risks, burdens and effectiveness of a new intervention must be tested against those of the best proven intervention(s), except in the following circumstances: Where no proven intervention exists, the use of placebo, or no intervention, is acceptable". The intervention, therefore, should be weighed up against the current best option available in order to determine its effectiveness such that it can be implemented in the future or discarded as appropriate. This, in combination with the welfare of the subject themselves being paramount, forms *clinical equipoise*, the genuine uncertainty within the scientific and medical community as to which of the two interventions is clinically superior, and thus the provision of either one is not deliberate harm.

25.7.4.9 Post-trial Provisions

> *"In advance of a clinical trial, sponsors, researchers and host country governments should make provisions for post-trial access for all participants who still need an intervention identified as beneficial in the trial. This information must also be disclosed to participants during the informed consent process"*.

25.7.4.10 Research Registration and Publication and Dissemination of Results

"Researchers, authors, sponsors, editors and publishers all have ethical obligations with regard to the publication and dissemination of the results of research. Researchers have a duty to make publicly available the results of their research on human subjects and are accountable for the completeness and accuracy of their reports. All parties should adhere to accepted guidelines for ethical reporting. Negative and inconclusive as well as positive results must be published or otherwise made publicly available". Ensuring documentation of not just benefits, but also

harms, or even a lack of difference in outcome, is vital. Failure, for example, to document an increased risk of death in a trialled surgical technique could result in the trial being repeated at a later date and participants coming to unnecessary harm.

25.7.4.11 Unproven Interventions in Clinical Practice

"In the treatment of an individual patient, where proven interventions do not exist or other known interventions have been ineffective, the physician, after seeking expert advice, with informed consent from the patient or a legally authorised representative, may use an unproven intervention if in the physician's judgement it offers hope of saving life, re-establishing health or alleviating suffering. This intervention should subsequently be made the object of research, designed to evaluate its safety and efficacy. In all cases, new information must be recorded and, where appropriate, made publicly available". Importantly here, the physician must judge the intervention as having the potential to provide benefit, and that this benefit outweighs harms. This final principle does not provide a platform for random experimentation that serves no conceivable benefit, nor for a patient to demand such a treatment.

This too came into effect before the end of the Tuskegee Experiment. Perhaps the most relevant change to this study implemented by the Declaration was that it specifically stated that any greater good must not be at the expense of the trial participants, which as previously discussed was clearly breached by the study.

In conclusion, medical research is primarily different from clinical practice in that the participants are not necessarily the group intended to benefit. Ethical research should aim to maximise benefits while minimising harms, should champion autonomy and should not weigh the knowledge to be gained as being of greater value than the lives of the participants. *Clinical equipoise* helps to justify the need for and value of the research to take place, such that there is clear evidence that harms are neither intended nor suspected. The Belmont Report provides a brief outline of the principles upon which ethical research should be based, and the Declaration of Helsinki further details the requirements that must be met. In emergency surgery, where lives arguably hang in the balance at a greater rate than other clinical fields, it is particularly important that these values are adhered to.

References

1. Beauchamp TL, Childress JF, editors. Principles of biomedical ethics. 5th ed. Oxford: Oxford University Press; 2001.
2. Kipnis K. Triage and ethics. Virtual Mentor. 2002;4:19–21.
3. Ryan JM. Triage: principles and pressures. Eur J Trauma Emerg Surg. 2008;34:427–32.
4. American College of Surgeons. Committee on Trauma. Advanced trauma life support. 9th edn. Chicago; 2012.
5. Repine TB, Lisagor P, Cohen DJ. The dynamics and ethics of triage: rationing care in hard times. Mil Med. 2005;170:505–9.
6. Netters S, Dekker N, van de Wetering K, Hasker A, Paasman D, de Groot JW, Vissers KCP. Pandemic ICU triage challenge and medical ethics. BMJ Support Palliat Care. 2021;11:133–7.
7. Oxford English Dictionary, 2nd ed. Oxford: Oxford University Press; 1989.

8. Mental Capacity Act, UK Public General Acts, United Kingdom Government. 2005. https://www.legislation.gov.uk/ukpga/2005/9/contents. Accessed 16 Mar 2022.
9. Faden RR, Beauchamp TL. A history and theory of informed consent. 1st ed. New York: Oxford University Press; 1986.
10. Benn P. Ethics. 1st ed. London: UCL Press; 1998.
11. Pavlikova B, van Dijk JP. Jehovah's witnesses and their compliance with regulations on smoking and blood treatment. Int J Environ Res Public Health. 2022;19:387.
12. Gillick v West Norfolk and Wisbech AHA. 1985. https://www.lawteacher.net/cases/gillick-v-west-norfolk.php. Accessed 14 Mar 2022.
13. Yefimova M, Aslakson RA, Yang L, Garcia A, Boothroyd D, Gale RC, Giannitrapani K, Morris AM, Johanning JM, Shreve S, Wachterman MW, Lorenz KA. Palliative care and end-of-life outcomes following high-risk surgery. JAMA Surg. 2020;155(2):138–46.
14. Pawlik TM, Curley SA. Ethical issues in surgical palliative care: am I killing the patient by "letting him go"? Surg Clin North Am. 2005;85:273–86.
15. Ferguson HJM, Ferguson CI, Speakman J, Ismail T. Management of intestinal obstruction in advanced malignancy. Ann Med Surg. 2015;4:264–70.
16. Krouse RS, Easson AM, Angelos P. Ethical considerations and barriers to research in surgical palliative care. J Am Coll Surg. 2003;196:469–74.
17. Pearse W, Oprescu F, Endacott J, Goodman S, Hyde M, O'Neill M. Advance care planning in the context of clinical deterioration: a systematic review of the literature. Palliat Care. 2019;12:1178224218823509.
18. Lichtenthal WG, Kissane DW. The management of family conflict in palliative care. Prog Palliat Care. 2008;16:39–45.
19. Sales E, Schulz RM, Biegel DE. Predictors of strain in families of cancer patients: a review of the literature. J Psychosocial Oncol. 1992;10:1–26.
20. Asadi-Lari M, Tamburini M, Gray D. Patients' needs, satisfaction, and health related quality of life: towards a comprehensive model. Health Qual Life Outcomes. 2004;2:32.
21. Ghandourh WA. Palliative care in cancer: managing patients' expectations. J Med Radiat Sci. 2016;63:242–57.
22. Lilley EJ, Cooper Z, Schwarze ML, Mosenthal AC. Palliative care in surgery: defining the research priorities. J Pall Med. 2017;20:702–9.
23. Tulsky JA. Beyond advance directives. Importance of communication skills at the end of life. JAMA. 2005;294:359–65.
24. Karnik S, Kanekar A. Ethical issues surrounding end-of-life care: a narrative review. Healthcare. 2016;4:24.
25. Aghabarary M, Dehghan Nayeri N. Medical futility and its challenges: a review study. J Med Ethics Hist Med. 2016;9:11.
26. Reilly BM. Don't learn on me. Are teaching hospitals patient-centered? N Engl J Med. 2014;371:293–5.
27. Moore FD. Ethical problems special to surgery. Surgical teaching, surgical innovation, and the surgeon in managed care. Arch Surg. 2000;135:14–6.
28. Bhanot K, Chang J, Grant S, Fecteau A, Camp M. Training surgeons and the informed consent discussion in paediatric patients: a qualitative study examining trainee participation disclosure. BMJ Open Qual. 2019;8:e000559.
29. McAlister C. Breaking the silence of the switch. Increasing transparency about trainee participation in surgery. N Engl J Med. 2015;372:2477–9.
30. Kocher MS. Ghost surgery: the ethical and legal implications of who does the operation. J Bone Joint Surg. 2002;84:148–50.
31. New Jersey. Supreme Court. Perna v. Pirozzi. Rep Cases Argued Determ Supreme Court N J N J Supreme Court. 1983;92:446–66. https://law.justia.com/cases/new-jersey/supreme-court/1983/92-n-j-446-0.html. Accessed 16 Mar 2022.
32. Lin YK, Liu KT, Chen CW, Lee WC, Lin CJ, Shi L, Tien YC. How to effectively obtain informed consent in trauma patients: a systematic review. BMC Med Ethics. 2019;20:8.

33. Adedeji S, Sokol DK, Palser T, McKneally M. Ethics of surgical complications. World J Surg. 2009;33:732–7.
34. Girdler S, Girdler J, Tarpada S, Morris M. Nonmaleficence in medical training: balancing patient care and efficient education. Indian J Med Ethics. 2019;4:129133.
35. Tarpada SP, Morris MT, Burton DA. E-learning in orthopedic surgery training: a systematic review. J Orthop. 2016;13:425–30.
36. Aggarwal R, Mytton OT, Derbrew M, Hananel D, Heydenburg M, Issenberg B, MacAulay C, Mancini ME, Morimoto T, Soper N, Ziv A, Reznick R. Training and simulation for patient safety. Qual Saf Health Care. 2010;19(Suppl 2):i34–43.
37. Hurwitz B. Legal and political considerations of clinical practice guidelines. BMJ. 1999;318:661–4.
38. Tebala GD. History of colorectal surgery. A comprehensive historical review from the ancient Egyptians to the surgical robot. Int J Colorect Dis. 2015;30:723–48.
39. Watson A. Medical malpractice law in ancient Rome. In Watson A. Failures of the legal imagination. University of Pennsylvania Press; 1988. https://www.degruyter.com/document/doi/10.9783/9781512821574-006/html. Accessed 13 Mar 2022.
40. Bal BS. An introduction to medical malpractice in the United States. Clin Orthop Relat Res. 2009;467:339–47.
41. Price K. The art of medicine. Towards a history of medical negligence. Lancet. 2010;375:192–3.
42. Tebala GD, Slack Z, Fantini V, Masato S, Parla M, Cirocchi R, Di Saverio S. Professional responsibility between guidelines and customary practice. A conflict of interest? Med Hypotheses. 2022;158:110737.
43. Hurwitz B. How does evidence based guidance influence determinations of medical negligence? BMJ. 2004;329(7473):1024–8.
44. Albrighton vs Royal Prince Alfred Hospital, 1980 2 NSWLR 542(CA), 562. https://nswlr.com.au/view/1980-2-NSWLR-542. Accessed 16 Mar 2022.
45. Montgomery vs Lanarkshire Health Board [2015] UKSC 11. https://www.supremecourt.uk/cases/docs/uksc-2013-0136-judgment.pdf. Accessed 16 Mar 2022.
46. Colbrook P. Can you ignore guidelines? BMJ. 2005;330:s143.
47. Tebala GD. The Emperor's new clothes: a critical appraisal of evidence-based medicine. Int J Med Sci. 2018;15:1397–405.
48. Sartelli M, Weber DG, Kluger Y, Ansaloni L, Coccolini F, Abu-Zidan F, et al. 2020 update of the WSES guidelines for the management of acute colonic diverticulitis in the emergency setting. World J Emerg Surg. 2020;15:32.
49. Hall J, Hardiman K, Lee S, Lightner A, Stocchi L, Paquette IM, Steele SR, Feingold DL. The American Society of Colon and Rectal Surgeons clinical practice guidelines for the treatment of left-sided colonic diverticulitis. Dis Colon Rectum. 2020;63(6):728–47.
50. Okamoto K, Suzuki K, Takada T, Strasberg SM, Asbun HJ, Endo I, Iwashita Y, Hibi T, Pitt HA, Umezawa A, Asai K, Han HS, Hwang TL, Mori Y, Yoon YS, Huang WS, Belli G, Dervenis C, Yokoe M, Kiriyama S, Itoi T, Jagannath P, Garden OJ, Miura F, Nakamura M, Horiguchi A, Wakabayashi G, Cherqui D, de Santibañes E, Shikata S, Noguchi Y, Ukai T, Higuchi R, Wada K, Honda G, Supe AN, Yoshida M, Mayumi T, Gouma DJ, Deziel DJ, Liau KH, Chen MF, Shibao K, Liu KH, Su CH, Chan ACW, Yoon DS, Choi IS, Jonas E, Chen XP, Fan ST, Ker CG, Giménez ME, Kitano S, Inomata M, Hirata K, Inui K, Sumiyama Y, Yamamoto M. Tokyo guidelines 2018: flowchart for the management of acute cholecystitis. J Hepatobiliary Pancreat Sci. 2018;25:55–72.
51. Sackett DL, Rosenberg WMC, Gray JAM, Haynes RB, Richardson WS. Evidence-based medicine: what it is and what it isn't. BMJ. 1996;312(7023):71–2.
52. Charlier P, Huynh-Charlier I, Poupon J, Lancelot E, Campos PF, Favier D, Jeannel G-F, Bonati MR, de la Grandmaison GL, Hervé C. A glimpse into the early origins of medieval anatomy through the oldest conserved human dissection (Western Europe, 13(th) c. a.D.). Arch Med Sci. 2014;10:366–73.
53. Baker SM, Brawley OW, Marks LS. Effects of untreated syphilis in the negro male, 1932 to 1972: a closure comes to the Tuskegee study, 2004. Urology. 2005;65:1259–62.

54. Gray FD. The Tuskegee syphilis study: the real story and beyond. Montgomery: NewSouth Books; 1998.
55. Friesen P, Kearns L, Redman B, Caplan AL. Rethinking the Belmont report? Am J Bioeth. 2017;17:15–21.
56. Shuster E. Fifty years later: the significance of the Nuremberg code. N Engl J Med. 1997;337:1436–40.
57. World Medical Association. World Medical Association Declaration of Helsinki: ethical principles for medical research involving human subjects. JAMA. 2013;310:2191–4.
58. Skloot R. The immortal life of Henrietta Lacks. New York: Crown; 2010.

Printed by Printforce, the Netherlands